Transforming the Culture of Dying

The Work of the Project on Death in America

DAVID CLARK

OXFORD
UNIVERSITY PRESS

OXFORD
UNIVERSITY PRESS

Oxford University Press is a department of the University of Oxford.
It furthers the University's objective of excellence in research, scholarship,
and education by publishing worldwide.

Oxford   New York
Auckland   Cape Town   Dar es Salaam   Hong Kong   Karachi
Kuala Lumpur   Madrid   Melbourne   Mexico City   Nairobi
New Delhi   Shanghai   Taipei   Toronto

With offices in
Argentina   Austria   Brazil   Chile   Czech Republic   France   Greece
Guatemala   Hungary   Italy   Japan   Poland   Portugal   Singapore
South Korea   Switzerland   Thailand   Turkey   Ukraine   Vietnam

Oxford is a registered trademark of Oxford University Press in the UK and certain other countries.

Published in the United States of America by
Oxford University Press
198 Madison Avenue, New York, NY 10016

© Oxford University Press 2013

Library of Congress Cataloging-in-Publication Data
Clark, David, 1953–
    Transforming the culture of dying: the work of the Project on Death in America/David Clark.
      p.; cm.
    Includes bibliographical references and index.
    ISBN 978–0–19–931161–3 (alk. paper)
    I. Title. [DNLM: 1. Project on Death in America.   2. Palliative Care—United States.
    3. Attitude to Death—ethnology—United States.   4. Program Development— United States.
    5. Program Evaluation—United States.   6. Terminal Care—United States. WB 310]
    616.02´9—dc23
    2012047605

9 8 7 6 5 4 3 2
Printed in the United States of America
on acid-free paper

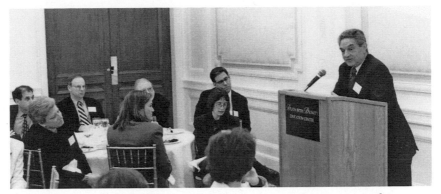

Photograph 1. George Soros giving the Alexander Ming Fisher Lecture in the Columbia Presbyterian Medical Center in New York at the launch of the Project on Death in America, on November 30, 1994.

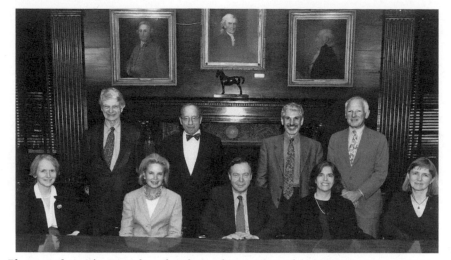

Photograph 2. The PDIA board with Aryeh Neier (president, Open Society Institute) at a faculty scholars retreat, New York, July 1996. Back row, left to right: Robert Butler, William Zabel, Robert Burt, David Rothman. Front row: Patricia Prem, Kathy Foley, Aryeh Neier, Susan Block, Joanne Lynn. The original board included Velvet Miller who was replaced by Ana Dumois. Just ten individuals served on the board through the lifetime of PDIA, five of them for the full duration of nine years.

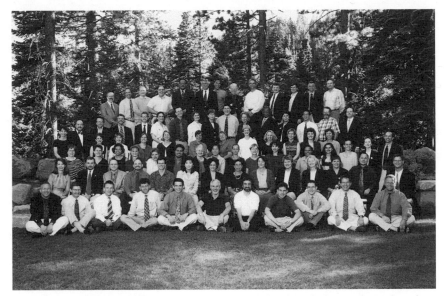

Photograph 3. PDIA board members, staff, guests, faculty scholars and social work leaders at the Granlibakken retreat, California, July 2000.

CONTENTS

No human being escapes death. We encounter it over the course of our lives, through the experiences of family and loved ones, and in time, we confront our own. Yet in our time and place, even for such a universal experience—so ubiquitous in popular culture and the nightly news—the subject has long been shrouded in taboo in the lives of most people, and in institutions such as hospitals where death frequently takes place.

This book chronicles the beginnings of a change in that picture. In the late 1980s, George Soros, whose philanthropy is grounded in a belief in "open societies," established the first of his series of foundations in the former Soviet sphere. His goal was to foster debate and discussion and establish and strengthen independent civil society groups in countries long constricted by censorship and other forms of state control. When Soros turned his attention to the United States, in 1994, the first issue he focused on was dying, a field he viewed as a kind of "closed society"—a zone in which there was scarce public discussion and virtually no philanthropic investment.

When I came to the Open Society Foundations (then called the Open Society Institute) a few years later to expand and direct its US Programs, the Project on Death in America (PDIA), which resulted from Soros's concern, was already well underway, and I and my colleagues learned a great deal from it. PDIA provided a template for the best of Soros's philanthropy, which we strived to reflect in the other programs we launched over time dealing with criminal justice, immigration, democracy, and professions like medicine and journalism.

David Clark's book tells two intertwined stories. One is about a shift in attitudes and practice about death and dying—in medicine, law, culture and other arenas. Clark captures a time in American life when the taboo on discussion of death and dying, first tested by pioneers like Elisabeth Kübler-Ross, started to crack, as the hospice movement began to grow, and there were intense public debates about the Terri Schiavo case, the practices of Dr. Jack Kevorkian, and the Oregon law on physician-assisted suicide. The nine years in which the Project on Death in America operated, from 1994–2003, were highly eventful ones in which real shifts began to occur.

That is no mere coincidence, of course, for the other story Clark tells is one about strategic philanthropy—about what George Soros and the Open Society Foundations did to catalyze change in this field. For the last one hundred years, since Andrew Carnegie and John D. Rockefeller established, just one year apart, their eponymous foundations, vast sums of money have been deployed by philanthropy to improve health and education, to affect public policy, to create organizations, and to recognize and foster leadership in various fields. Yet for all its desired and actual impact, philanthropy is rarely written about, rarely well, and rarely in detail for a nonspecialized audience. Most books on the subject are biographies of wealthy donors where the actual work of the philanthropy is off-stage, or highly technical tracts, or practically focused "how-to" books.

David Clark drills deep down into how a highly engaged board and staff, charged by a visionary donor like George Soros with making a difference in a vast field but with virtually no instruction or limits (except financial: Soros gave them a budget of up to $5 million a year), chose what to focus on and how to determine whether they were making an impact.

We see a distinguished board of half a dozen leaders—chaired by the palliative care physician Kathleen Foley—working hard to determine the best ways to use money and other forms of philanthropic leverage to make real change in a field long resistant to it. We see them devise and widely circulate a "request for proposals" that brings in applications by the thousands. We see the Project on Death in America trying and jettisoning approaches like arts and culture awards to photographers and theater companies, and grants to pastoral leaders, before settling on a more avowedly "elite" approach aimed at the hospitals where so much death takes place. Creating a prestigious "faculty scholars" program, the PDIA used powerful incentives in medicine—professional recognition and money—to forge changes in practice, particularly in the country's largest and best-known teaching hospitals, which have a huge influence on the rest of the field. Since death, no matter what its circumstances, connotes failure for most physicians, PDIA did what it could to make the way that people die—whether their pain is properly managed, whether they are in a setting that is comfortable to them, surrounded by those they care about most, able to say a proper goodbye—a core element of best medical practice, not an idiosyncratic preference or accident.

Indeed, it was just this desire—sparked by the death of his father, alone and in suffering, followed by the passing of his mother, her pain under control, with family at the bedside—that motivated George Soros to launch a philanthropic initiative on death in the first place.

In time the physician scholars were joined by more nurses and social workers, but the heart of PDIA's approach was always through professionals. Clark includes an impressive catalog of their recognition by professional associations, their many peer-reviewed articles in professional journals, and the other forms of recognition that continue to mount for the PDIA scholars and for the field of palliative care as a whole.

While Clark is highly laudatory of the PDIA's work, he doesn't flinch from pointing out where it could have made a stronger contribution. The professional focus left little room for significant work on broader policy issues, particularly health-care financing, where changes can have a wide impact on a great many people. It could probably could have done more, sooner in its limited life, to focus on the particular concerns of racial minorities, who in pain management as in all other forms of medical treatment, lag far behind whites in access to the best standards of care. But on the whole, this is a story of a thoughtful and tenacious route to success.

At the Open Society Foundations, there was always a lot of black humor about the "exit strategy" of the Project on Death in America. It actually lives on in an International Palliative Care Initiative (IPCI), and its legacy goes well beyond geographic borders. George Soros has a preference for making a strong impact in a concentrated period of time. He's under no illusions that philanthropy can "solve" every problem, certainly not forever, but he is a big believer in seizing the "revolutionary moment" and making the best of it.

This he did with PDIA. It is hard to measure the change in our culture around dying, though it has undoubtedly altered in the last twenty years, but the growth in the legitimacy and reach of palliative care is undeniable. PDIA drew new institutions and partners into the field that have continued to make an impact long after it is gone. The faculty scholars continue their influence, in some cases through important new institutions like the Center for Palliative Care, to which Soros made a significant contribution. Among many other things, PDIA built a community of thought leaders that will long outlive it.

Those concerned with philanthropy will learn much from Clark's account of the reflectiveness with which PDIA went about its work, its capacity for self-examination and criticism, and its ability to learn from its mistakes and failures. In an age of increasing mega-philanthropy, where hundreds of millions of dollars can be spent in vast fields like health and education, and fail to make them better—and sometimes make them worse—what PDIA was able to do with just $5 million a year is worth study and emulation.

Humility is more than a virtue; it is essential to clear thinking that can sort promising approaches from dead ends. Leadership matters, and connecting leaders to one another amplifies their impact. Small amounts of money can be transformative, if used well. Philanthropists seeking change and impact should spend some time with David Clark's book. If they come away with these lessons, they're more likely to get what they're looking for.

Gara LaMarche
December 2012

In July 2003, I sat on the train from San Francisco, climbing high through the Sierra Nevada to the small town of Truckee. As the train ascended into the sharp air of the mountains, so my sense of expectation increased. I was to spend the next few days in the company of a group of experts with a special interest in the care of seriously ill and dying people. The faculty scholars of the Project on Death in America (PDIA) were meeting in California for their annual "retreat" at the resort of Granlibaaken, close to Lake Tahoe. I was there as a researcher who had been asked to write a history of the PDIA, covering the nine years of its active existence. The retreat was my first opportunity to spend time with the PDIA board and a selection of its grantees.

I felt daunted by the task. How does one of the most death-denying cultures in the world go about reforming its care of the dying? I had been reading about PDIA on its website, and there seemed to be so many projects, personnel, and linked initiatives. How could they be grouped, explained, scrutinized? Where did PDIA end and other work begin? Would a non-American be at an advantage or a disadvantage in making sense of it all? It is often said that Britain and America are two cultures separated by the same language. How would this impact my study? Would my own expertise in the global history and development of hospice and palliative care help me forge a *special relationship* with PDIA that would overcome the barriers of distance, jurisdiction, and culture? I felt confident that I knew *how* to go about this study, but remained tentative about engaging with the subject matter. I reminded myself that this was appropriate in a sociologist and historian. The study would be a journey and only by the destination would all become clear.

Lake Tahoe would prove to be the first of five research visits to the United States in which I was able to meet with key personnel involved in the PDIA, conduct a range of interviews, join in meetings and discussions, and have access to all of the files and documentation associated with PDIA activities from inception to closure. I spent time at other retreats and also in the New York offices of the PDIA, working with staff and meeting major collaborators. I came to look forward to the visits and to enjoy the excitement of gathering data, developing hunches and ideas about where it was leading and, over the period 2003–2004, capturing some of the key aspects of PDIA just as it ceased operations. I shall explain here something of the aims, scope, and methods of the study, but first PDIA and the source of its funding require some introduction.

In the America of the 1990s, private philanthropy was moving in new and controversial areas. This book gives an account of a philanthropic intervention which sought to "transform the culture of dying" in the United States. The Project on Death in America ran from 1994 to 2003 and formed part of the work of the Open Society Institute, founded by the billionaire financier George Soros.[1] Born in Budapest on August 12, 1930, Soros survived the Nazi occupation of his home city and left communist Hungary in 1947 for England, where he studied at the London School of Economics. Here he found inspiration in the work of the philosopher Karl Popper and established a lifelong preoccupation with the value of pluralist, multicultural "open societies."[2] After years of financial success on the international markets and on the basis of a huge personal fortune, he established the Open Society Institute in the United States in 1993, building on the work of a network of foundations that became active across more than fifty countries with a combined annual budget of some $400 million.

George Soros first became engaged as a philanthropist in 1979, giving support to help black students attend Cape Town University in apartheid South Africa. During the 1980s, he funded Eastern European dissidents and organizations including Solidarity in Poland and Charter 77 in Czechoslovakia. He established his first foundation in Hungary in 1984, two years after creating the Central European University in his native city. The foundations are dedicated to building and maintaining the infrastructure and institutions that characterize an open society. Soros then channeled more than $2 billion into his philanthropic networks during the 1990s. His focus on the former communist world of Eastern Europe and Central Asia centered on the creation of a civil society and a viable third sector between the state and private enterprise. Later, his philanthropic activities spread into southern Africa, Haiti, Guatemala, and also across the United States itself.

Established in 1994, the Project on Death in America was Soros's first US-based philanthropic initiative. It sought to promote a better understanding of the experience of dying and bereavement in ways that would lead to a transformation in the culture of dying. It was quickly followed by the creation of the Lindesmith Center, focusing on harm reduction in the area of drugs and located within the US programs division at OSI—the home from then on for many more US-based initiatives and projects. "Death" and "drugs" were controversial topics for private philanthropy. We shall see here how George Soros, drawing on

---

1. See, for example, George Soros, *Soros on Soros: Staying Ahead of the Curve* (New York: Wiley, 1995); M. T. Kaufman, *Soros, The Life and Times of a Messianic Millionaire* (New York: Vintage Books, 2003); George Soros, *George Soros on Globalization* (New York: Public Affairs, 2002).

2. See Karl Popper, *The Open Society and Its Enemies*, Vols. 1 and 2 (Routledge: London, 1945).

personal experiences with the death of his parents, gave rein to a group of experts to address the issue of end-of-life care and, in the process, to tackle many barriers–within the public imagination, among the professions, in the architecture of policy, and ultimately among dying people themselves in their communities and families.

The purpose of this book is to capture the history of PDIA and to produce an account of its development, situated in the wider context of end-of-life issues in the United States over a decade starting in 1994. I have come to regard this as a "document of record" in the sense that it seeks to be a comprehensive account of PDIA activity. At the same time I have sought to make it more than a catalog of programs and grants. These can be found in PDIA's own publications and reports. My purpose instead has been to capture how and why PDIA came into being, the manner in which it was organized and run, and something of its legacy and impact. In doing this I have set out in detail the work of those supported by PDIA and tried to show the issues and challenges faced by its grantees and scholars. I do this by tackling the work of PDIA thematically—not in relation to the structure of its funding programs nor in relation to the chronology of its development. The first chapter contains a brief history of PDIA, to set the context and mode of operation. Chapter 2 examines PDIA-funded work that focused on illuminating the cultural dimensions of dying, death, and bereavement in modern America. It leads into a discussion in chapter 3 of projects that aimed to highlight direct experiences of care at the end of life—and some of their deficiencies. Chapter 4 deals with a range of service and practice innovations that were developed by individuals and organizations with PDIA funding in a variety of settings and circumstances. In chapter 5, I examine how PDIA addressed the barriers to improved care, particularly for underserved communities. This sets the scene for a discussion in chapter 6 of the policy implications surrounding improvement in end-of-life care, notably in relation to ethical, legal, and financial matters. Chapter 7 offers an extended consideration of how PDIA influenced the field of palliative and end-of-life care through the promotion of research, education, and training activities. Chapter 8 contains an assessment of how PDIA was structured and organized and the legacy it created, exploring the challenges of transforming a culture and the opportunities to influence a professional field. The final chapter sets out some of the developments that have take place in palliative and end-of-life care in the United States in the decade following the closure of the PDIA in 2003. I finished writing this book in the summer of 2012.

The study was conducted using a variety of methods. Case studies of particular programs within PDIA draw on a range of documentary sources, from original grant applications and progress reports to publications, reviews, and wider commentaries. I have made extensive use of work in the public domain that has been generated by PDIA grantees in the form of publications, as well as other outputs—from poetry to film, from essays to needlework. I spent several weeks working in the PDIA offices in New York shortly before the material was removed to the OSI archives. I was given unlimited access to files and records that included financial data, minutes of board and other meetings, background reports, correspondence, publications, and press cuttings. These visits also provided me with extensive opportunities to talk with PDIA staff, to learn more about OSI, and to get a direct sense of how George Soros's philanthropy was organized on a day-to-day basis. In total I conducted 59 individual and group interviews with many of the key grantees and scholars who received PDIA support. I attended retreats of scholars (2003, 2004) and of social workers (2004), and I was able to sit in on sessions, conduct interviews, and have extended conversations with those involved. Although the field visits were relatively short, they did provide a wealth of anthropological insight into the culture and norms of PDIA. Interviews, conducted "on the record" were also invaluable in teasing out individual perceptions, experiences, and assessments of PDIA programs. Later, as I drew my primary data together, I also made extensive use of Internet searches, reviews of the literature, and, in particular, a close reading of many publications that had been produced from work funded by PDIA. In the chapters that follow I draw on all these sources and try to use the interviews to highlight specific points and interpretations.

The work was commissioned by OSI. I have been conscious that it would have to do a lot of "heavy lifting" as the major summative statement about almost ten years of activity and an investment of $45 million. I have also been aware that my human subjects are all still alive, actively engaged in the field in many cases, and often with strong opinions about PDIA, in its many aspects. I have questioned how analytical or objective I could be in such circumstances. Yet I have not felt constrained in accessing material or people. I have been free to write as I will, forming my own judgments and piecing together the evidence in my own way. I have approached PDIA in the same manner that has oriented my research on palliative care more generally—as a "critical friend" to the enterprise, wanting to see how palliative care can be improved and access to it made more available, but also concerned about some of the approaches adopted, and hoping to apply the perspective of the academic researcher in order to highlight strengths and weaknesses, as well as new ways forward. In short, this is a piece of applied social research intended to benefit the field but not at the expense of robust analysis. I hope it will be read by anyone with an interest in improving palliative and end-of-life care, as a record of a major project that may have lessons and applications that are relevant elsewhere. If it can inspire further philanthropic interest in the subject, that will be a wonderful bonus.

David Clark
Dumfries, Scotland
September 2012

ACKNOWLEDGMENTS

There are many people I must thank for their encouragement, support, and facilitation of my efforts in writing this book. Kathy Foley and Mary Callaway had the idea of asking a British academic to write the history of a project that had meant so much to them and to the Project on Death in America (PDIA) board. The Open Society Institute (OSI, now the Open Society Foundations) went on to fund the work. Over several years various members of the OSI team dealt with my inquiries and requests with efficiency and charm. I am grateful too for the space and resources that were made available to me at OSI's head office in New York, where I worked on documentary sources associated with PDIA. My thanks also go to all the people I interviewed for the study, who gave their time, experiences, and reflections so readily; I am particularly grateful to those who responded so willingly and swiftly to my requests for information and references while I was writing the final chapter of the book. Likewise I thank those PDIA board members, especially Joanne Lynn, Bo Burt, Patricia Prem, David Rothman, and Kathy Foley who commented so helpfully and in detail on the first draft of the book. In addition, the anonymous reviewers engaged by Oxford University Press provided numerous helpful insights and concrete suggestions, many of which I have been able to implement. I also thank Abby Gross at OUP for seeing the potential of the book and Rebecca Suzan, Emily Perry, and Andrea Seils for shepherding it through the various stages to publication. Margaret Jane transcribed the interviews with considerable skill. Tom Lynch and Michelle Winslow kindly conducted some extra interviews for me. Nic Hughes read the whole first draft and gave much encouragement. A special word goes to Lynda Crawford for her meticulous copyediting, immaculate timekeeping, and supportive reflections on the whole manuscript. At the University of Glasgow various colleagues helped to shape my thinking and connected the work to other endeavors. Recognizing all these contributions, any errors of fact or interpretation remain mine alone.

A Brief History of the Project on Death in America

Like many innovative ideas, the Project on Death in America started from modest beginnings, and these burgeoned beyond the earliest imaginings of those involved. For George Soros, it grew out of personal experience, which led in turn to an interest in the wider scenario of death and bereavement in American society. For those who took up his challenge, it set in motion an exhilarating journey that encompassed diverse communities and cultures across the United States, as it sought to engage with complex ethical and legal issues and to tackle questions of public policy, finance, and professional regulation. It brought with it a heady mix of surprise, opportunity, and innovation, coupled with a determination to embrace the scale of the task and a commitment to getting on with the job in the best way possible. It called for difficult decision making in the face of grant seekers from so many backgrounds and with varying levels of expertise. In turn it required vision, energy, and strategic planning in order to make the biggest impact with the available resources in the time available. Ultimately it called for a willingness to take hard decisions about the focus of the project and, in due course, to decide how it should end.

This chapter provides a portrait of the Project on Death in America from its pre-beginnings to its closure. It explains how the initiative came about, how it was resourced, structured, and governed—and the programs that it developed and supported. This in turn sets the scene for more detailed analyses of PDIA activities and provides a roadmap and timeline with which to navigate the many initiatives and activities that are described.

WHY A PROJECT ON DEATH IN AMERICA?

In 1992, Patricia Prem, a psychiatric social worker in New York, had recently retired from private practice. She contacted an old friend, George Soros, whom she had known since the 1960s when he and her first husband had played tennis together.

> I called him and asked if there wasn't something constructive I could do. He had started all these foundations a number of years earlier. His reach was getting very big and grand. He talked about the death of his mother, which I think occurred two-to-three years before. How sad, of course, but how gratifying it had been to him and his family because he knew what to do. She was a cancer patient and her dying was protracted. He described how he knew enough to gather his family around to be with her, hold her hand, and talk about where she was going and her life. It was a memorable event for his family. He talked about the time years earlier when his father was dying. He was at home in his own room. The family knew he was dying, but they didn't know what to do. Like many families, they didn't talk about it. He forgave himself, he said, because he didn't know any better.
>
> The transition was immediate. "Let's see how old people die in America. Why don't you run around and find out what's going on across the country?" And typical of George that he would take on such a grand, open-ended project like this. I took it seriously and I ran around for about a year interviewing people I could find in the field. I would talk to one and they would send me on to another. This way I eventually got to Kathy Foley, Balfour Mount, Joanne Lynn, Susan Block, and Andy Billings, all of whom were very helpful and deeply involved with end-of-life issues. I pulled this information together and met with George, claiming that this is the state of dying in America. He was impressed with the pages of information, but felt there was something more out there.[1]

At the time, Kathy Foley had no knowledge of George Soros but had been struck by Patricia Prem's quiet determination to find out what she could. A neurologist, Foley already had a global reputation for her expertise in palliative care and pain management. Many years at New York's Memorial Sloan-Kettering Hospital had developed her clinical, management, and leadership skills, and since the early 1980s she had played a major role in the development of the World Health Organization's strategy for cancer pain and palliative care.[2] When Prem reported back to Soros, he sensed that there were experts available who could help, and he was encouraged enough to take things further. He proposed a meeting to take

---

1. Patricia Prem, interview by David Clark, July 23, 2003.

2. Kathleen Foley, is an attending neurologist in the Pain and Palliative Care Service at Memorial Sloan-Kettering Cancer Center in New York City, and a professor of neurology, neuroscience, and clinical pharmacology at the Weill Medical College of Cornell University.

place at his home in Southampton, Long Island, over a weekend in September 1993. It would be a gathering of experts, activists, and sharp thinkers likely to be capable of tackling an issue of this scale and complexity. Kathy Foley recalls the makeup of the group and the atmosphere at the gathering:

> We were invited for the weekend, starting on Friday night and leaving on Sunday. The group that came included Susan Block; Andy Billings; Bob Butler; Patricia [Prem]; Charles Sabatino, then liaison for the American Bar Association and the Care of the Elderly; and Jack Gordon, at that point the head of the Hospice Foundation, and Jack had been a congressman from Florida, a major advocate for hospice care, and an expert advisor on that topic. And there was Ron Pollock, head of Families USA; and Chris Cassel, now the president of the American Board of Internal Medicine; and Victor Osiatynski, a human rights activist lawyer from Poland who happened to be visiting George and who spent a little time with us in the beginning of the discussions. And Aryeh Neier, who at that point was in the process of being appointed president of what eventually was called the Open Society Institute. When we were meeting, the Open Society Institute had not been named as such...There was also a woman who was a leading expert on geriatrics from California...[3] George was quite engaged: he played tennis on Saturday morning, and then in the afternoon sat with us and sat through dinner with us. And then on Sunday, by the time we were going to close the meeting, he said, "OK, well what would you like to do?" And he really wanted us to tell him what to do...As this was a rather disparate group of people—we had not all worked together—it didn't seem to me that there was a way that all of us were going to easily come to one decision. But our sense was that, yes, there was an important issue, that there was an important need, that there were a variety of things that could be done, and that the next step probably should be to put together a group of people to work on further defining what could be done. So coming out of that meeting...Aryeh was given the task of moving it forward.[4]

That process led to some individuals from the weekend dropping out of the picture and others coming in. Those who remained involved were Patricia Prem, Kathy Foley, Susan Block, and Bob Butler. Those joining were the social historian David Rothman (a student of the closed spaces of asylums and prisons and a writer on the contemporary history of medical practice in the United States); academic lawyer Bo Burt (who had sat on an Institute of Medicine Committee with Kathy Foley); health policy expert Veronica (known as "Velvet") Miller; and lawyer and colleague of George Soros, William Zabel. Joanne Lynn, a prominent palliative care activist and physician was also quickly appointed to the board, just as the results were emerging from a major study she had conducted on

3. Joanne Lynn also was invited, but was unable to attend.

4. Kathy Foley, interview by David Clark, July 22, 2003.

end-of-life care in American hospitals. Kathy Foley soon emerged as the person that Aryeh Neier wanted to chair the group.[5] There was a sense of pressure to move things forward, despite the absence of a clear modus operandi. Mr. Soros seemed in a hurry to see things happen.

Meetings took place in March and June of 1994, and at the second meeting, Aryeh Neier introduced a framework for operations and details of the available resources. The experience of being given a budget to disburse was uniquely energizing for this group of board members, weighted toward academics and clinicians who saw themselves at that time as primarily grant getters rather than grant makers.[6] Bo Burt captures something of their reaction:

> We sit down and Aryeh says, "Well, I'm sorry that George isn't here," and I wonder, gosh, why would he *be* here? "But here is what he wants me to tell you and that is that he has set aside $15 million to be paid out over three years and his goal is to improve the way that we deal with death and dying in the United States." He then explained about how the philanthropy worked, which was setting up these independent boards with public-spirited citizens to whom he gives money; he identifies the problem and then he gives the money to the board, and they spend it as they see fit. And [what has] passed into the lore of this group is that my mouth dropped to the floor...I had no idea...I just thought he was asking for advice and that would be just fine. I just couldn't believe it. It reminded me...there was a program, a television program...called *The Millionaire*...so I *think* I said at that point "This is like John Beresford-Tipton. This is like *The Millionaire*...what are we to do with the money?" So then, kind of calming myself a bit to be more lawyer-like, I said to Aryeh, "Well, but surely, you know, there are *conditions*. You know, he can't just give us this money." So Aryeh said, "Well, actually there are two conditions: the first condition is that you can't give the money to yourselves..." I thought, well, that's reasonable..."and the second condition is that you can't parcel out the money so that each of you dictates a little piece of it. You have to come to agreement amongst yourselves...You decide." He said..."We leave it to you. We trust *you* [with] what to do." So that was very exciting. I mean, just the *challenge* of it. And then our next meeting as a board was in Dartmouth...and what we all agreed very quickly was $15 million was *nothing*! [laughter] I mean, the problems were so *huge*, we couldn't *begin* to make a dent. [We went] from being kind of staggered—"Wow, $15 million!"—to suddenly, "It's not going to *begin* to

---

5. Joanne Lynn had also been interested in this role but was happy to work with Foley: "Kathy was sort of in my pantheon of stars, and I'd never had a chance to work any with her." Joanne Lynn, interview by David Clark, July 14, 2004.

6. The PDIA staff felt the same way. Mary Callaway, the long-time administrative colleague of Kathy Foley at Memorial Sloan-Kettering Hospital and member of the PDIA team from the outset commented: "For 16 years at Memorial, we had been trying to raise money from philanthropy and grants. Now we were on the other side. Developing a funding initiative at

scratch the surface!" But the excitement that I felt, we all felt, about this opportunity [has] just persisted to this day.[7]

The sense of responsibility was palpable. Susan Block, an internist and psychiatrist and, at that time, junior faculty member at Harvard Medical School recalls her reaction:

> I remember thinking...I don't play in those circles. I'm not a New Yorker. I'm not a fancy-pants person...I mean it was just *amazing* to me to be in that kind of a setting, and with autonomy and responsibility and...it was a really pretty extraordinary opportunity. It's very moving to think about having that kind of opportunity and the trust he put in us...And I think the board collectively felt that and shared that, and it created a sense of bonding and connection, and specialness, and real dedication and commitment. We just felt like we had to use this money really very well.[8]

Joanne Lynn described the process rather differently—as one of "being handed a job of a board of a foundation and not knowing how much money there would be, how long it would run, or even what would count as good outcomes."[9] Of major significance, however, was not simply the level and duration of the resource, but also the manner in which it would be deployed. Here was a program being forged by a group chiefly composed of academics and clinicians. Kathy Foley's view is that "from the beginning, there was a very elite perspective on our model of social change, and the elite perspective was that we were not going to be a grass-roots movement."[10] She further elaborates:

> The perspective was that...one of the major problems identified was in medicine itself and that...hospitals were places where most people died, and physicians were those engaged in their care [and] had in a way lost their way and that our focus of change should be at a very elite level of engaging the health-care professionals. Going to the public with this discussion...the amount of money we had was just hardly enough to begin any kind of a public campaign. Not to suggest that the heavily weighted board of academics didn't in a way influence the thinking of this kind of a process, because we were not public communicators, we were not activists. We were academics who thought about change in a rather academic fashion.[11]

---

the Foundation was like going to the other side of the world." Mary Callaway, interview by David Clark, July 22, 2003.

7. Bo Burt, interview by David Clark, July 23, 2003.

8. Susan Block, interview by David Clark, July 21 and 24, 2003.

9. Joanne Lynn, interview by David Clark, July 14, 2004.

10. Kathy Foley, interview by David Clark, July 22, 2003.

11. Kathy Foley, interview by David Clark, July 22, 2003.

By the end of the June 1994 board meeting, the initiative had a name: "The Project on Death in America."[12] That too had been a product of deep searching, as David Rothman remembers:

> Aryeh had joked with me that somehow or other we had to try to get *rights* into the title, punning on *rites* versus *rights*. I think he would have been happy with some kind of "Final Rites." ... My own favorite was "The Way Out Foundation," but this was black humor. Everybody felt very strongly that we would not mince words, that it was going to be about death in America, and we weren't going to do "passing on" or "lost" or any other euphemism. This is terribly important. It would be "Death in America." We were going to use the *D* word—staunch determination about that. And so: the Project on Death in America—not an accidental frame or phrase, but reflecting a real sense, in keeping with the original Soros intention, that we were going to take death out of the closet by putting it first and foremost right into our title ... It was I think one of the first markers for me that we were onto something really important, that ultimately, by using death in the title and announcing ourselves as interested in death in America, we were allowing people to open up and talk about a subject that heretofore had been cloaked and camouflaged. So I was genuinely proud of that and very, very alert to the importance of what we were doing.[13]

It soon became clear that the board was an "extraordinary cast of people."[14] It worked together in a manner akin to evangelists dedicated to the promotion of a cause. The members were open to the many proposals and suggestions that came to them. But they also put in a huge amount of their individual concerns and interests. In the early days, they spent time together on retreats and shared personal experiences; for some of them the involvement proved to be life changing. They had a great deal to draw on as the group encompassed high level achievers in academic and clinical medicine and health-related research; they included a distinguished historian and social critic, a social worker and social activist, a geriatrician and a lawyer. The talents of the board were indeed extensive and they needed to be, for as one member put it, the mission they had been given by Soros "was breathtakingly open-ended."[15]

---

12. Subsequently one board member had reservations and wrote: "My domestic critics—my wife and eldest daughter—didn't much like 'Project on Death in America.' It didn't seem adequately communicative to either of them, and they fanned my misgivings: were we about violence and gun control? What anyway did we intend to do about death in America? Have less of it? My daughter then suggested a variation that all of us liked: *Facing Death in America: A Project of the Open Society Institute*." Bo Burt, letter to Kathleen Foley, 6 June 1994. (The name was not changed.)

13. David Rothman, interview by David Clark, March 31, 2004.

14. Kathy Foley, interview by David Clark, July 22, 2003.

15. Susan Block, interview by David Clark, July 21 and 24, 2003.

It could be observed that there were some distinct biases in the composition of the PDIA board: American, mostly East Coast, specifically New York, weighted toward medicine and other elite professions, predominantly white. From the outset, there were also issues about conflicts of interest and a concern that external perceptions of these "should not mar our project."[16] So, for example, board members recused themselves in certain selection procedures when an applicant was known to them,[17] and in April 1995, three such applications were refereed externally. For the most part their dealings were harmonious, but at times the discussions got heated, as at the board meeting of March 13, 1998, when feelings ran high over the merits of some proposals, tempers flared, and subsequent email and fax correspondence fanned the debate over several days.

The papers for the meeting of Thursday, September 24, 1998[18] are a fine example of the range and volume of activity the board would take on. Over an inch thick and neatly divided by brightly colored tags, the materials are arranged into nineteen sections. They contain a detailed update from Professor Christine Cassel about work to "strengthen the palliative care code" at the Mount Sinai Medical Center in New York. There is a funding application from Richard Heffner (of *The Open Mind* weekly television program). Bill Moyers writes enthusiastically about his plans for a four-hour documentary special, *A Better Way to Die*, that will feature examples of PDIA-funded work. There are numerous applications and letters of intent for a range of proposals, including a children's bereavement project, a community bioethics initiative on the end of life, a conference on health and spirituality, work on the epidemiology of dying among Native Americans, and a proposal for town meetings across America on death and dying. There are plans to be discussed for a forthcoming PDIA meeting on economic issues in end-of-life care; updates on the work of the faculty scholars, and several other PDIA initiatives—on nursing, social work, arts and humanities, economics, and litigation. And there is a detailed program for a forthcoming conference on death and dying in prisons and jails. Finally, there is the budget to be agreed for 1999. The eight-hour meeting, in other words, contained a remarkable spectrum of PDIA issues, from the mundane and administrative to questions of major importance for the promotion of end-of-life care across the United States.

Over time, the composition of the board changed, but only slightly. In the first three years it comprised Foley, Block, Burt, Butler, Lynn, Prem, Rothman, and Zabel. The early departure of Velvet Miller, as a result of work pressures, took away the only African American on the board. At about the same time, Bill Zabel, a lawyer working in Trusts and Estates for George Soros, was interested in becoming a part of the board, and he served for about two years before other commitments forced him to leave. Zabel's departure was followed during the second three-year cycle by that of David Rothman, who had begun developing

---

16. K. M. Foley, memo to Velvet Miller and Bill Zabel, March 28, 1995 (PDIA files).

17. K. M. Foley, summary of minutes of board meeting, March 10–11, 1995 (PDIA files).

18. Box 734907: Meetings 1998 (PDIA files).

his own Open Society Institute program on Medicine as a Profession, and left to concentrate his efforts in that direction. Joanne Lynn, according to Foley, "was a very strong force on the board,"[19] but in a context where PDIA wished to support the kind of policy work in which she was engaged there appeared to be a conflict of interest, and so she was to leave the board and take her policy-related work forward with PDIA support. It then became apparent that the issue of diversity on the board still remained and, in this context, the Cuban-born social activist Ana Dumois was invited to join in 1999, just as she was retiring from her position with the Community Healthcare Network in New York. She was eager to get involved.

> What struck me when I met the board was the very optimistic perspective with which they approached the subject...You didn't walk into a room of very somber people with funeral faces. They actually were a very happy group of people: scientists, lawyers, physicians, psychiatrists...a group of very accomplished professionals in many diverse fields, dealing with a very difficult subject. But at the same time, the mandate was an awesome mandate—to try to change the culture of death in America. They approached it with a realistic view of how difficult it was, but, at the same time, with an optimism that we could do something.[20]

From that time onward a decision was made not to add any more members to the board, which had the same composition up until the project ended in 2003. Just ten individuals served on the board through the lifetime of PDIA, five of them for the full duration. Kathy Foley held the unusual position of being a member of the board and the director of the project throughout. In 2003, she reflected on some of the dynamics of the PDIA board over its nine-year lifetime:

> The board has continued to operate...at times like a dysfunctional family, at times like a highly functional family. I think we all have learned to become tolerant of each other and tolerant of our opinions. I don't think I would recreate the kind of situation that I found myself [in], being a member of the board *and* director of the project, because that's a hard thing to do and I wouldn't advise it...I would keep the executive director and the members of the board separate...I've grown up a lot in understanding how to listen to lots of different opinions and to understand how initiatives happen and don't happen. I think that the more people you have on a board, the more you can dumb down the program, and the more confined you get to doing ordinary things rather than extraordinary things; and so I think that the smaller the board, the more rapid [in] responding they are.[21]

---

19. Kathy Foley, interview by David Clark, October 27, 2003.

20. Ana Dumois, interview by David Clark, July 23, 2003.

21. Kathy Foley, interview by David Clark, July 22, 2003.

The modus operandi of the board is recognized in the following observations from Gara LaMarche, vice president of the Open Society Institute from 1996 on and director of US Programs:

> It has been a hands-on board, and in a sense the board has been playing more of a staff role than a board role...I think that's worked pretty well. They've been compensated for their time, which is not what we generally do with board members, because it's recognized that they played an operational role.[22]

There is no doubt that the board of PDIA crossed boundaries and hybridized some otherwise functionally separated roles. We shall see more evidence of this in later chapters. The board was a group of colleagues and, to an extent, of friends. They invested more time in their PDIA activities than almost any of them had ever done on other committees of similar kind. They fostered a close personal identification with the goals of the PDIA and, at times, they used the board as a vehicle to promote individual projects and professional goals. The board meetings were frequent, often long, but apparently never tedious. Throughout the lifetime of the project, the board was the key driver, shaping programs, seeking out new opportunities, setting policy, and reviewing progress. It was a level of activity that was breathtaking at times and which demanded huge commitment. It resulted in a rich, varied, and extensive program of initiatives over almost a decade.

PROJECT ON DEATH IN AMERICA: PROGRAMS AND GRANTS, 1994–2003

The Project on Death in America was unveiled publically on November 30, 1994, when George Soros gave an Alexander Ming Fisher Lecture in the Columbia Presbyterian Medical Center in New York.[23] The lecture began with an account of the death of each of his parents—his father in 1963 and his mother more recently. These more reflective elements led on to a hard-hitting critique of the culture of dying in modern America:

> We have created a medical culture so intent on curing disease and prolonging life that it fails to provide support during one of life's most emphatic phases—death. Advances in high technology interventions have deluded doctors and patients alike into believing that the inevitable can be delayed almost indefinitely.[24]

---

22. Gara LaMarche, interview by David Clark, October 28, 2004.

23. The lecture was arranged by PDIA board member, David Rothman, professor of Social Medicine at Columbia University.

24. George Soros, Reflections on Death in America, *Project on Death in America, July 1994–December 1997* (New York: Open Society Institute, 1998), 5.

He identified three major recommendations. First, improved training for professionals involved in the care of the dying. Second, the adoption of a comprehensive Disease Related Group (DRG) for terminal care in hospitals. Third, the increased availability of hospice services for terminally ill patients, without restrictions on admission and reimbursement. With 2.2 million people dying in America every year, the task seemed enormous and those taking forward the Project on Death in America would, he remarked in passing, "have their work cut out for them."[25] Susan Block captures something of the urgency of the early days as well as the enormity of the agenda:

> When I look back to the very beginning of this enterprise, what I remember most is a sense of something being really broken in the system of how we cared for the dying. There was no road map. No one really knew how to approach it. There were few real experts. We also sensed that doing things better was a very real possibility—that we could create a system that addressed the real needs of dying patients and families.[26]

With such a challenging mission, the PDIA board sought from the outset to foster cooperation and collaboration among the various professionals with cognate interests already working in nursing, medicine, social work, ethics, policy, and financing, as well as in philanthropy and the media. Encouraged by Kathy Foley, the board developed a regular practice of identifying experts from different disciplines and convening meetings to map the field and determine the most pressing needs. They held a two-day symposium on this basis at the Stanhope Hotel in New York in January 1995. Sherwin Nuland, author of *How We Die*, was meeting with them on February 9, 1996.[27] Two months later they were joined by drug availability expert David Joranson. The board members approached these meetings with a sense of deep conviction, but also one of working without a net—as naïve neophytes in the world of major philanthropy.[28] Patricia Prem reflects on the decisions made during this time:

> Some of it was trial and error... seven years later after we learned our lessons about how to spend money, we probably wouldn't have funded some

---

25. Soros, Reflections on Death in America, 6.

26. *Transforming the Culture of Dying: The Project on Death in America, October 1994 to December 2003* (New York: Open Society Institute, 2004), 17.

27. Sherwin B. Nuland, *How We Die. Reflections on Life's Last Chapter.* (New York: Vintage Books, 1993).

28. "Our earnestness, our naiveté, our enthusiasm, our belief that we might really be able to do something about this issue—all of this was central to our work. The grandiose mission to "transform the culture" was there from the start, and each of us had a can–do attitude that helped us pursue a dream that we knew was possible. Supporting other individuals who shared that dream—and could actually make it a reality—was what PDIA was all about." Kathy Foley in *Transforming the Culture of Dying*, 9.

of these proposals...That is not a veiled criticism. I just think that we've had second thoughts about some of our funding...and that's the downside, I guess, of that kind of philanthropy. We had people who were prominent in the field, not necessarily people experienced in grant making. So we had to learn as we went along. I still think it has been enormously successful and...we've had enormous impact.[29]

The early discussions on the board were extensive and probing. External experts also helped shape thinking and strategy. So it was that in 1995 PDIA announced a grants program to address seven priority areas for funding, hoping to cast a broad enough net to address the many significant areas of need. It was in a context of "complete freedom to formulate our own agenda for transforming the culture of death and care of the dying"[30] that the program emerged and in which two interlocking themes were dominant: the harms inflicted by the medical system on dying people, and the harms caused by public attitudes about death itself, the so-called "denial of death."

The areas to be covered were as follows:

- The epidemiology, ethnography, and history of dying and bereavement in the United States
- The physical, emotional, spiritual, and existential components of dying and bereavement
- The contribution of the arts and humanities
- New service-delivery models for the dying and their families and friends
- Educational programs for the public about death and dying
- Educational programs for the health-care professions
- The shaping of governmental and institutional policy

Robert Butler recalls the implication of the first Request for Applications (RFA):

There were nine of us originally on the board and I *think* it's accurate that every one of us read every proposal that came in the first round. It was something like 1,500 proposals [chuckles], but it was terrific, because it was like "open sesame." We learned a whale of a lot about what was going on in America, about what people were thinking at this time. So in terms of the funding cycles, I think in those first ones we really devoted an enormous amount of time to getting a feel for what was out there and what the field was all about.[31]

In both its size and range the response to the RFA was overwhelming. With hindsight, it was viewed as the perfect tool to assess the range of interest in

---

29. Patricia Prem, interview by David Clark, July 23, 2003.

30. *Transforming the Culture of Dying,*17.

31. Robert Butler, interview by David Clark, July 23, 2003.

death-related topics across America. But in practice, it was to lead to a very broad range of initial investments, some of which bore fruit while others did not, as Kathy Foley remembers:

> It was the best survey we could have done of the field, because these were individuals who had to only send in a letter of intent. They could be relatively unsophisticated; they could be quite sophisticated. But as letters of intent, you judge them more on concept, novelty, originality, or the need, or how it fits your criterion, more than you judge them on the great details of the application per se. So it was extraordinary. I think it was an incredibly democratic process. People that wrote at that time ranged from [members of] local communities who were in need of a bereavement counselor, to individuals who wanted to just give us advice, to [people with] very sophisticated ideas of what would be important and how [these ideas] should be moved forward. And we had to take that list of 1,500 and bring it down to a list of 300 or 400 that would be manageable and then ask for full applications... it was pretty extraordinary.[32]

Something like 80,000 copies of the initial RFA were distributed to announce the program. There was little preparation for the response that would result. The volume was phenomenal, as Mary Callaway explains:

> We had no system. We had no idea how we were going to catalog them. We had no database to enter them into. So it was a development process that was quite a challenge. We finally got the first cycle of grant awards made in June of '95. But during a part of that, when the board was meeting and setting up the structure... they decided that they were really going to focus on a grants program and a professional development program, with particular emphasis on faculty scholars. The board laid out the seven program areas where they wanted to target their funding, and that's what went out in the first program announcement. And that was to fund grants on epidemiology and ethnography of death and dying; projects in the arts and humanities that would give language and voice to the experience of death and dying; service delivery; research; and public policy. So the announcement went out and we requested grant letters of intent back. Then the board met and... they selected letters of intent that they were going to request full proposals from. That's basically how it started.[33]

In its first three years, PDIA received more than 2,000 grant requests over four grant cycles and funded 122 projects in the seven priority areas. The grant amounts ranged from $5,000 to $400,000 and represented many different approaches to the subject of dying—from the medical to the philosophical to the political. The

---

32. Kathy Foley, interview by David Clark, October 27, 2003.

33. Mary Callaway, interview by David Clark, July 23, 2003.

board chose to fund a broad range of initiatives to reflect the complexity of the medical and societal challenge of providing appropriate, compassionate care to dying people and those close to them.[34] Eventually, three grant cycles unfolded as the PDIA was extended from three years to six years and then to nine years. Kathy Foley explains:

> So the first three years we had a vague strategic plan, which was based in our RFA for a grants program and our RFA for a faculty scholars program. Then our next three years became much more focused and our...last three years became more focused, in which we took projects that hadn't risen to the top in those other [years], or that needed some special help, and we focused on them and devoted...money to each of those projects.[35]

From an early stage, the PDIA board began to forge the view that it was essential to change the culture of medicine in hospitals and nursing homes, where 80 percent of Americans die. The creation of the Faculty Scholars Program proved pivotal in addressing this and absolutely fundamental to the outcome of the project as a whole. Immediately after the Long Island weekend, Susan Block had begun to sketch out an idea of what it might look like, building on a discussion about "the problems that are not being taught in medical schools."[36] The idea was to identify and support outstanding clinical and academic leaders in medicine and nursing who could change medical culture from the inside. The board envisioned a national network of health-care professionals—nurses, physicians, and social workers—who would be role models and serve as champions of palliative care in their institutions. More than half of PDIA's funds were eventually to be used to support professional education initiatives.

The Faculty Scholars Program was the single largest investment of PDIA funds. It was established to identify outstanding faculty and clinicians committed to working in end-of-life care and to support them in disseminating good models of organization and practice and in developing new approaches for improving the care of the dying. It also emphasized the promotion of education for health-care professionals about the care of dying patients and their families. The program was to promote the visibility and prestige of clinicians committed to this area and sought to enhance their effectiveness as academic leaders, role models, and mentors for future generations of health professionals. Participants were offered the knowledge and skills necessary to develop innovative programs in clinical care, research, education, and advocacy, and to take leadership roles at their institutions as well as more widely. The program aimed to develop an intellectually vibrant, mutually supportive, and cross-fertilizing network of colleagues involved in multiple facets of work with dying and bereaved people.

---

34. For a listing of all PDIA grants, see Open Society website, http://www.soros.org/initiatives/pdia.

35. Kathy Foley, interview by David Clark, July 22, 2003.

36. Susan Block, interview by David Clark, July 21 and 24, 2003.

Interaction among the scholars fostered new interdisciplinary approaches to key issues related to death in America. The first cohort of scholars began its activities in 1995 and the final group was selected in 2002. (A full listing of the faculty scholars appears in appendix 1.)

In total, eighty-seven individuals (fifty-two men and thirty-five women) in a set of eight cohorts were supported by the PDIA faculty scholars program.[37] Just five were African American and three were Asian. Three were from Canada. The medical professions dominated the program overwhelmingly. Medicine, oncology, geriatrics, and psychiatry were the prominent disciplinary backgrounds, with just ten nurses and three social scientists taking part. The scholars represented a total of fifty-nine medical schools, ten nursing institutions, and two universities. For the most part, each scholar was funded for three years. Despite its eventual heavy emphasis on medicine, the Faculty Scholars Program began life with an interdisciplinary orientation. When the applications came in, however, there were few from outside medicine that seemed credible and of an appropriate standard. In response to a question about whether the program was only intended for physicians, Susan Block makes a number of important points:

> No, we had in mind nurses, we had in mind social scientists, we had in mind ethicists—it was very open. I think we hoped…that there would be a lot of doctors in it. I think what happened early on was, and maybe this was our bias, I think we felt that the applications from some of the non-doctors were not as strong, and so we didn't fund them. And then it became perceived that we didn't fund them, so they didn't apply so much, so it became this sort of self-perpetuating cycle. But the other piece that I was going to say was that there was this recognition that the biggest chunk of the power to create change was in the hands of the doctors, not in the hands of the social workers, not in the hands of the nurse as much, not in the hands of the social scientists as much. And we wanted to create change. We didn't want to *understand* stuff like social scientists do [chuckles]; that was good but that was not what the aim was. The aim was to create change and, in that sense, we thought doctors had the most power to do that.[38]

The Faculty Scholars Program became hugely influential and was widely regarded on the board as being the single most successful aspect of PDIA. For their part, some faculty scholars almost regarded the program as being *synonymous* with the PDIA. Led by PDIA board member Susan Block, the program was committed to improving care for dying patients through the support of talented individuals with a demonstrable potential to change clinical practice and create innovations in service delivery. Five to eight scholars were chosen each year to receive awards of up to $70,000 per year. All scholars conducted a clinical,

---

37. Susan Block, presentation: *PDIA Faculty Scholars Program, 1995–2004.* Granlibakken, California, July 13, 2004.

38. Susan Block, interview by David Clark, July 21 and 24, 2003.

research, educational, or advocacy project for the period of their award, and participated in individualized professional development and a collaborative faculty development program with the other PDIA scholars. The program enhanced the professional visibility of the faculty scholars, enabling them to become more effective leaders and moving them into more influential positions within their institutions. As we shall see, the eighty-seven faculty scholars selected during the program's nine years became among the most prominent and active leaders of palliative care in the United States.

There were those on the board who considered that the faculty scholars model could be extended to other professions and that, indeed, there was a need to address the heavy physician dominance of the program by promoting the work of other groups involved in end-of-life care. Most obvious among these was the nursing profession. As noted, ten of the faculty scholars were nurses and, in addition to their involvement, PDIA also supported nurses through support for a Nursing Leadership Institute in End-of-Life Care. The initiative was first developed by Cynthia Rushton at Johns Hopkins University, together with Betty Ferrell and Colleen Scanlon, and was supported with some initial funding from PDIA. Nurses in all practice settings and roles are faced with quandaries about the provision of humane and dignified end-of-life care. The project sought to promote the development of a Nursing Institute on End-of-Life Care to advance the profession's agenda to improve care at the end of life by increasing the relevant leadership capacity of nurses.

Some board members also argued—in the face of resistance—for greater prominence to be given to social work perspectives in end-of-life care.[39,40]

Eventually Kathy Foley talked with Grace Christ, a former social work colleague at Memorial Sloan-Kettering, and in 1998 invited Christ to produce a white paper to review the issues affecting social workers in their work in end-of-life care. Under Christ's careful guidance, the result was the Social Work Leadership Program, which began in 2000 and encouraged applicants to submit proposals addressing a critical issue in the care of the dying; proposals must have institutional support and the potential for integration into existing structures. In particular, they sought projects that could be generalized to other settings, populations, and institutions, and which represented an innovative approach to care, education, research, or advocacy. Especially encouraged were initiatives that addressed the design, implementation, and dissemination of research

---

39. As Patricia Prem noted in an interview: "This is a board that's very science oriented. I mean that's their training—they're doctors—and so it's hard for them to accept the fact that this [social work] is a strong enough discipline to be involved at this level ..." Patricia Prem, interview by David Clark, July 23, 2003.

40. Susan Block explains her skepticism: "The reason I wasn't enthusiastic was that I didn't think they were going to create change, and we had a very short window to create change. If we had all the money in the world and all the time in the world, *absolutely* I'd want to bring social workers in, but I thought it was a strategic error to bring them in at the point we did and to put the resources we did into them, given what a small window we had to make things happen." Susan Block, interview by David Clark, July 21 and 24, 2003.

on new social work service-delivery models for the dying and their network of family and friends. The result was a late rally for social work within PDIA and a program involving forty-two social workers—50 percent academicians with PhDs and 50 percent with master's qualifications and working in direct practice.[41] (A full listing of members of the Social Work Leadership Program appears in appendix 2.)

These major professional development programs took a significant share of the PDIA budget, but funds were also used in innovative ways to support a variety of other activities, which speaks to the board's inclusive approach to transforming the culture of dying within American society. One approach was to make alliances with other foundations and philanthropic groups to raise awareness about end-of-life issues and to promote more interest in grant making for improved end-of-life care. Following the first publication to appear from the landmark study SUPPORT (Study to Understand Prognoses and Preferences for Outcomes and Risks of Treatment)[42] in 1995, the Robert Wood Johnson Foundation held a conference in March 1996 which explored many dimensions of the end-of-life care issue, particularly bringing together clinicians with consumer organizations, and this led to the formation of the Last Acts Partnership, which was launched in 1997 and ran alongside an extensive program of grant making in the area of end-of-life care that totaled some $150 million over the period to the mid-2000s. In this climate of growing interest among private foundations in the subject of end-of-life care, the PDIA had joined forces in 1995 with the Robert Wood Johnson Foundation, the Nathan Cummings Foundation, the Rockefeller Family Office, and the Commonwealth Fund to form Grantmakers Concerned with Care at the End of Life. This coalition organized conferences and shared information in order to inform funders about major social, economic, and medical issues in end-of-life care and to encourage them to address those issues in their grant making. A similar initiative occurred when in 2002, PDIA and the Emily Davie and Joseph S. Kornfeld Foundation formed the Funders' Consortium to Advance Palliative Medicine. This alliance supported existing and new palliative care fellowship training programs with the goal of increasing the numbers of physicians with advanced training in palliative medicine, and thereby contributing to the wider goal of obtaining formal recognition of palliative care as a medical subspecialty with the Accreditation Council for Graduate Medical Education and the American Board of Medical Specialties.

PDIA launched an arts and humanities initiative in 1998, chaired by board member David Rothman. Grantees produced video, photography, poetry, essays, dance, and artwork to express individual and community experiences of illness, death, and grief and encourage conversation and thoughtful reflection.

---

41. Grace Christ, interview by David Clark, October 27, 2004.

42. The SUPPORT Principal Investigators, "A Controlled Trial to Improve Care for Seriously Ill Hospitalized Patients: The Study to Understand Prognoses and Preferences for Outcomes and Risks of Treatments (SUPPORT)," *Journal of the American Medical Association* 274 (1995): 1591–1598; and see below, chapter 4.

Again, there was little unanimity on the board about the success of this initiative, as Rothman notes:

If I had to put it in a provocative phrase: a series of people never got it... How can you measure the impact of a photographic essay? How can you measure the impact of a narrative? How can you measure the impact of... a literary analysis of elegies? I all too often felt that a narrow-minded commitment to outcome measures got in the way of people actually being able to think broadly about what it means to open up a project in arts and humanities in and around death and dying.[43]

Nevertheless, the arts and humanities initiative funded an innovative range of projects, capturing cultural expressions of death and dying in exhibitions, theatre, film and video documentary, poetry, photographs and essays, performance work, and even the unusual medium of fabric and thread. It made fourteen grants to thirteen grantees and highlighted the role of creative artists in giving form through language and image to experiences at the end of life. This initiative sought to promote expressions of illness, death, and mourning, and thereby to help "identify leverage points for change within our society."[44]

In 1999, a community grief and bereavement initiative was led by Bo Burt. From interfaith, community-based, and school-based programs to programs for special groups, such as incarcerated youth or union home health-care workers, grantees created programs to support individual and community bereavement.

We solicited grants for [bereavement] and we ended that program after I think two years because we were very disappointed in the applicants that we got. It was amazing to us that bereavement was a totally underdeveloped field... But the money that we spent on bereavement was I think a quarter of a million, maybe $300,000, and again nothing lasting came from that. I mean they were nice projects, but there was no growth that came out of them, so they were kind of disappointing.[45]

PDIA also chose to address challenging legal and economic barriers, and to improve access to care for particularly vulnerable populations, as well as for those socially excluded and denied access by the health-care system. These underserved groups included children, the elderly, non-English speakers, those incarcerated, the homeless, ethnic and cultural minorities, and people with physical or developmental disabilities. Ana Dumois highlights one of the projects:

We developed a specific emphasis at some point in trying to reach the African American community. We were very concerned with the fact that that community by and large doesn't use hospice care... and that there is

43. David Rothman, interview by David Clark, March 31, 2004.

44. *Project on Death in America, January 1998–December 2000, Report of Activities* (New York: Open Society Institute, 2001), 40.

45. Bo Burt, interview by David Clark, July 23, 2003.

some bias on their part against using hospice care...So the effort to reach into some African American communities and professionals to try to get them to develop proposals aimed at getting to the black physicians, the clergy...we identified areas where proposals were not coming from and significant populations that were not being involved, and we tried to identify actors who could really access those communities.[46]

Little data existed to explain why members of the African American community used relatively few palliative and hospice services, although historical denial of access to health care and past abuses in medical research may have contributed to a general mistrust of the health-care system. Indeed, from this perspective, palliative and hospice care may well appear to pose further barriers to full medical treatment—a problem compounded by the relative scarcity of physicians trained to deliver culturally competent end-of-life care. Led by Richard Payne, MD, chief of the Pain and Palliative Care Service of Memorial Sloan-Kettering Cancer Center, PDIA launched its initiative to improve palliative care in the African American community, seeking to define and promote a research, education, and policy agenda, and to build coalitions among organizations and stakeholders working in the African American community to promote palliative care.

In 1998, when 1.83 million men and women were incarcerated in prisons and jails across America, more than 2,500 prisoners died of natural causes in state and federal correctional facilities. Longer sentences and fewer paroles, coupled with the increasing age of prisoners, contribute to an increasing numbers of terminally ill inmates. In response, PDIA and the Center on Crime, Communities, and Culture, another Open Society Institute program, cosponsored the first-ever meeting devoted to the growing problem of caring for the dying in prisons and jails in order to define the issues and explore possible solutions. PDIA also supported the production of a compelling video documentary on one of the nation's first prison hospice programs at Angola Prison in Louisiana, in which inmate volunteers are trained to care for other dying inmates. As a result of these efforts, a series of ongoing initiatives was developed to advance the care of dying prisoners through educational initiatives for prison health-care professionals and associated policy changes. In collaboration with the Robert Wood Johnson Foundation, PDIA supported the development of national guidelines for palliative care in America's prisons and jails.

If this array of activities was not enough, in the late 1990s PDIA also extended its reach into areas outside of the United States that were of concern within the network of Open Society foundations. In 1998, Kathy Foley and Mary Callaway attended a meeting of the OSI Public Health Network Program, bringing together their Public Health Coordinators from each of the OSI foundations in Eastern Europe and central Asia—some twenty-eight countries in all. They gave a plenary lecture and a workshop on palliative care. Soon afterwards, many of

---

46. Ana Dumois, interview by David Clark, July 23, 2003.

the coordinators contacted the Public Health Network program director and expressed an interest in taking things further. Mary Callaway explains:

> So funding started in 1998... It ended up being a collaboration between the OSI Network Public Health Program and the Project on Death in America.... The international palliative care initiative really grew out of that collaboration.... We had the foundations identify two potential leaders, or two people in their countries that were interested in hospice and palliative care, and we brought these people together for two and a half days in Geneva, in advance of the European Association for Palliative Care meeting,[47] and we met with them to find out what their needs were in their country... So they said that they had an enormous need for professional education, that their doctors and nurses and social workers, if they had social workers, weren't receiving training on end-of-life care in medical schools and nursing schools; that the public wasn't aware of end-of-life care or that they were entitled to pain management or decision making at the end of life, so there was an enormous need for public education; that drug availability was a huge issue in all of these countries; that there weren't opioid analgesics available for basic pain management; and that there needed to be changes in health-care policy and in the systems in each of these countries. So we went back and basically developed a program to address those issues... $500,000 a year which we were given for three years. So the first year that was how it was announced... we got about 275 or 300 applications back. We ended up funding five resource training centers and then a series of national education programs, about seventeen translation grants, and then a series of travel grants and scholarships.

Funding for this program was subsequently secured to go to 2005. In 2003 the international program was further extended, to include a program of grants for South Africa, initially at a funding level of $300,000 a year over three years.

The various programs of PDIA were described in a 2001 publication in the *Journal of the Royal Society of Medicine*[48] and can be summarized as follows:

- Arts and Humanities: encouraging individuals from the literary, visual, fine arts, and performing arts to use their creative skills and insights to identify and convey meaning in facing illness, disability, and death.
- Community Support for Grief and Bereavement: enhancing the capacity of individuals and of communities to grieve and to support one another in the experience of grief.

---

47. This meeting took place in September 1999.

48. F. Aulino and K. Foley, "The Project on Death in America," *Journal of the Royal Society of Medicine* 94 (2001): 492–495.

- Grants Program, 1994–97: funding a diverse range of organizations aimed at understanding and transforming the culture and experience of dying in America.
- Palliative care for African Americans: defining and promote a research, education, and policy agenda for the improvement of care for African American patients facing serious illness.
- Social Work Leadership Development Awards: promoting innovative research and training projects that advance the ongoing development of social work practice, education, and training in the care of the dying.
- Faculty Scholars Program: supporting researchers, educators, and practitioners of palliative care.
- Palliative Care Fellowships: supporting the training of physicians in the principles and practice of palliative care, to help build the capacity of fellowship programs, and to help establish palliative medicine as a recognized subspecialty of medicine (jointly funded with the Emily Davie and Joseph S. Kornfeld Foundation).
- International Palliative Care Initiatives: enhancing hospice and palliative care programs in Central and Eastern Europe and the former Soviet Union.

The PDIA was funded over a series of three-year budgetary cycles. Toward the end of year two of the first cycle, the PDIA board put forward a tapering budget totaling $12 million, which would lead to closure after two cycles and a total of six years. Kathy Foley explains how this was presented to the full board of OSI:

> We decided in the proposal that we gave to the [OSI] board that we would ask for $5 million, $4 million, and $3 million, and we would use the time in this second three-year period to come up with an exit strategy.[49] So we went to the board meeting with George, it was being held in Baltimore. We met and presented the strategy and it was quite a lively discussion…the board got quite engaged…. Clearly [we] were the most loved group there that day, and [George] said, "Well, why would you be closing?" I said, "Well, we thought that this is going to be a reality, we had to deal with it, and we should be a model to you and other programs of how to do this." He said, "Well, I don't see any reason for you to do this now." So basically when we asked for 12 million; he gave us 15 million.[50,51]

---

49. This coincided with a time when Soros's investment fund was doing less well and the OSI board had been advised by the head of US programs, Gara LaMarche, to put forward a tapering budget toward an exit strategy and closure at six years.

50. Kathy Foley, interview by David Clark, July 23, 2003.

51. In his biography of George Soros, Michael T. Kaufman notes of the meeting: "Soros made it clear how pleased he was with the project and its director, Dr. Kathleen Foley, and quite casually he approved its budget. He never mentioned the reorganization of the fund or the losses he had spoken of so publically twenty-four hours earlier, and neither did anyone else." M.T. Kaufman, *Soros: The Life and Times of a Messianic Millionaire* (New York: Vintage Books, 2003), 315.

In fact, PDIA in due course entered a third funding cycle, again at $15 million, making a period of nine years in all—from1994 to 2003, with total funding at $45 million.

EXIT STRATEGY

During the final year of operation, the staff and board of PDIA reviewed the original funding strategies, goals, and individual initiatives. They hosted round-table discussions and individual meetings, actively engaging palliative care leaders—former board members, faculty scholars, nursing and social work leaders, grantees, cognate organizations, associations, experts in the field, and other funders—to help frame a comprehensive exit strategy for PDIA. The overwhelming consensus was that this should be consistent with the project's long–standing focus on supporting health-care professional development. This strategy centered on strengthening the capacity of existing professional associations to impact upon health policy, financing, education, research, and clinical training in palliative care. It also recognized the importance of encouraging other funders to include palliative care on their funding agendas.

The need for an exit strategy, albeit one that had been postponed, proved a painful experience for board members and staff, Kathy Foley remembers:

> Well, I think that first of all, it was very hard for the board to understand that the project was going to end, and so there was a great deal of discussion of how could we continue the project? And where could we potentially find other funders? And should we...spin off as an independent entity and find funding to do that? But it became very clear in our discussions that maybe that wasn't the right approach. We knew for sure we were closing [from] May of 2002. So we had that amount of warning.... We knew we had about $2 million that had not been [allocated].... As a group we eventually came to the decision to engage a lot of people in what they thought the field needed and what needed to happen. We wanted to emphasize our role in professional education, and we wanted to stay with that as our major focus, recognizing that there wasn't any grant that we could make that could begin to change it, and there was no public engagement that we could [begin] with this small amount of money. Could we support the capacity of individual organizations to be sustainable in the future? The more we talked with these different groups, it became apparent that we weren't going to have one group that we could give money to that would move forward and take on all of the issues that PDIA had done. And there was no NGO out there that met the sort of criteria that we...were focusing on, that is advancing professional education...and so we made a decision to fund about six programs and take the $2 million and split it up.[52]

---

52. Kathy Foley, interview by David Clark, July 23, 2003.

The exit strategy focused around support for a number of key organizations active across the United States in the field of end-of-life care.[53] One major beneficiary stood out, however, and this was the American Academy of Hospice and Palliative Medicine, a physician-based professional organization dedicated to advancing practice, research, and education in palliative medicine. PDIA awarded a $1.2 million grant to the Academy to support its infrastructure and to strengthen its ability to serve the needs of palliative care professionals through the creation of an academic college to house the legacy and leadership of the PDIA faculty scholars, as well as to strengthen the Academy's capacity to support and nurture academic leaders in all fields and to expand its role in the promotion of interdisciplinary professional education in palliative care.

In contrast, other exit grants were relatively modest. Four groups each received a grant of $200,000. The 5,500 member Hospice and Palliative Nurses Association received support to advance professional nursing education by building on the work of the Johns Hopkins Nursing Leadership Academy on End-of-Life Care and the End-of-Life Nursing Education Consortium (ELNEC). A further sum was earmarked to support a Social Work Summit on Palliative and End-of-Life Care with the goal of helping the field of social work to build professional consensus, create interdisciplinary partnerships, further a research agenda, collaborate on program initiatives, and construct the educational structures needed to train future generations of social workers in palliative and end-of-life care. The National Hospice and Palliative Care Organization received support to strengthen its organizational infrastructure and expand its reach into diverse communities, as well as its relationships with long-term care providers, also to extend the work of the Veteran's Administration Hospice and Palliative Care Initiative, and to establish an office of diversity to expand access to end-of-life care and reach out to underserved communities.

Finally, two grants of $100,000 each were awarded. The first of these was to the Harvard Medical School's Program in Palliative Care Education and Practice to support scholarships to enable health-care professionals from minority or underserved communities to attend the Harvard's faculty development program. The second grant was to the American Board of Hospice and Palliative Medicine to implement standards for fellowship training programs in palliative care and to begin the application process to make palliative medicine a subspecialty.

In addition to these specific grants, PDIA undertook to support the activities of Grantmakers Concerned with Care at the End of Life through 2004, based at OSI and serving as a resource center for other funders who might need information or advice about funding in the field.

With this program of exit funding, PDIA completed all grant making at the end of 2003. In October 2004, the project issued a special report, *Transforming the*

---

53. Chapter 11 contains an evaluation of the extent to which these organizations were successful in fulfilling the goals associated with their exit grants.

Culture of Dying, in which its activities over a nine-year period were reviewed.[54] The PDIA invested $45 million in improving care available to patients and their families at all stages of serious illness. The report highlighted examples of strategic grant making and included specific funding recommendations focused on areas of special opportunity where philanthropic investment might make a dramatic difference to the lives of dying people and their families. It also emphasized the enormous impact of private philanthropy on the development of palliative and end-of-life care services in the United States and highlighted OSI's interest in sharing with the greater funding community those lessons learned over the lifetime of the PDIA. Gara LaMarche, vice president and director of US Programs at the Open Society Institute, was quoted as follows:

> Over the past decade, foundations have had an enormous impact on the development of palliative and end-of-life care services in the United States. Thanks to grant makers across the country, people with life-threatening illnesses are now more likely to be cared for by health-care professionals— nurses, clergy, social workers, and doctors—trained in pain management, knowledgeable about advance care planning, and respectful of how religion or culture can affect a patient's experience of illness and dying. Caregivers and patients are learning that isolation, pain, and inadequate care need not define the dying process.

The report also asserted that all people with serious or advanced illness should expect and receive reliable, skilled, and supportive palliative care in order to relieve pain and other physical symptoms and promote the highest quality of life possible at all stages. It acknowledged that palliative care can be delivered alongside potentially curative treatments and is best delivered by an interdisciplinary health-care team that can address physical, psychological, and practical problems. It recognized that palliative care supports families throughout the patient's illness and is sensitive to the importance of religious, spiritual, and cultural responses to death and bereavement.

The report was in part aimed at funders who might use it to consider how the communities they serve will benefit from improved palliative and end-of-life care services, and how they might integrate palliative care into funding priorities. PDIA was by no means the only grant maker concerned with improving end-of-life care. Several other funders had begun to devote significant resources to the field. In fact, PDIA was part of a consortium of grant makers that came together—formally and informally—to share information and ideas. The Nathan Cummings Foundation paid particular attention to spirituality at the end of life, an area that PDIA could not fully address. Likewise PDIA could never equal the Robert Wood Johnson Foundation's impact on public education and community outreach. The Emily Davie and Joseph S. Kornfeld Foundation joined

---

54. *Transforming the Culture of Dying: The Project on Death in America, October 1994 to December 2003* (New York: Open Society Institute, 2004).

PDIA in supporting palliative care fellowship training programs. This collaborative approach, fostered by PDIA, undoubtedly gave a greater voice and impact to efforts to enhance attention for end-of-life care grant making.

Around 2.4 million individuals die in the United States each year. Many more tens of millions are affected as bereaved relatives, companions, friends, and caregivers. The Project on Death in America drew attention to this remarkable set of social circumstances and sought to explore the consequences and implications and, most important, what might be done about it. From its beginning, PDIA focused on the vulnerable and voiceless individuals who had, in a sense, been abandoned by the health-care system. Their suffering suggested ways in which modern high-technology medicine had lost its way. PDIA took the view that palliative care and treatment can enhance the field of medicine and can demonstrate the importance of both competence and compassion in modern health-care practice.

In the chapters that follow we examine the work of the PDIA in more detail, focusing on an exploration and analysis of its programs, initiatives and activities. We shall look in depth at grants and grantees, and activities and projects, exploring a wide range of innovations and seeking to make sense of their impact. We shall see how PDIA held a mirror up to questions about mortality and end-of-life care in modern America. And we shall try to reach some assessment of its overall impact and long-term legacy.

2

Exploring the Meanings
of Death

There were some on the board of the Project on Death in America (PDIA) whose primary orientation was toward action to improve care, and there were others who felt more at ease in reflective mode, standing back and trying to make sense of things from the distance imposed by an academic orientation. From the beginning, however, the board was willing to take a wide view of the problem of death in American culture and this led to some inspired grant making across a range of projects and studies.

Central to this approach, and certainly the most coherent example of it, was a program of contributions from the arts and humanities, in which PDIA encouraged persons from the literary, visual, and performing arts to undertake projects that would "identify, create and convey meaning in facing disability and death, and ... invoke and deepen understanding of the diverse myths and metaphors that shape the experience of suffering in dying and bereavement."[1] But this was achieved by first building on the experiences of the initial grants, where the objectives were to tease out cultural aspects of death, dying, and bereavement in order to promote interpretation, reflection, and debate. This earlier potpourri of projects gave way to a more coherent and longer lasting arts and humanities program, which undoubtedly had a meaningful and sustained long-term impact.

In this chapter we shall look in some detail at the PDIA-funded work that emerged from the arts and humanities program, as well as activities exploring the meaning of death that were supported from generic grants and through a number of other special initiatives. We shall see examples of community

---

1. F. Aulino and K. Foley, "The Project on Death in America," *Journal of the Royal Society of Medicine* 94 (2001): 492–495.

engagement projects, artistic endeavors, and some research studies. These activities show how PDIA gave expression to a range of work that allowed for the elucidation of meanings relating to death, dying, and bereavement in modern America—and in turn how it provided a framework for thinking about the configuration of end-of-life care services.

CONTEMPORARY MEANINGS AND PRACTICES RELATING TO DEATH AND DYING

From the first request for applications in 1995, PDIA had been committed to a broad approach for elucidating aspects of death, dying, and bereavement in American society. This could be seen within several strands of work: the epidemiology, ethnography, and history of dying and bereavement in the United States; the physical, emotional, and existential components; as well as in contributions from the arts and humanities.

A grant of $90,000 was given to the Strong Museum for an exhibition entitled *Memory and Mourning: American Expressions of Grief,* which combined historical artifacts and documents, images, and interactive stations to examine the cultural history of grief and its expression in America from the middle of the nineteenth century. A particular feature of the exhibition was to highlight the enduring nature of postmortem photography within American culture, and this was further enhanced with some striking artifacts and objects, from Elvis Presley and James Dean coffee mugs to funeral wreaths, memorial cards, and mourning attire. The exhibition had opened in 1993, before the commencement of PDIA, and during a 15-month run was seen by an estimated 130,000 visitors. The PDIA grant contributed to the costs of taking the exhibition to nine locations[2] over a three-year period, with support for public conferences, school lessons, and other educational programs at each of the host museums. Through this support, it was seen by another 158,000 people.[3] The Strong Museum, with its powerful emphasis on everyday and family life in America, was the ideal vehicle for this work. Scott G. Eberle, vice president for Interpretation at the museum, commented in 2005 as follows in a detailed account of the development of the exhibition:

> *Memory and Mourning* performed its most valuable public service by providing a quiet space for decompression and reflection—a resource center and a secluded spot to record thoughts and feelings. Seemingly obvious and essential now, this small space at the time represented a thoroughgoing change in thinking, one arrived at by degrees at the Strong Museum and over a broad range of subjects, both grave and buoyant. This exhibit,

2. An itinerary was listed in the *PDIA Newsletter,* no. 2 (September 1996), 9.

3. S. G. Eberle, "Memory and Mourning: An Exhibit History," *Death Studies* 29, no. 6 (2005): 535–537.

like some others, functioned as a device to generate involvement and record reflection by enhancing awareness and drawing on personal experience.[4]

The exhibition made a powerful impact on Kathy Foley, chair of the PDIA board:

> I think that the exhibition from the Strong Museum particularly was very moving. As it traveled around the country, people were given books in which they could write and then they moved to an exhibit that showed body bags, funereal dress, clips from various movies, and really an extraordinary potpourri of things that America identified with death and loss.[5]

One visitor wrote in the comment book that this was the second time he had attended in a year, because two days after his previous visit, the friend who had accompanied him was killed in a road accident. Another saw the exhibition and returned the following week with her husband and children, on the anniversary of the death of her youngest child.[6] Here then was a fine example of good grant making by PDIA that added value to an already excellent product. In parallel with the work of the Strong Museum, PDIA also supported a second exhibition, initiated by the National Hospice Foundation, entitled *Hospice: A Photographic Enquiry*,[7] which opened at the Corcoran Gallery of Art in Washington, DC, in early 1996 to favorable reviews and large audiences. It toured seventeen museums and galleries in the United States through 2000 and used hospice volunteers as docents.[8] Organized jointly between the Corcoran and the National Hospice Foundation, the exhibition contained the work of five internationally recognized photographers—Jim Goldberg, Nan Goldin, Sally Mann, Jack Radcliffe, and Kathy Vargas—who created a range of images of the experience of living and working in hospices. The exhibition was captured in a large and beautifully presented book[9] and accompanied by a documentary film, *Letting Go: A Hospice Journey*, directed and produced by Susan Froemke, Deborah Dickson, and Albert Maysles. In the book, the photographers describe their individual projects and introduce the powerfully visceral images of care at the end of life, seen close up in all its mundanity, messiness, and emotion. The images are often to hard to bear,

---

4. Eberle, "Memory and Mourning," 535–537.

5. Kathleen Foley, personal communication, 11 May 2004.

6. "Memory and Mourning: Exhibition Helps People Cope with Loss," *PDIA Newsletter*, no. 2 (September 1996), 8–9.

7. PDIA was just one of several foundations that supported the exhibition; others included Warner-Lambert Company; the Prudential Foundation; the Glen Eagles Foundation; and the National Endowment for the Arts.

8. *PDIA Newsletter*, no. 1 (March 1996), 6.

9. Dana Andre, Philip Brookman, and Jane Livingston, eds., *Hospice. A Photographic Exhibition* (Boston: Bullfinch Press, 1996).

and not because they shock or are intended to do so, but rather because they bring to the public gaze a deeply observed preoccupation with an otherwise sequestered world—hospice care settings where families, friends, patients, and relatives make intense encounters with one another in the face of imminent death.

Documentary film and photography were also the chosen media of PDIA grantees Bastienne Schmidt and her husband Philippe Cheng. The couple built on earlier work in Latin America to explore the evolving culture of death in America through the emotional, spiritual, and practical experience of mourning, grief, and loss, uncovering through meticulous observation how social and cultural environments impact and shape these responses. The project explored the traditional rituals surrounding the process of dying, death, and mourning, but also the emerging cultural and social responses to more recent trends in dying—for example, where diverse segments of the population deal with premature death due to AIDS or inner-city violence. The range of subject matter covered by Schmidt and Cheng was extraordinary, as was its geographic extent. The two documented Veterans Day in Washington, grieving African American women in Alabama, funeral directors in Louisiana, and rural cemeteries in Mississippi. They worked with a Navajo community and with the Pasqui Yaqui tribe, and they visited the first Native American hospice. They explored the Day of the Dead among the Latino community in San Francisco and the Russian community's remembrance of the dead on the Sunday after Russian Easter in New York. They traveled to the state penitentiary in Angola, Louisiana, to document a groundbreaking prison hospice program (see chapter 5). They wrote of their intent in all this work in their final report:

> During the past two years we have collected a wide range of imagery that documents many rituals and rites of the death and dying experience in America. This archive of images was created not only to encourage and stimulate debate … but also to place this debate in a context. A context that is not only emotional and physical, but also geographical.[10]

The work of Schmidt and Cheng was widely used in exhibitions, in PDIA publications, and in conference activities, and it also led to a documentary trailer of the project.

During the summer of 1995, PDIA board member Bo Burt entered into various discussions and began preparing briefing documents on the theme of *dying and the inner life*. Burt's idea was to explore through a conference the question of suffering in dying as a way to approach the inner life. As he noted, there was a need to explore "the basic vocabulary for talking about the way that dying or seriously ill people and their families think about themselves when death becomes transformed from an abstract inevitability into a currently confronted reality."[11]

---

10. B. Schmidt and P. Cheng, *Remembrance and Mourning. On Death and Dying in America: Exploration though Documentation*, PDIA, September 1999.

11. Bo Burt, memorandum (no title), 30 August 1995.

There were initial explorations of this with the Nathan Cummings Foundation and, eventually, some common ground was found upon which to move forward, though at one point the PDIA approach (led by Burt) was described as "too intellectualized, too academic."[12] Nevertheless, at the end of May 1996, a meeting of some twenty-five invited participants took place at the conference center of the Fetzer Institute, outside Kalamazoo, Michigan, to explore the theme of dying and the inner life. The letter of invitation was signed by Kathleen Foley (PDIA), Charles R. Halpern (Nathan Cummings Foundation), and Arthur Zajonc (Fetzer Institute), and it described how the three groups were committed to improving the care of dying people and their families in the United States. But it also acknowledged the difficulties encountered when approaching "the spiritual/emotional/ psychological aspects of dying," described in shorthand as "the inner life". The letter bore the typical hallmarks of early PDIA concerns to avoid the strictures of a narrowly defined and medical model of dying, death, and bereavement:

> Outside this narrowly medicalized perspective, there are different traditions for considering the inner life issues of dying. From some perspectives, the approach of death is an opportunity for heightened spiritual awareness and insight—whether drawn from the ritual practices and underlying philosophic premises of eastern contemplative traditions or from western religious practices and premises. Some dying people today, as well as those close to them or working with them, find guidance and support in these traditions; others find those traditions opaque and unhelpful in facilitating or even defining a "good death."[13]

Held over a weekend, the program of the meeting was ambitious and wide-ranging. Some sessions were led by board members: Robert Butler on life review, Susan Block on videotaping interviews with dying patients, Bo Burt on the modern self. There were also sessions of guided meditation and an exploration of death narratives, the latter led by Canadian palliative care expert Balfour Mount. Delegates were presented with a detailed program and accompanying literature. It was a good example of an in-depth exploration of key issues, facilitated by PDIA and others. Yet the follow-up and "product" are less easily identified. The event took much organization but left little in its wake.

Bo Burt also took a particular interest in the development of a program of activities on grief and bereavement. During a fertile period of innovation and energetic pursuit of new ideas in the early years of the PDIA, a key meeting took place on January 28, 1998, at which participants were invited to explore the following questions that had been put to them in advance:

- What community resources are needed in the areas of grief and bereavement?

---

12. Bo Burt, memorandum, "Update on Inner Life," 29 September 1995.

13. Letter of invitation from Kathleen M. Foley, Charles R. Halpern, and Arthur Zajonc, 25 January 1996.

- What are the barriers to developing these resources?
- What strategies have worked or might work to overcome these barriers?
- What are the reasons for their actual or potential success?
- How can a foundation most effectively support proven approaches and stimulate the development of innovative strategies?

Once again, the PDIA was able to gather noted luminaries in the field to this meeting, such as sociologist and member of the International Work Group on Death, Dying, and Bereavement, Charles Corr, and psychologists Robert Neimeyer and Wiliam Worden, as well as a couple of dozen participants active in the delivery of frontline services, along with policy makers and other PDIA notables.[14] The letter of invitation described the purpose of the meeting: "to solicit your advice to help us in the preparation of our small funding initiative to develop community resources to support grieving individuals and resources for grieving communities."[15] It was another example of careful and sensitive consultation with provider agencies and experts prior to targeted grant making.

The program was rooted in a particular PDIA construction of grief and bereavement[16] that saw the inadequacy of contemporary support for the experience and expression of grief as a source of needless suffering. These problems were thought to be exacerbated by the impersonalized nature of modern hospital deaths, by geographic mobility and age-segregated living arrangements, and by the erosion of family bonds. Grief for many was seen as something to be endured alone. The goal of the initiative was therefore "to enhance the capacity of individuals and of communities to grieve and to support one another in the experience of grief."[17]

It was an ambitious program that awarded thirteen grants. Some quite large awards were made. The American Hospice Foundation received $80,000 toward a grief-at-school training program to prepare teachers and others working with young people to offer appropriate bereavement support,[18] an additional grant of $52,876 was awarded to test the program in fourteen schools. Other grants ranged from $65,000 to 75,000, with a range of recipients: a religious foundation, hospitals and universities, and various health-care providers. In Florida, Maryland, Hawaii, and South Carolina, there were projects to establish networks of bereavement support groups led by volunteers and with the purpose of creating resource centers. In a poor area of Boston's South End, a university

---

14. Box 734881: Grief and Bereavement Meeting, 28 January 1999 (PDIA files).

15. E. M. Sunderland and K. M. Foley, letter of invitation to Grief and Bereavement Meeting, 6 January 1999. Box 734881: Grief and Bereavement Meeting, 28 January 1999 (PDIA files).

16. *Project on Death in America, January 1998–December 2000, Report of Activities* (New York: Open Society Institute, 2001), 47–53.

17. *Project on Death in America, Report of Activities,* 47.

18. H. Fitzgerald, *Grief at School: Training Guide* (Washington, DC: American Hospice Foundation, 2001).

department of pediatrics focused on the needs of bereaved children and their families through peer support groups, trained volunteers, community outreach, and counseling services. In Duluth, an educational program in bereavement was set up to reach out to some 2,500 professionals in local, regional, and state agencies. An innovative project in Los Angeles sought to offer education in grief and bereavement to home-care workers caring for low-income elderly, disabled, and terminally ill people to better equip them to deal with regular encounters with death and loss. In Washington, DC, the William Wendt Center for Loss and Healing worked with the Office of the Chief Medical Examiner to reduce distress among families and individuals in the identification of a person after a sudden fatality. There were also projects concerned with bereavement needs assessment in Alabama and with incarcerated youth.

The projects were geographically widespread and engaged with a number of organizations hitherto unlikely to have made grief and bereavement a high priority in their work. Despite this, when interviewed in 2003, Bo Burt himself was critical of the grief and bereavement program:

> We set up a bereavement program that would be community-based, and we solicited grants for that, and we ended that program after, I think, two years, because we were very, very disappointed in the applicants that we got. It just was amazing to us that bereavement was a totally underdeveloped field. So we had people coming in saying, "Well this is a program I'm putting together …" "Well why do you think it will succeed?" "Well I don't know, because I've been doing it this way." … We actually thought about doing something aimed at church groups and didn't do it in the end, but we explored with different church organizations, and we felt that they were too unfocused in what it was that they saw themselves doing in end-of-life care. So we never put any money there. But the money that we spent on bereavement was I think a quarter of a million, maybe $300,000, and, again, nothing lasting came from that. I mean they were nice projects but there was no growth that came out of them, so they were kind of disappointing.[19]

One year after the meeting on grief and bereavement, a similar event took place on June 8, 1999 and involved four overlapping groups of leaders in the field of pastoral care: educators, chaplains, counselors, and coalitions. The goal of the meeting was to "identify ways to improve pastoral care offered at the end of life,"[20] and this time the leading board member was Patricia Prem. She comments on the events of that evening:

> We had one meeting … things did happen, but it was very clear fairly early on that the board as a group was not willing to fund, and in retrospect

---

19. Bo Burt, interview by David Clark, July 23, 2003.

20. Box 734881: Pastoral Care Meeting, "The Field of Pastoral Care," memo from Patricia Prem to Ed Sunderland, June 8, 1999 (PDIA files).

I agree with them … And I really understand that it's the soft end of the deal and so I sort of backed off … maybe wrong…. We had our one meeting out there, which was very nice … it awakened us to what's there and what's possible, but we didn't seem to have the energy or the conviction yet, at that point, that we could run with anything. So we didn't.[21]

Some projects on spirituality were funded, however, such as a piece of work by the Park Ridge Center for the Study of Health, Faith, and Ethics, which focused on retrieving spiritual traditions in long-term care for the elderly. The project had three goals: (1) to understand the nature of aging within the major world religions, (2) to conduct a qualitative study of nursing home residents and their religious values, and (3) to develop educational models for use in lay ministry and by health professionals.[22]

From time to time opportunities arose to link PDIA to other programs within the Open Society Institute. In July 1999, the OSI's Youth Initiatives Program, led by Erlin Ebrek, combined forces with PDIA to support a joint venture on teenage experiences of death. A meeting between the two groups, involving key community leaders in the youth field, was held on May 24, 1999 and set the scene for a "summer media project" that would have three objectives: (1) design a project that would allow young people to investigate issues of loss and its impact on teenagers in their communities, (2) document the results using one or more mediums (video, radio, photography, writing, or music), and (3) present the outcome to the public.[23] Eight New York City youth media organizations were funded to document young people's perspectives on death and bereavement and to contribute to a broader debate. Grants were really very small—no award was made for more than $6,000—and they were to support work in video, print, radio, photography, and on the Internet. The return on investment was high. Sixty young people from New York's inner city communities took part.[24] The results were disseminated throughout the year 2000 on public television and in communities across the United States.[25,26] The Arthur Ashe Institute for Urban Health in the Bronx worked on a peer-focused newspaper called *Urban Health Chronicles,* which contained a number of articles on death, dying, and bereavement. The Downtown Community Television Center produced a documentary about teenagers who

---

21. Patricia Prem, interview by David Clark, July 23, 2003.

22. The review paper and the study were also supported by the Nathan Cummings Foundation, the Mather Foundation, the Pritzker Foundation, and Emily Davie and Joseph S. Kornfeld Foundation.

23. Box 734881: Youth Initiatives (PDIA files).

24. "Talkin' Death: Inner-City Teenagers Tell Their Stories of Loss," *PDIA Newsletter,* no. 7 (April 2000), 3–4.

25. "Summer Media Project: An Exploration of Teenage Experiences of Death," *PDIA Newsletter,* no. 6 (December 1999), 8–9.

26. *Project on Death in America, Report of Activities,* 55–58.

had lost a friend or family member. The Educational Video Center ran a workshop to help students develop the technical, artistic, and emotional capacities needed to create a documentary about death. Youth Communications New York worked with teenagers to write stories about death, grief, and loss for publication in *New York Youth Connections*, a city-wide magazine with a readership of 200,000 young people and adults. The Global Action Project was supported in running an eight-week workshop in which young people explored urban youth perspectives on death and bereavement and created a website. Young people in the Harlem Writers Crew carried out an ethnographic study about local rituals and ceremonies relating to death, and the Photographic Center of Harlem ran a workshop for young people recently or soon to be bereaved.

Most notable of all perhaps was the radio diary created by Laura Rothenberg, working with Joseph Richman at *City Lore: The NY Center for Urban Folk Culture and Radio Diaries*. Her broadcasts, which later appeared on CD,[27] aired under the title *My So-Called Lungs* on NPR's *Radio Diaries*, and her story was also featured in the *New York Times* and *U.S. News and World Report*. She went on to write a book-length memoir about her experience of living from birth with cystic fibrosis.[28] Building on these youth initiatives, a $35,000 grant was awarded to the weekly PBS series *In the Mix* ("Your issues. Your interests. The national award-winning TV series for teens"),[29] which produced the 30-minute program *Dealing with Death*, enhanced by a discussion guide and a website that included youth-produced writing, photography, contact information, and resources. The program included excerpts from several of the summer 1999 projects. There seemed little doubt that the goal of the youth initiative was achieved: to document through various media the texture and variety of teenage experiences of death in New York City. Laura Rothenberg observes the following in her radio diary:

> I definitely think about after I am gone. I've always been scared that people will forget about me, but I'm also here right now. So it's about trying to come to a place where I can just accept that things have gone the way they've gone, and accept that it's never going to be perfect.[30,31]

There were several other small projects, unconnected to one another and not framed within the structure of a given PDIA program or initiative, which from various perspectives illuminated the theme of dying, death, and bereavement within modern American culture.

In the South Bronx in New York City, a group called *Health Force: Women and Men Against AIDS* undertook a peer education community intervention

27. My So-Called Lungs (CD) (New York: Radio Diaries, nd), first broadcast August 5, 2002.

28. L. Rothenberg, *Breathing for a Living* (New York: Hyperion, 2003).

29. See *In The Mix*, PBS, http://www.pbs.org/inthemix/ (accessed May 18, 2007).

30. My So-Called Lungs (CD).

31. Laura Rothenberg died on 21 March 2003, after rejection of a lung transplant.

project that was also documented by Bastienne Schmidt and Philippe Cheng. Generally known as the "Dear Mr. Death" project, the work was presented at the XII International AIDS conference in Geneva in 1998.[32] In a context where adults and children in the South Bronx—the poorest area in the United States with the highest AIDS rate in New York City—experience multiple deaths of parents, relatives, and friends, and where outlets and rituals for helping people cope with grief are almost nonexistent, the project explored accessible ways to help overwhelmed communities cope with unrelenting grief while documenting the ongoing impact of death in a poor environment. Dear Mr. Death used letters addressed directly to "death," enabling individuals to express their feelings and release their emotions about what death has done to them and their community. More than 200 HIV-positive people and their family members wrote letters. Letter-writing was accompanied by discussion with a grief counselor. Interest in writing the letters was intense. Reflecting the community's diversity, letters were written in English, Spanish, French, Swahili, and Arabic. The letters were blown up and displayed at places ranging from churches to courthouses to the United Nations Headquarters in New York City. An accompanying survey showed that, on average, letter writers had lost six people close to them in the past ten years, over a third from AIDS.

On the whole, the letters were extraordinarily eloquent. The participants not only found solace in writing the letters, but many stated that the letter writing had, for the first time, helped them deal with overwhelming emotions. This was particularly the case with teenagers. Exhibits of the blown-up letters were seen by more than 50,000 people, helping them also understand the impact of AIDS deaths. Efforts to deal with massive deaths are imperative for AIDS-stricken communities. The writing and display of letters provide a means of expressing deep emotions about death that are widely accessible, even for people unaccustomed to writing. In a poor community like the South Bronx, people seemed to feel that writing their thoughts signaled that they were being taken seriously (for once). Based on participants' feedback, the project leaders concluded that this had more immediate therapeutic impact than standard counseling.[33]

The letters were striking in their directness and unusual in providing a vehicle for the expression of thoughts and feelings, particularly on the part of young people, on a topic rarely explored in day-to-day public discourse:

Dear Mr. Death,

You have come into my life on many occasions. You were not welcomed. Each time you came, you took a part of me with you when you left. In my mind I know why you exist although in my heart there is a deep hatred of

32. D. Greene et al., "Dear Mr. Death": Community Bereavement for Multi-Grieved Adults and Adolescents in a Poor AIDS Stricken Area, *International Conference on AIDS* 12 (1998): 488 (abstract no. 24246).

33. Greene et al., "Dear Mr. Death."

your existence. I fear you, not because of death, but because of what's left when you leave.

Felicia Coleman
April 16, 1996[34]

A handful of PDIA projects relating to the cultural aspects of death, dying, and bereavement were undertaken by academic researchers. At a time when increasing numbers of Americans live well into their eighties and nineties, Dr. Paul Wink, assistant professor at Wellesley College, identified the need to understand better the psychological processes that influence the role of the diverse social contexts of social mobility, gender, and participation in war on bereavement, resiliency, and healthy adaptation to the process of aging. A grant of $150,000 over two years allowed him to draw upon existing archival data from two longitudinal studies of men and women (The Oakland Growth Study and the Berkeley Guidance Study), which included a rich array of personality, cognitive, and health data gathered in childhood, adolescence, and at three points in adulthood. The project investigated adaptation, influence of past and present religious beliefs and spirituality, long-term and interpersonal factors, and integrity in health, old age, death, and bereavement.

Following up study participants now in their seventies, he was able to conduct in-depth interviews with older people. Successful adaptation to life in the post-retirement age is commonly assumed to require a "life review" in which the individual takes stock of his or her life and arrives at a new level of self-understanding. Wink's data challenged this assumption. While a minority of the study's participants ("seekers") did undertake and benefit from reviewing their life, the majority of the men and women in the study ("dwellers") did not show signs of life review in old age and did not appear to suffer any negative consequences.[35] He also found that religious belief does not necessarily ease fears about death. Those who take their religion seriously have little fear of the great beyond, yet atheists also report they are unafraid to die since they fear no retribution awaiting them. However, people who believe in an afterlife, but don't often attend religious services—a large proportion of Americans, according to Wink— are most afraid of dying.[36] This was a more conventional piece of grant making by PDIA, which supported a mainstream academic study, but a large number of papers and publications resulted and the investment was worthwhile.

---

34. "Writing Letters to Death Helps South Bronx Deal with Chronic Grief," *PDIA Newsletter*, no. 2 (September 1996), 6.

35. P. Wink and J. Scott, "Dwelling and Seeking Post-Retirement Pathways," WBGH Forum Network, http://forum.wgbh.org/wgbh/forum.php?lecture_id=1245 (accessed June 16, 2007).

36. P. Wink and J. Scott, "Does Religiousness Buffer Against the Fear of Death and Dying in Late Adulthood? Findings From a Longitudinal Study," *Journal of Gerontology:Psychological Sciences* 60 (2005): P207–214.

The PDIA also supported an American–Canadian collaborative work between the medical humanities professor David Barnard and palliative care physician Anna Towers, who worked with oncology nurse Patricia Boston and doctoral student in folklore and ethnography Yanna Lambrinidou. The resulting work, *Crossing Over*, provides a unique set of narratives of patients, families, and their caregivers as they strive to maintain comfort and hope in the face of incurable illness.[37] Using a variety of qualitative research methods, including participant-observation, interviews, and journal keeping, the book comprises a rich set of multi-textured accounts of specific patients, families, and those caring for them. Described by one reviewer as a set of "rich, nuanced portraits of several patients facing the end of their lives,"[38] the book has been widely used in palliative care education. It contains twenty beautifully written accounts of palliative care patients and families in a variety of settings and circumstances and provides a vivid exploration of the relationship between the formal goals of palliative care and the lived reality. *Crossing Over* can be regarded as a classic work within the palliative care narrative genre and contains a foreword by Cicely Saunders, who noted: "It is 'the essence of man' that we meet in this book and I believe we will be wiser and more confident in both our service and our living because of what we have learned here."[39]

These PDIA grants seem to have produced some remarkable work of lasting value. They also represented a relatively small portion of the total PDIA spending over the full nine years of its duration. Yet most board members and staff seem to have evaluated the work in a rather poor light. Patricia Prem sums up a common attitude:

> Trying to be objective ... [now], we probably wouldn't have funded some of those people ... as far as our mission to move the field forward and be more visible [is concerned], we would have been more discriminating and tougher.[40]

---

37. D. Barnard et al., *Crossing Over: Narratives of Palliative Care* (New York: Oxford University Press, 2000).

38. John L. Shuster Jr, review of *Crossing Over: Narratives of Palliative Care.* In *Psychosomatic Medicine* 63 (2001): 511–515.

39. C. Saunders, "Foreword," In D. Barnard et al., *Crossing Over: Narratives of Palliative Care* (New York: Oxford University Press, 2000).

40. Patricia Prem, interview by David Clark, July 23, 2003. She is referring to work done by Continuing Support Services, Inc., which was given a small PDIA grant for two musical traveling puppet shows for children, addressing the grief associated with loss of a loved one and HIV/AIDS, titled "Good Grief, It's Sky Blue Pink" and "Birds of a Feather ... Learn about HIV/AIDS Together." A workshop was given in conjunction with the shows that provided children with the opportunity to discuss disease, death, and grief with their teachers, counselors, and fellow students.David Rothman recalled that PDIA took some "flak" for the puppet shows. There was also some mild fun made of them in the board itself: "I can remember

David Rothman gave voice to a concern of some board members, even those who supported this work:

> The board came haltingly to this and I think missed the fact that using the arts and humanities wasn't going to give you a one-to-one outcome. Of course, supporting fellows isn't going to give you a one-to-one outcome, but it's a little easier to measure, right? How many publications? Did they get promoted? Did they get grants? That's a little easier. What do you do? Count reviews, or changing people's lives? What does it mean to go through an exhibit? We supported some work in the Rochester museum; we supported a gallery of photographs—what impact did it have on the viewers? ... What did it allow them to say to each other? What did they take home from it? How did it change their attitudes when their next of kin were gravely ill? I thought we did some really important things, even though this was I think, for the most part, too hard-headed a board to be able to appreciate the importance of opening up spaces within the humanities and the arts to take on death and dying.[41]

ARTS AND HUMANITIES GRANTS PROGRAM

Despite the unease of some board members about such approaches to grant making, by late 1997 plans were in place for a meeting to bring together a number of individuals with a special interest in social and cultural issues related to human mortality, dying, and bereavement. The meeting was structured around nine presentations that were summarized in detail in a report by Kathleen Woodward, director of the Center for Twentieth Century Studies at the University of Wisconsin-Milwaukee.[42] The meeting was held in January 1998 and the participants came from the fields of literature, women's studies, theatre, history, performance studies, anthropology, media studies, filmmaking, photography, and creative writing.[43] Speakers and presenters included the photographer and filmmaker Eugene Richards; medical anthropologist Sharon Kaufman; literary critic Sandra Gilbert; and performance theorist Barbara Kirshenblatt-Gimblett. It was out of these discussions that a commitment emerged to support a special grants program in the arts and humanities with its own particular focus, call

---

being teased ... I don't remember being such a great supporter of the puppet show, but I think there was a certain amount of teasing that "David was onto another one of his puppet shows." David Rothman, interview by David Clark, March 31, 2004.

41. David Rothman, interview by David Clark, March 31, 2004.

42. K. Woodward, *Forms of Feeling: Death in America*, report on a meeting of January 30–31, 1998; Box 73892: Humanities and Arts, January 30–31, 1998 (PDIA files).

43. The meeting was coordinated by Kathleen Woodward, professor of English at the University of Wisconsin-Milwaukee and was reported on in some detail by her in "The Art of Creating Meaning in Our Dying," *PDIA Newsletter*, no. 3 (September 1998), 6–7.

for applications, and review process. This was never going to be an easy venture. The professionally dominated board of PDIA found it hard to reach universal agreement on the value of a program focused on the arts and humanities. There were arguments in favor of free thinking and risk taking and the value of cultural explorations of death, dying, and bereavement; but there was also a growing commitment to narrowing the focus onto the field of palliative care. The mix could be problematic.

The PDIA Arts and Humanities Program was first announced in 1998 and awarded a total of fourteen grants over four grant-making cycles which brought in a total of 262 applications. Overwhelmed by the level of interest, the program made extensive use of external reviewers, who were asked to rate the applications against questions relating to the strengths and weaknesses of the proposal and the applicant's ability (based on credentials, expertise, capabilities, past performance) to carry out the project. They were also asked to consider whether the project would make a significant contribution to the PDIA mission, whether the intended results could be achieved within the timetable set forth, the adequacy of the dissemination plan, and the appropriateness of the budget and time frame. By cycle four, a special card had been printed to acknowledge receipt of applications.[44] Again, as with other PDIA board work, there were huge files of individual applications to go through, upon which the board made the final decisions, albeit guided by the recommendations from external reviewers. Most grantees received around $50,000. The competition was fierce and the total sum awarded was just $684,451 dollars, arguably a modest investment for what was achieved.

Several grants were for filmmaking. Other projects made use of photography, craft work, exhibitions, and the written word, and sometimes combinations of these.

Ellen Bromberg and Douglas Rosenberg were supported to produce *Singing Myself a Lullaby*, a video documentary that chronicles the creation and performance of a multimedia stage work, which was developed in collaboration with performer John Henry. A west coast dancer with AIDS, Henry wanted to make his own life the subject of his final work. An investigation of identity, both the documentary and the stage work of *Lullaby* presented vignettes from Henry's life, along with more universal movement rituals. The intention was to share the belief that creativity and metaphor can facilitate understanding and acceptance of the dying process. Choreographer Ellen Bromberg, formerly of the Bay Area, was commissioned by Henry to make a dance about AIDS. Henry did not reveal that he was suffering from the disease at first, but soon into the process Bromberg understood that he was and that this was to be Henry's final stage work.[45] For the documentary, Bromberg collaborated with director Douglas

---

44. Some unsuccessful applicants complained about a lack of feedback; one applicant, twice unlucky, wrote: "With no enclosure or response or even reaction on the part of your decision-making committee, it seems spurious for me to even consider let alone attempt to apply for a third year or another time in the future." Letter to PDIA, June 2, 2000.

45. John Henry died on 8 April 1996, in San Francisco, California, age 49.

Rosenberg and incorporated interviews with family members, fellow dancers, friends, a psychologist, a critic, and the collaborators themselves. Bromberg and Rosenberg received an Isadora Duncan Dance Award for the work. The contribution of PDIA was to ensure that *Lullaby* was captured for the future, following a series of live performances. In a paper presented in 2000, Bromberg explained the process:

> We premiered the work in Tucson in 1995, and during the next year it was performed at New Performance Gallery in San Francisco, at P.S. 122 in New York City, and again in San Francisco at the Cowell Theater, as part of The Edge Festival for New Performance in the spring of 1996. John died two weeks after the final performance. Each performance of the work was different as video footage was used increasingly to replace John's live performance, as he grew weaker from the illness. It was our intention that the final work would result in a video piece, which has indeed come to pass. The Open Society Institute's Project on Death in America (part of the Soros Foundation) has funded the creation of this video/dance/documentary and it has also been supported by Wisconsin Public Television, which will broadcast the work some time this year ... As the illness progressed and John's body diminished in size and vitality, the contrast between his real image and his video image was striking. We realized that embedded within the artistic vision of the work was a visual chronicle of a dying man, and that with each performance, that chronicle became more complete. Like an extended cross-fade from flesh to projected image, the ultimate completion of the work was predicated on the death of the performer. The irony of this experience was that as a friend, watching John's body diminish in size and vitality was devastating. And yet at the same time, as an artist, I was fascinated by the gradual displacement of his corporeal being by his projected image on stage ... The video also allowed us to see aspects of his illness that might not have been readily visible from a proscenium stage. It was of critical importance that we make a work of art that defined John not simply as a dying man for whom we feel mainly sympathy, but rather as a man offering us an opportunity for our own self-reflection. And, by participating in this way with John, we experienced the work not only as a meditation on death, but an affirmation of life.[46]

Eugene Richards of New York also took up a biographical theme in the twenty-seven-minute video documentary *But, the Day Came*, which details the complex lives of the "oldest old" (those 80 and over) in the town of Auburn, Nebraska. Central to the story are an 84-year-old still-practicing physician and a

---

46. E. Bromberg, "Re-corporealizing the Body via Screen Dance," paper presented to the *Dance for the Camera Symposium* (UW Madison, 2000), http://www.dance.utah.edu/uploads/forms/misc/recorporealizing_the_body_via_screen_dance.pdf (accessed May 15, 2007). I am grateful to Professor Bromberg for bringing this paper to my attention.

92-year-old farmer fighting to keep out of a nursing home, their lives set against the backdrop of the rolling eastern Nebraska landscape. Coproduced with Janine Altongy, the work was named Best Short Film at the DoubleTake Documentary Film Festival, and won the Eastman Kodak Cinematography Award and the Best Documentary Award at the Hope Film Festival. Eugene Richards went on to get further support from PDIA for two further works (*Long as I Remember* and *All that's Sacred*). The latter took the viewer inside Good Samaritan, the same nursing home the aged farmer in the earlier film had wished so passionately to avoid. Inspired by the death of his father-in-law, Richards's film documents the lives of the residents of Good Samaritan and explores the circumstances that led them to the home.

Thomas R. Cole[47] was supported by the program to make a film *Still Life: The Humanity of Anatomy.*[48] This work for medical education and public broadcasting was an official selection at the Double Take Documentary Film Festival in April 2002 and explores the special yet unstated relationship between medical students in the anatomy lab and the people who donate their bodies for dissection. Medical humanities expert Sandra Bertman comments on the project:

> Film clips of Cary Grant as the consummate anatomy professor ... are interspersed with comments from contemporary gross anatomy students, two medical school faculty intimately connected with dissection and the body donation tradition, and a live body donor. In what ways "yes" and "no" could both be proper responses to the statement, "A cadaver in the classroom is not a dead human being," is the key premise, beautifully presented in the cutaways, organization, and editing of this piece. The structure of the film is an as-if dialogue between young dissectors and soon-to-be cadaver (the body donor). Interviews heighten and explore the relationship between the living and the dead—and not just medical students and body donors. The medical students do not speak directly with the future donor, though we see him shaking hands with them, visiting (and speculating on) the spot where his remains will eventually be deposited. The video concludes with a moving annual ritual, the disposition of body donors' cremated remains at sea.[49]

Another related work funded by PDIA was that of New York–based documentary photographer Meryl Levin, entitled *Anatomy of Anatomy in Images and*

---

47. Thomas R. Cole is the Beth and Toby Grossman Professor and Director of the McGovern Center for Health, Humanities, and the Human Spirit at the University of Texas and Professor of Humanities in the Department of Religious Studies at Rice University.

48. Distributed by Fanlight Productions, Boston, 2001. Directed by David Thompson and Randy Twaddle. ttweak Productions, Houston, TX, 2001. Video, color, 27 minutes.

49. NYU School of Medicine—Literature, Arts, and Medicine Database, "Still Life: The Humanity of Anatomy," http://litmed.med.nyu.edu/Annotation?action=view&annid=10151 (accessed May 13, 2007).

Words, which took the form of a book[50] and travelling exhibition on the place of anatomy in the training of medical students. Published in December 2000, the book combined photographs of first-year medical students at Cornell during their dissection of cadavers in gross anatomy class with excerpts from journals kept by the students during the course. Levin's exhibition went on to tour medical education centers across the country, where it was accompanied by discussion meetings involving local faculty and students and Levin herself and was later made available as a Web exhibit.[51] It also found its way into the content of college programs on medicine and humanities.[52] Unadorned by textual commentary, in this work the words of the students interplay with compellingly busy images to create a riveting tableau of the anatomy class. The photographs abound with a sense of concentration, energy, and sheer hard work that never overcomes a feeling of respect for the cadavers as persons. One student (Rajiv) writes the following:

> Our professors have made a special point to emphasize what a unique privilege it is to be able to dissect a human cadaver. Not too long ago, doctors had to pay off gravediggers to acquire them. But we are lucky. Contrary to lay belief, our cadavers have not been pulled out of the East River. They were willed by their owners, while they were living, to be used for scientific purposes. I feel a sense of awe for these brave souls.[53]

Sandra Bertman linked the works of Cole and Levin in terms of value and saw the two as excellent companions.[54] Levin's project was also reviewed at length in *The Journal of Palliative Medicine* by the associate dean of student affairs at Dartmouth College, where the exhibition had been displayed and where Levin had held a discussion group. The reviewer observes:

> Just over a week into the [anatomy] course, the students gathered, and Meryl showed her images as student volunteers read excerpts from the reflections from Cornell. First-, second-, and fourth-year Dartmouth students gave their reflections, and several faculty (including me) did so, too. We gathered

---

50. M. Levin, *Anatomy of Anatomy in Images and Words* (New York: Third Rail Press Inc., 2000).

51. For the Web exhibit, see http://litmed.med.nyu.edu/poems/anatomy_of_anatomy/p2.html (accessed May 15, 2007).

52. See, for example, Georgetown University, "Interacting with the Medical Humanities," http://www.georgetown.edu/faculty/wellberc/imh/unit2/unit2Sec1i.htm and Fanlight Productions, "Still Life: The Humanity of Anatomy," http://www.fanlight.com/downloads/Still_Life.pdf (accessed May 15, 2007).

53. M. Levin, *Anatomy of Anatomy in Images and Words*, 11.

54. NYU School of Medicine—Literature, Arts, and Medicine Database, "Still Life: The Humanity of Anatomy," http://litmed.med.nyu.edu/Annotation?action=view&annid=10151 (accessed May 13, 2007).

afterwards as a group to share refreshments and further reflect, and this whole session got anatomy off to the best start in years.[55]

One grant within the PDIA Arts and Humanities Program was for an interactive art installation work, The Waiting Room, by San Francisco-based Richard Kamler. Built to the exact specifications of the death row visiting room at San Quentin Prison in California, the installation sought to initiate a conversation into the various ways that the death penalty contributes to collective cultural perceptions of death and dying. The work toured the United States extensively and was widely and positively reviewed.[56]

The visual arts were also represented through photography and craft media. The exhibition *Aging in America* by San Francisco–based photographer Ed Kashi and interviewer and writer Julie Winokur is a compilation of seventy photographs and accompanying essays exploring the unprecedented strains placed on the elderly and their caregivers and covering the experiences of elderly prisoners, older persons who have followed their children to the United States from other countries, and even the impact of natural disasters upon seniors. From a 90-year-old heavy machine operator to a foster care program for older adults, from burlesque dancers in their seventies to geriatric prison wards, the exhibition was described as follows by the James A. Michener Art Museum, where it was again on view to the public some ten years after its original creation:

> A powerful and realistic portrayal of what it means to be an older person in our culture. This compassionate, often surprising account dares viewers to see old age through a new lens; it confronts our stereotypes about aging and asks whether society is truly prepared to handle an increasingly elderly population. *Aging in America* ... uses vivid storytelling, endearing characters and stunning imagery to defy expectations.[57]

Kashi and Winokur's work on rural hospice care had also appeared in the *New York Times Magazine*, as well as accompanying a story on Alzheimer's in the December 2000 edition of *Scientific American*. *Aging in America* began touring in November 2002. The authors published a book in 2003, containing some 200 black-and-white photographs and with a preface by PDIA board member and geriatrician Dr. Robert Butler.[58] In the same year they released an accompanying

55. J. Harvey, review of M. Levin, *Anatomy of Anatomy in Images and Words*. In *Journal of Palliative Medicine* 5, no. 1 (2002): 165–167.

56. Melody Ermachild Chavis wrote an extensive review for Media Channel, in which she described the installation in detail and reported on an associated community meeting, held in Huntsville, Texas. See Melody Ermachild Chavis, "To Die For ..." *The Media Channel* (June 7, 2001).

57. The Art & Soul of Buck's County, "Aging in America: The Years Ahead," http://www. michenermuseum.org/exhibits/aging.php (accessed May 14, 2007).

58. E. Kashi and J. Winokur, *Aging in America: The Years Ahead* (New York: Powerhouse Books, 2003).

fifty-six-minute documentary film and an updated Web exhibit of additional striking photographs and commentary. There can be no doubt that their PDIA grant, together with support from the Robert Wood Johnson Foundation, was key to their successful foray into the areas of aging and death. Julie Winokur noted in 2000 how PDIA had provided "a rare opportunity in our creative lives to follow our vision without financial constraints holding us back."[59]

If the range and immediacy of their images were the hallmarks of Kashi and Winokur's endeavors, Deidre Scherer by contrast worked in fabric and thread panels to produce a subtly understated work, *Surrounded by Families and Friends*. The abiding features of this approach were a sense of intimacy and of entry into a private world. The collection is made up of six panels, each depicting a domestic scene of care at the end of life. *Surrounded By Family and Friends* evolved from a series of nine fabric and thread works, *The Last Year*, in which Scherer chronicles the final months in an elderly woman's life. Scherer noted, "Families and friends who support a loved one at the end of life witness the most powerful of life's events. These are images of death that present dying as a natural part of life and that start a cultural dialogue and deeper reflection."[60] Scherer built on her experience as a hospice volunteer, and one familiar with visiting hospitals and nursing homes to portray archetypal images of death and dying so finely nuanced as to betray the craft medium in which she works. As the Canadian palliative care physician and leader Balfour Mount noted: "The captivating expressiveness of her creations speaks of an artist in complete command of her medium. We come away enriched by a renewed understanding of our transience."[61]

Between May and July of 2001, the inaugural exhibition was on display at the Brattleboro Museum & Art Center before touring to various locations, including Montreal. There were favorable reviews in newspapers across the United States, as well as in various professional journals and magazines. The enduring interest in these works is well demonstrated; seven years after completion, they were still being exhibited successfully—for example, at the Hebrew Union College–Jewish Institute of Religion Museum, New York, from November 2006 to February 2007. Deidre Scherer's major book, *Work in Fabric and Thread*, which preceded the PDIA grant, had already established her reputation as an artist interested in matters of human mortality and was reviewed extensively in medical journals, including *JAMA*.[62] Likewise, images from *Surrounded by Families and Friends* were widely used subsequently in palliative care reports and presentations, as well as in materials produced by departments of medical humanities.

---

59. Julie Winokur to Michael Pardy, cover letter with grant report, December 13, 2000.

60. See Hebrew Union College, "Deidre Scherer: Surrounded by Family & Friends," http://www.huc.edu/newspubs/pressroom/2006/11/scherer.shtml (accessed May 16, 2007).

61. B. Mount, A commentary. In D. Scherer, *Surrounded by Family and Friends* (Williamsville, VA: Grinswold Printing Inc., nd).

62. See J. Olshansky, Review of *Deidre Scherer: Work in Fabric and Thread*. In *Journal of the American Medical Association*, 284 (2000): 2524.

Meredith Monk's *Magic Frequencies*, by contrast, is an interdisciplinary performance work (subtitled "a science fiction chamber opera".) examining life and death through visitations of beings from other realms. In the work, the celebrated vocalist, composer, filmmaker, and choreographer deals with the idea of several different realities existing simultaneously. PDIA provided funding for a series of post-performance conversations on death and dying that became part of the touring component of this piece. These were facilitated by PDIA recommended experts, including James Cleary, Susan Seats, and Maren Monsen. A critically acclaimed performer who has made extensive international tours, Meredith Monk's work has also been the subject of scholarly analysis.[63] *Magic Frequencies* was performed widely in the United States and also on a tour of Eastern European countries in 2001. The PDIA folder on the Monk grant contained a file almost one-inch thick, packed with reviews of *Magic Frequencies* in newspapers and journals, including the major broadsheets from all over the United States.[64] The *Los Angeles Times* dubbed it "a wonder opera."[65] But on opening at the Joyce Theater in November 1999, the *New York Times* gave *Magic Frequencies* a cautious welcome:

> There is some classic Monk here. In the opening scene, Ms. Monk captures the dynamics of a couple's dinner conversation through wordless vocal counterpoint, then brings in a trio of extraterrestrials to examine the diners as they eat corn on the cob … The evening's only entirely nonhumorous vignette, a deathbed scene with a choreographed out-of-body experience, comes early in the work … Still, apart from some pleasantly consonant, moderately quirky chord progressions, a few invitingly tactile percussion interludes written and played by John Hollenbeck, scattered moments of interestingly manipulated film and electronic sound, and the humor inherent in Ms. Monk's compositional and choreographic style, a listener doesn't take much away from this work.[66]

In the final grant report, however, value from the work is observed:

---

63. N. P. Smithner, "Meredith Monk: Four Decades by Design and by Invention," *TDR* (sic) 49, no. 2 (Summer 2005): 93–118. Smithner wrote: "The kitchen table setting in *Magic Frequencies* was part of what Monk called 'the earth scenes,' tableaux depicting everyday life while other performers portrayed aliens peering into the domestic world. The aliens sang in a kind of hiccupping counterpoint. Sometimes, driven by curiosity, they reached toward the kitchen table to sample some corn on the cob. Other scenes in *Frequencies* alternate the humorous and the disturbing, ranging from a duet in a shopping mall to the sickbed of a dying man who sees people from his life passing before him. Typical of Monk, the piece is nonlinear and surrealist, creating a sense of childlike wonder and play" (108).

64. Box 191652705, 1999 (PDIA files).

65. See Mark Swed, "The Wonder of 'Magic Frequencies,'" *Los Angeles Times* (February 29, 2000), http://articles.latimes.com/2000/feb/29/entertainment/ca-3619.

66. A. Kozinn, "Wordless Singers and Other Sendups," *New York Times* (November 4, 1999).

Through this project, Monk hoped to present an image of death and dying that is in harmony with the values of dying with dignity, integrity, comfort, spirituality, and compassion. Art can offer endless possibilities for gaining a greater understanding and appreciation of death and dying. James Cleary, a specialist in palliative care, remarked during one of the conversations that music and art therapies can have an extraordinary relevance to caring for the dying. Ultimately, the *Magic Frequencies* tour and the conversations that followed some of the performances helped to stimulate thoughtfulness and a meaningful discussion on the subject of death and dying in America within a creative context.[67]

There were several works of literary criticism, of theoretical exploration, of personal narrative, and of poetry funded by the PDIA Arts and Humanities Program.

Sandra M. Gilbert, a professor of English at UC Davis was supported to write *Inventions of Farewell: A Book of Elegies*.[68] Death has always served as one of the most powerful catalysts for poetry and so *Inventions of Farewell* collects English-language poems of mourning from the late Middle Ages to the present. The work shows how poetic styles have altered over the centuries, yet the great and often terrifying themes of temporality, change, age, and death remain timeless. The poems in Gilbert's collection trace the trajectory of grief, and illustrate how the deepest sorrow has produced countless poignant and resonant works of art, works that can aid us as we struggle with our own farewells.[69] This work seemed to inspire Gilbert to further endeavors related to human mortality. Her book *Death's Door: Modern Dying and the Ways We Grieve*[70] took several years to write and was not published until 2006, three years after the PDIA had come to a close, but it clearly builds on a legacy of work started some years earlier. There were intellectual and personal struggles in the process, but the result proved to be a searching exploration of death in modern American culture. One interviewer comments as follows:

> In undertaking *Death's Door*, Gilbert set out to write a study of the elegy but wasn't satisfied with the result. "I had to write something more directly personal," she said. "I had to bear witness, in the way that people do when they bear witness to their grief" … *Death's Door* is very personal; Gilbert returns again and again to her own loss as she surveys Western attitudes

---

67. Box 191652705, 1999 (PDIA files).

68. S. M. Gilbert, *Inventions of Farewell: A Book of Elegies* (New York: W.W. Norton & Company, 2001).

69. New Publications from Arts and Humanities Grantees, *PDIA Newsletter*, no. 9 (December 2001), 17.

70. S. M. Gilbert, *Death's Door: Modern Dying and the Way We Grieve* (New York: W. W Norton & Company, 2006).

toward death. But her examination, including the institutionalization of the dying and the medical and technological attention given to a passage that once took place in the home, always returns to poetry. "We're always struggling to control death," she said. "Poetry reminds us that we can't."[71]

Poet and essayist Nancy Mairs built on a long writing career and her own experiences of illness and disability in preparing *A Troubled Guest. Life and Death Stories*.[72] Her personal essays are centered on the theme of how the living cope with death and by these means she explores the early, sudden death of her father and her mother's lingering illness and passage into old age. She reveals her own attempted suicide and tells of her growing relationship with a young man on death row, of her unsuccessful appeal on his behalf, and of hearing of his death. In a tragic coda, Mairs recounts the shooting of her son, Ron, which occurred while she was writing the book, and the agonizing decision to take him off life support. The book explores some of modern America's most controversial current debates, including assisted suicide and the death penalty.[73] A 2004 CD of the spoken word entitled *Essays Out Loud* includes the first piece from *A Troubled Guest*. One reviewer writes as follows:

> Mairs notes that Catholics are still called upon to observe All Souls' Day on November 2 and to devote a whole month to reflections on mortality. *A Troubled Guest: Life and Death Stories* is just the right resource to use during this sober period.[74]

Mairs' commitment to the enterprise is highlighted in her final grant report where she states: "This is plainly not a project that ends when the fellowship runs out. As I point out in the first essay in *A Troubled Guest*, death seems to have become my life's work."[75]

Lisa Schnell, a teacher of English at the University of Vermont, received PDIA funding for *Learning How to Tell*, a book which would explore the brief life and death in 1998 of her youngest daughter, Claire, who had suffered from a rare birth defect, lissencephaly. The experience introduced Schnell to a world of suffering that initially produced in her a sense of exile from her own life story. She later observed the following:

---

71. See NewsReview.com, Ken Munger, "Death Is the New Sex," http://www.newsreview.com/ sacramento/Content?oid=oid%3A55892 (accessed May 15, 2007).

72. N. Mairs, *A Troubled Guest. Life and Death Stories* (Boston: Beacon Press, 2001). See http:// maskink.com/mairs/works.htm#troubled (accessed May 15, 2007).

73. Publications from Arts and Humanities Grantees. *PDIA Newsletter*, no. 9 (December 2001), 17.

74. F. and M. A. Brussat., review of N. Mairs, *A Troubled Guest. Life and Death Stories*. In *Spirituality and Practice* (n.d.), http://www.spiritualityandpractice.com/books/books. php?id=3455 (accessed May 15, 2007).

75. Box 193288626, 1999 (PDIA files).

Having learned to live, albeit tenuously, with the grief associated with her life, we were in some ways entirely unprepared for the grief that accompanied her death. The eighteen months of her life, however, had given me time to begin to find my way through our story. So when, six months after Claire's death, Andrew came home with an application for a grant from an institution with the unadorned name "Project on Death in America," I knew I had found my opportunity to try to say what we were learning from Claire about the encounter of life and death. I applied for a grant to write a book I had been thinking about. The writing of the proposal itself convinced me that, grant or no grant, I needed to write this book. One part of my need came from my growing understanding of the redemptive power of language. I knew that words could not have made Claire healthy, that they could not bring her back now; but I recognized that the struggle to find the words to tell my grief was itself leading me to an understanding and an intense appreciation of the many things Claire had taught me about life, and that was saving me from the bitterness that I knew was always lurking around the corner ... But also, as I wrote the proposal for the grant, and as I continued to think about the book I was conceiving, I found myself going back to the conversation I had had with my colleague on the day I returned to work in February of 1997. He had said that my life as a literary critic would help me to find my way through the minefield of despair and bitterness and unrelenting sadness that was ahead of me. And I could see now how very right he had been.[76]

This project captures Lisa Schnell's story of her intellectual and spiritual journey. In a PDIA newsletter she writes the following:

In writing about Claire, in writing about *me*, I struggle with what death teaches us, what as Jacques Derrida says "gives us to think beyond the giving and the taking, in the *adieu*." And while there can be no simple synopsis of the lessons death has taught me, I recognize there is much I know now that I could not have known before I loved Claire. In carefully setting down before others what I have learned myself, in getting beyond the adieu, I am still Claire's mom.[77]

She wrote further about the experience in an article in the journal *Literature and Medicine*[78] and also presented her work to wider audiences, including a conference on *The Social Context of Death, Dying, and Disposal*, held in London

---

76. See *Vermont Quarterly*, "The Language of Grief," http://universitycommunications.uvm.edu/vq/VQFALL00/language.html (accessed May 15, 2007).

77. L. J. Schnell, "A Lament and a Lesson: I Am Still Claire's Mom," *PDIA Newsletter*, no. 7 (April 2000), 9.

78. L. J. Schnell, "Learning How to Tell," *Literature and Medicine* 23, no. 2 (Fall 2004): 265–279.

in 2000 and another on Narrative Medicine and Psychoanalysis in Gainesville, Florida, held in 2004.[79,80]

Poet, translator, novelist, critic, and journalist David R. Slavitt is the author of more than seventy works of fiction, poetry, and drama in translation. His honors include a Pennsylvania Council on Arts award, a National Endowment for the Arts fellowship in translation, an award in literature from the American Academy and Institute of Arts and Letters, and a Rockefeller Foundation Artist's Residence. He lives in Philadelphia and is on the faculties of Bennington and Yale.[81] Slavitt was given support by PDIA[82] to provide a translation of and meditation on the *Book of Lamentations*, the biblical account of the destruction of the Temple in Jerusalem in 587 BC, on the ninth day of the Jewish month of *Av*: *Tish'a b'Av*. Most of the Jewish population was deported to Babylon, and the ensuing period came to be known as the Babylonian Captivity. According to tradition, the *Book of Lamentations* was written in response to this political, social, and religious crisis. The five poems composing the book express Israel's sorrow, brokenness, and bewilderment before God. *Tish'a b'Av* is the day on which observant Jews fast, pray, and mourn. Slavitt notes how the day is viewed in his meditation:

> It is forbidden on *Tish'a b'Av* even to study the Torah, except for the *Book of Job* and the *Book of Lamentations*. This is the day on which we grieve for every terrible thing that happens in this world. It is the worst day of the year.[83]

Slavitt's meditation provides a context for reading the scriptural text. Cast in the same style as the Hebrew poetry, his meditation recounts how sorrow and catastrophe have characterized so much of the history of the Jewish people, from their enslavement in Egypt to the Holocaust of Nazi Germany. There is praise for this work from arts and medicine expert Sandra Bertman:

> Slavitt, self-revealing and humble in his assertion about the benefits as well as the costs of grief, hopes "that there may be people who will see in what is here my love for the work and that they may come to feel that love themselves" (xiv). This reviewer did.[84]

---

79. See The Social Context of Death, Dying, and Disposal, "Authors and Titles of Papers," http://www.srgw.demon.co.uk/deathcon/2000.html (accessed May 15, 2000).

80. Her book was "still in the works" in Spring 2007. Lisa Schnell, personal communication.

81. See Poets.org, "The Social Context of Death, Dying, and Disposal," David R. Slavitt, http://www.poets.org/poet.php/prmPID/448 (accessed September 25, 2012).

82. Publications from Arts and Humanities Grantees, *PDIA Newsletter*, no. 9 (December 2001), 17.

83. D. R. Slavitt, *The Book of Lamentations* (Baltimore: Johns Hopkins University Press, 2001), 6.

84. See NYU School of Medicine—Literature, Arts, and Medicine Database: "The Book of Lamentations: A Meditation and Translation," http://litmed.med.nyu.edu/Annotation?action=view&annid=12075 (accessed May 15, 2007).

Alan Shapiro, a National Book Critics Circle finalist and Los Angeles Times Book Award winner, was supported by the program to work on a collection of poetry, *The Dead Alive and Busy*.[85] This work built on his 1997 collection, *Vigil*, exploring his relationship with his sister before her death from breast cancer. Shapiro, at the time a teacher at the University of North Carolina, Chapel Hill, deals with contemporary experiences of sickness, love, and loss, with an eye toward the mythic and literary worlds of cultures that once viewed death as an intimate part of daily life. *The Dead Alive and Busy*, Shapiro's sixth book of poetry, won the 2001 Kingsley Tufts Poetry Award for emerging poets, administered at Claremont Graduate University in California.[86] The New York Times comments as follows:

> What has got loose in Shapiro's sixth collection is the dead—in all their guises and disguises. Shapiro like a kind medium, offers these loose souls his hand so that he might know them and, in the process, give those of us on this side of the great divide a new way of seeing.[87,88]

How would you make sense of such a rich and diverse collection of works as that which comprised the PDIA Arts and Humanities Program? Sandra Bertman brought them all together in an interesting website that captures the range and vibrancy of the various projects.[89] Her project, End of Life: Visions and Voices, had the goal of providing ongoing access to the PDIA arts and humanities projects and to create lasting benefits from the program as a whole, making it available to community groups and professionals alike.

It would be a mistake to see the totality of works described here as solely the product of PDIA funding. Part of the astuteness of PDIA was that it saw work in progress and gave it further support. It spotted innovative ideas and made them better known. It built on worthwhile projects and added value. Occasionally it found something that no one had noticed and enabled a work to develop and become known.

The Arts and Humanities Program grew out of a potpourri of initiatives that reflected the board's desire to address death, dying, and bereavement through a

---

85. A. Shapiro, *The Dead Alive and Busy* (Chicago: University of Chicago Press, 2000).

86. See University of North Carolina at Chapel Hill, Katie Blixt, "UNC Poet Alan Shapiro Receives Award for Best Poetry by a North Carolinian," http://www.unc.edu/news/archives/nov02/shapiroaward112502.html (accessed March 19, 2007).

87. M. Hainey, review of *The Dead Alive and Busy, New York Times* (April 9, 2000).

88. Alan Shapiro was killed on 16 May 2005 when he was hit by a truck while out jogging in Las Vegas, http://www.alanshapiro.org/ (accessed October 17, 2007).

89. Sandra Bertman, "End of Life: Visions and Voices," http://www.sandrabertman.com/visionsandvoices/index.html (accessed October 12, 2007).

cultural lens. The program itself was the centerpiece of PDIA's engagement with cultural issues. Sometimes this was done by grant making in association with others. The support it gave to documentary photography can also been seen in relation to the wider interest in this approach within the Open Society Institute itself. For example, in 2003, OSI launched the Documentary Photography Project, building on an established tradition of supporting documentary photographers, whose work has long been on prominent display in the organization's New York City offices.[90]

Looking back, key staff members were stretched by the question of how effective the PDIA engagement with the arts and humanities had been, as Mary Callaway commented in 2003:

> I think that we never quite knew what to do with it, and we didn't have an art-type person on the board, or a staff person, that was strong enough in it that we were really able to communicate the importance of what the arts and humanities initiatives are. I think also because ... it took a long time to write a book, it wasn't like doing a research project or doing some study that could be done in a year or two years. In many cases ... these books or projects took three or five years to complete. So I'm not sure that we know what the effect has been or the value added by the arts and humanities project yet. I know in my heart there has been, but ... we haven't been able to verbalize it yet.[91]

There was a sense of vision about these aspects of PDIA grant making that was not accompanied by a matching clarity of purpose and outcome. A relatively inexperienced board was bold (if divided) in supporting arts and humanities ventures. It then found itself unable to meet its own evaluation criterion: measureable impact on the culture of dying in America. Yet those individuals and groups it supported often remained grateful to PDIA several years later, and some of their works remained in the public domain and continued to resonate with audiences and critics even after PDIA had ceased to exist. The charge that these grants produced little of lasting impact seems unfounded. More salient in understanding this internal assessment of the arts and humanities projects is that they seemed to the board, in retrospect, to have been merely a preliminary to the central work of PDIA, which came about through a narrowing of focus—into care settings, professional practice development, and the education of staff responsible for the care of those facing death. These latter efforts would in time be seen as the key successes of PDIA and its more visible and long-lasting legacy. A key step toward them was in projects that drew attention to and highlighted the diversity of American experiences in care at the end of life, to which we now turn.

---

90. See, for example, the exhibition Moving Walls, http://www.soros.org/initiatives/photography/about (accessed October 12, 2007).

91. Mary Callaway, interview by David Clark, July 23, 2003.

3

Highlighting Experiences of Care

Through its attention to the role of culture, and by engaging with the arts and humanities as vehicles for exploring the meanings of death, dying, and bereavement in modern America, the interest of the PDIA board was able to focus with increasing sharpness on the lived experiences of care at the end of life. Early grant making in this area occurred across a broad contextual spectrum, which quite quickly narrowed onto experiences of giving and receiving care in different settings. As these projects came on stream, they underlined the range of places and spaces in which the dying process is played out in America and the many challenges that confront patients, families, clinicians, and those responsible for the organization of services. Also noted were the importance of community factors that impact upon debates about end-of-life care as well as the manner in which such issues are expressed in media representations. In this chapter we explore these aspects of PDIA grant making and see how they were to set the scene for further work that brought about innovations in policy and practice.

As board chair Kathy Foley observed to a journalist in 1996, "What we want to do is get death out of its hiding place in the intensive care wards, and bring it back into our homes and everyday life."[1] The PDIA agenda here, as elsewhere, was unequivocally reformist. It sought to highlight the fact that, while death is inevitable, few Americans make plans for dying. Grantee Frank Ostaseski of the Zen Hospice Project observed to *Time* magazine, "We have more preparation for how to operate our VCRs than we do for how to die."[2] Against this background, PDIA was also concerned to highlight the fact that while most Americans wished to die at home, the majority end their lives in medical institutions, and a significant

---

1. J. Woodward, "Death Usually Belongs in the Home," *Western Report* (July 22, 1996): 38–39.

2. Quoted in: "A Kinder, Gentler Death," *Time* 18 (September 2000): 60.

portion spend time in an intensive care unit in the last six months of life. PDIA was seeking to generate a debate about appropriate pain medication and to dispel the myths and phobias that lead to the undertreatment of pain, even at the end of life. It asked the questions how will we die and how can we die more comfortably? It promoted activities that would shed light on these issues and capture the experience of end-of-life care in modern American society. Yet it did so with a sense of what could be learned as well as what could be taught. As the very first PDIA newsletter observed, "The many diverse cultural communities in this country offer a tremendous amount of wisdom about the ways death can be a less devastating issue for the dying person and his or her caregiver."[3]

GIVING AND RECEIVING CARE

Each stage of your decline, if it was hell
while you were in it, did it become too brief a heaven
once it had passed...?

—ALAN SHAPIRO, *"Hand"* [4]

PDIA supported some outstanding work on the elucidation of personal experience at the end of life, from the perspectives of patients, families, and caregivers. The collaborative work of Barnard, Towers, and colleagues on narratives of end-of-life care (described in chapter 2) exemplified an approach that was congenial to several PDIA grantees and faculty scholars. Notable among these in terms of wider impact was the work of Canadian physician David Kuhl. Beginning with a doctoral dissertation, PDIA faculty scholar Kuhl made the unusual transition of building on an academic orientation in order to write for a wider public. His book *What Dying People Want* proved to be a best-selling trade title that led to appearances on radio and television shows and extensive lecture and promotional tours across Canada and the United States.[5]

Based on interviews with people with cancer and AIDS, Kuhl set out to produce a guide for people with a terminal illness, or those caring for a dying person, as well as those seeking to deepen their understanding of the dying process. It was reviewed widely and positively by those who saw in it not only a powerful illumination of the experience of what it means to be dying, but also a sound guide to clinical practice.[6] He comments:

3. "An Exploration of Some of the Issues Surrounding the Experience of Dying," *PDIA Newsletter*, no. 1 (March 1996), 7.

4. A. Shapiro, "Hand." In *The Dead Alive and Busy* (Chicago: University of Chicago Press, 2000), 70–71.

5. D. Kuhl, *What Dying People Want: Practical Wisdom for the End of Life*. (New York: Public Affairs, 2002).

6. B. Evelyn Kelly, review of *What Dying People Want. Practical Wisdom for the End of Life*, by D. Kuhl, *AMWA Journal* 20, no. 2 (2005): 101.

> And my project in essence was...to ask people, what's it like to live with the knowledge that you're dying? What's it like to live with the knowledge that you've got cancer or that you've got AIDS? I'd ask the question and then I'd just let them talk. I transcribed those tapes, identified themes, and went back to them, and I said..."We don't need another doctor's perspective; I want to understand this from your experiences as much as is humanly possible."...After I finished the dissertation, the people who participated in this study...asked that I write a book and they had clearly stated that it not be directed at an academic audience, that it not be written for doctors or nurses, because they said they wouldn't read it. They said "We'd like you to write a book, but we want you to write the book for other people who have a terminal illness or for their families. So we want you to use our stories.... We know you have to disguise us, [but] we'd like you not to disguise us so much that our families don't recognize us, because we've said things to you that we've never said to anybody else...but hold to writing to the public, don't write to the university." So that was my decision then to move from academic writing to writing for the public.[7]

Sensitively written and full of the *phronesis* promised in its subtitle, Kuhl's book is packed with engaging narratives, case examples, and good advice on how individuals, families, and whole groups of people might proceed in the face of mortal illness. It also appears to be a tribute to the stimulating environment of PDIA, which did so much to nurture Kuhl's ideas and to encourage him in his doctoral research ambitions. Building on this, Kuhl wrote a well received follow-up, published in 2006, *Facing Death, Embracing Life: Understanding What Dying People Want*[8] in which he distilled the advice presented in his first book into concrete, step-by-step suggestions, as well as offering space for readers' private reflections. The guide included advice on talking to health-care providers about treatment and diagnosis; learning the right questions to ask specialists; finding out about alternative treatments; considering home care versus hospitalization; finding sources of financial support; and offering space and guidance for recording and reflecting on larger, more emotional themes. Kuhl's work did a huge amount to gain airtime for death and dying in the North American media and even gained coverage on the Oprah Winfrey show. It is a particular example of how one piece of work within PDIA could do so much to contribute to the wider goal, that of transforming the culture of dying in American society.

Based in the University of Virginia School of Medicine, physician and PDIA faculty scholar Carlos Gomez also made use of narrative methods but in this instance as a vehicle for the training of residents in palliative medicine. He describes in some detail how it worked:

---

7. David Kuhl, interview by David Clark, July 15, 2004.

8. D. Kuhl, *Facing Death, Embracing Life: Understanding What Dying People Want* (Canada: Doubleday, 2006).

[It's a project called] The Ethics of Lamentation, and part of what I've done is I've collected the narratives of our patients and the doctors taking care of them and tried to see what sorts of themes come out of it and tried to compare the themes that come out of the...oral histories with what's actually in the chart. It's two different stories: There's a meta story going on that never gets transcribed, deeply moving, very personal; it's the stuff that makes you get up in the morning and also the stuff that makes you cry at night, which I think contains a key to this somewhere. And part of what I found is that there is this lacuna...where "I have run out of things to give you for treatment of whatever you've got, and I don't have anything else to offer you verbally. I don't have anything that I've been trained to do for you, even though I want to continue to be your doctor. I want to continue to have the relationship."

The genesis for this came to me about three years ago. We had an Hispanic family in our service and I'm a Spanish native speaker, very familiar with the culture. And when I went in to give the bad news, there was wailing, there was keening...on and on and on. The staff were horrible. It was just, "What the hell? What's the issue?" I [said that I] just told them that their mother was going to die, "so what do you expect?" And they said, "Well, I don't know, but isn't this excessive?" And I said, "Well, better that; then I know that they've absorbed the information that I've given them. They're not asking me to put Mom in the ICU. They're not asking for more chemotherapy. They're not faulting me. They're not..." and I went on through things that they hadn't done, and I said, "If their way of dealing with what is in fact sad to them is to keen and wail, so be it." And it turned out to be quite a wonderful death where the family was called, the patient had time to say goodbye...I mean all the things that we say that we want for our patients. But the reaction of the staff and my colleagues, especially the ones that were covering that weekend was "Oh my God, the so-and-so family—aren't they a handful?" And I said..."No"...[chuckles]..."they're a handful for *you*; they're doing just fine." And that's where the notion of lamentation came in...Why in American medicine...is it the culture? Is it that we are the society that [because of] our industry and enterprise [we don't] understand the nature of defeat or compromise?...I don't know. I'm not a cultural historian. Other people will do a better job of it. But within my field, within my profession, this inability to give voice to lament, to accept it, to be present and bear witness to it—I think goes to some extent in explaining what I consider to be our errors or our weaknesses in palliative care.[9]

HIV disease specialist Jeffrey H. Burack at the University of California was supported as a faculty scholar to work on a project exploring the transition to terminal illness. His starting point was with a medical profession that most commonly emphasizes the search for diagnosis and curing, but which finds it difficult to

---

9. Carlos Gomez, interview by David Clark, July 23, 2003.

switch to palliative care when cure is no longer considered possible, or when trying to achieve it becomes excessively burdensome. He observed that more is at stake in this transition than a mere shift in therapeutic emphasis. For the patient, coming to view oneself, and coming to be viewed socially, as terminally ill, marks a life change of dramatic psychological, spiritual, and existential consequence. Burack's work explored this transition into terminal illness and into exclusively palliative modes of medical care, as seen from patients' perspectives as well as those of their physicians and caregivers.[10]

Building on the SUPPORT study, social scientist Marguerite Stevens of Dartmouth College used a multi-method research project to understand the experience of dying in 132 seriously ill adults. The study analyzed patient and family reports of severe pain and developed descriptive models of "good" and "bad" dying experiences from the viewpoints of the patient and family.[11] In a similar vein, social anthropologist Lesley Sharp of Barnard College, Columbia University, undertook an investigation into the cross-cultural dimensions of death and mourning and their specific relevance to professional versus lay attitudes in the context of organ donation and procurement in urban Manhattan.[12] The study showed that the donation process alters grieving, and it may, in fact, prolong and even intensify the period of grief and mourning.[13]

PDIA seemed to attract health-care professionals who were inspired to write openly about their own struggles in being involved in the care of those seriously ill and dying. This can be seen as part of a wider trend in American medical writing during the period, in which physicians reflect on their clinical experience in ways designed to reach a wider public.[14] In 1997, the year that he became a faculty scholar, Peter Selwyn published his book *Surviving the Fall* to wide general interest.[15] One reviewer notes the following:

> Physicians engaged in high-stress medicine often pay a hidden price for continuing their professional work. Trauma surgeons, oncologists, and AIDS specialists, among others, call it burnout, an exhaustion of the personal resources required for technically demanding procedures and humane medical care. *Surviving the Fall* is not really about burnout but the turmoil

---

10. *Project on Death in America, January 1998–December 2000, Report of Activities* (New York: Open Society Institute, 2001), 15.

11. *Project on Death in America, July 1994–September 1997, Report of Activities* (New York: Open Society Institute, 1998), 13.

12. *Project on Death in America, July 1994–September 1997, Report of Activities* (New York: Open Society Institute, 1998), 14.

13. There do not appear to have been any publications from the studies referred to in this paragraph.

14. For a discussion, see J. Coulehan and A. H. Hawkins, "Keeping Faith: Ethics and the Physician Writer," *Annals of Internal Medicine* 139 (2003) 307–311.

15. Box 734907: Selwyn Book Signing, 31 March 1998 (PDIA files).

engendered by the AIDS epidemic in a literate and sensitive physician who was already psychologically wounded. Under pressure, Selwyn's suppressed childhood hurts burst forth and merge with the trauma of watching young patients die of an infectious disease. *Surviving the Fall* tells an ennobling story of how one physician sorted out his professional obligations and his life.[16]

With the support of PDIA, others were able to use their personal experience of life-threatening illness as a vehicle for further exploration. Betsy McGregor's study of dying and the inner life, begun in 1998, interlocked with her own preoccupations as a person with breast cancer, and she made creative use of the ethnographic approach that PDIA board members had been eager to foster. During the project, people with terminal illnesses talked to her about how they handled their sense of pain and regret, about experiencing forgiveness, acceptance, love, and even freedom. The results of the in-depth qualitative study were published in 2001 and revealed the dominant themes characterizing patients' perspectives on death during their last months of life. Serial, in-depth, semi-structured interviews were conducted with thirty patients with a mean of 4.2 interviews per person, and each was followed as close to the time of death as possible. Patients were referred to the study by Beth Israel Medical Center clinicians if they had a diagnosis of a life-threatening condition of which they were aware; if they were likely to die within one year according to their physician; if they had experienced symptoms of the illness; if they were sufficiently alert to discuss the topics addressed in the study; if they conversed easily in English; and if they consented to participate. MacGregor and her colleague found that outlooks on dying were grounded in patients' frames of reference and were consistent with other major events in their lives. Seven motifs were distilled that characterized these perspectives on death: struggle (living and dying are difficult), dissonance (dying is not living), endurance (the triumph of inner strength), coping (finding a new balance), incorporation (belief system accommodates death), quest (seeking meaning in death), and volatility (unresolved and unresigned). These patients demonstrated a striking capacity for coherence, integrating their responses to dying with broader motifs in their life stories, and the authors concluded that health-care providers would be well advised to become more aware of such motifs so as to better understand patient preferences for care and responses to treatment recommendations:

For physicians and other health-care providers, neglect of this context— the patient's broader biography or narrative—may undermine efforts to implement an effective care plan. Well-intentioned but uninformed providers may fail to distinguish between Mary's openness to addressing unresolved issues (volatile motif) and Esther's resignation (struggle motif);

16. Robert S. Schwartz, review of *Surviving the Fall: The Personal Journey of an* AIDS Doctor, by Peter A. Selwyn. In *New England Journal of Medicine* 338 (19 March 1998): 846–847.

Angela's inner strength may be confused with denial; Bob's acceptance of his changing status (coping motif) may be interpreted as depression; and Arthur's contempt for his quality of life (dissonance) may suggest a need for aggressive rehabilitation. Some of these responses would culminate in missed opportunities and others in unwanted interventions...Awareness of the motifs underlying patients' perspectives may reveal opportunities for effective intervention and may minimize misunderstandings or discrepant expectations; such familiarity may be helpful in identifying existing coping mechanisms that merit support or enhancement, or in addressing patient resistance to recommendations that are incompatible with their organizing models.[17]

Studies of this type showed that at the end of life, suffering has special resonance for patients *and* physicians, and the relief of suffering becomes the fundamental goal of medicine. Yet physicians rarely evaluate suffering or discuss it explicitly with patients. University of Washington doctors Anthony Back and Robert Pearlman, working as faculty scholars, took on a two-part project that aimed to improve medical evaluation and amelioration of suffering for patients in the last year of life. The project team conducted a qualitative study involving longitudinal patient interviews to characterize suffering and its evolution over time. These patient narratives were then integrated into an education program for faculty physicians with inpatient medicine attending responsibilities. The goal was to improve patient–physician communication and to add to the growing body of medical research on suffering and its treatment. Back, Arnold (another PDIA faculty scholar), and Quill observe the need for a twofold approach to communication:

When patients and physicians discuss life-threatening illness by focusing exclusively on hope, they may miss important opportunities to improve pain and symptom management, respond to underlying fears and concerns, explore life closure, and deepen the patient–physician relationship. The difficulty for physicians is acknowledging and supporting the patient's hopes while recognizing the severity of the patient's disease, thus offering an opportunity to discuss end-of-life concerns.

Hoping for a cure and preparing for potential death need not be mutually exclusive. Both patients and physicians want to hope for the best. At the same time, some patients also want to discuss their concerns about dying, and others probably should prepare, because they are likely to die sooner rather than later. Although it may seem contradictory, hoping for the best while *at the same time* preparing for the worst is a useful strategy for approaching patients with potentially life-limiting illness. By acknowledging all the possible outcomes, patients and their physicians can expand their medical

17. M. J. Yedidia and B. MacGregor, "Confronting the Prospect of Dying: Reports of Terminally Ill Patients," *Journal of Pain and Symptom Management* 22, no. 4 (2001): 807–819.

focus to include disease-modifying and symptomatic treatments and attend to underlying psychological, spiritual, and existential issues.[18]

At the Mayo clinic, a small grant made to Mary E. Bretscher enabled some wider reflection on the understanding of suffering and the lessons from palliative medicine. She and a colleague made the important observation that the "healing" of people who are suffering requires attention to all dimensions of personhood, not just the physical aspects. Moreover, they argued that palliative care physicians have discovered how "being an agent of healing for another human being at the end of life confers a personal richness that is difficult to find elsewhere in medicine. It is not just the patient who is healed."[19]

These projects and the resulting publications demonstrate the remarkable range of collaborations and interconnections that were made by PDIA grantees, both during the lifetime of PDIA and subsequently. These works often led to complementary overlaps between individual projects or to new and shared ventures that grew out of the original grant applications. There was cross-fertilization and considerable interweaving of effort that made for a whole that was more than the sum of the parts. The effect of the faculty scholar retreats was particularly notable in this regard, as medical anthropologist Barbara Koenig notes:

> There are…scholars I work with regularly. For example, yesterday at breakfast I sat down with Tony Back and Bob Pearlman, and we did some comments on a manuscript review that we'd just gotten on the first—to our knowledge—interview-based qualitative study of…patients seeking physician-assisted suicide in the United States, not in Oregon but in an area where it's not legal, so the subjects are all from Washington State. We're trying to get that published at the moment, so that's the kind of thing we do at the retreat. We sort of sit down and we're together and we work and…there are a lot of connections like that.[20]

One example of this was a paper on the "good death," which saw two faculty scholars, Nicholas Christakis and James Tulsky, combine their efforts with other colleagues to address the question of how the good death might be defined. The purpose of the study was to gather descriptions of the components of a good death from patients, families, and providers through focus group discussions and in-depth interviews. Seventy-five participants, including physicians, nurses, social workers, chaplains, hospice volunteers, patients, and recently bereaved

18. A. L. Back, R. L. Arnold, and T. E. Quill, "Hope for the Best and Prepare for the Worst," *Annals of Internal Medicine* 138, no. 5 (2003): 439–444.

19. M. E. Bretscher and E. T. Creagan, "Understanding Suffering: What Palliative Medicine Teaches Us," *Mayo Clinic Proceedings* 72 (1997): 785–787.

20. Barbara Koenig, interview by David Clark, 15 July 2004. The study was not supported with funds from PDIA, but was published as H. Starks et al., "Why Now? Timing and Circumstances of Hastened Deaths," *Journal of Pain and Symptom Management* 30, no. 3 (2005): 215–226.

family members, were recruited from a university medical center, a veterans affairs medical center, and a community hospice.

Participants identified six major components of a good death: pain and symptom management, clear decision making, preparation for death, completion and closure, contributing to others, and affirmation of the whole person. The physicians' discussions of a good death differed greatly from those of other groups and offered the most biomedical perspective, while patients, families, and other health-care professionals defined a broad range of attributes integral to the quality of dying. The authors noted that "Although there is no 'right' way to die, these six themes may be used as a framework for understanding what participants tend to value at the end of life. Biomedical care is critical, but it is only a point of departure toward total end-of-life care. For patients and families, psychosocial and spiritual issues are as important as physiologic concerns."[21]

Some PDIA scholars and grantees took a special interest in the experiences of children with life-limiting illness. Joanne Wolfe of the Dana-Farber Cancer Institute recognized that although most children with cancer survive, 40 percent eventually die of their disease and many of these experience substantial suffering. Her multi-institutional study aimed to critically evaluate the quality of care provided to children with advanced cancer and to assess the impact of implementing a symptom assessment tool on the integration of a palliative care service in the management of medical problems. As Joanne Wolfe explains, this study built on earlier work that had identified some of the deficiencies in the care of dying children:

> Our research, which was primarily based on a survey of 103 parents of children who died of cancer, showed that while there were high levels of satisfaction with providers, when it came to asking specifically about the experience of the child, parents reported that their children experienced substantial suffering in the last month of life...like fatigue, pain, dyspnea, and poor appetite. Eighty-nine percent of children experienced significant suffering from at least one symptom...parents reported while there were efforts to treat certain symptoms such as pain and shortness of breath, those efforts were not successful, or minimally successful in the majority of situations. So...suffering, physical suffering, became a big theme of what we were trying to change, and then with regard to communication issues, we found that parents came to understand that their child had no realistic chance for cure...if physicians came to that understanding about seven months before the child died, parents came to that understanding...at three-and-a-half months before death on average. So there is this gap, and we tried to look at factors that were related to smaller differences between physician and parent understanding...If there was a psychosocial clinician involved, like a psychologist or social worker, then there was better overlap in that understanding, perhaps suggesting that an interdisciplinary

21. K. Steinhauser et al., "In Search of a Good Death: Observations of Patients, Families, and Providers," *Annals of Internal Medicine*. 132, no. 10 (2000): 825–832.

approach to communication would lead to more effective communication. We also found that when parents and physicians came to the understanding that their children had no realistic chance of a cure earlier on together, there were differences in the patterns of care, so children were less likely to receive cancer-directed therapies, they were more likely to have the support of a home-care program, parents were more satisfied with that home-care program, and most importantly, the physician and parent goals were aligned at primarily relieving suffering as opposed to extending life—the theory being that if you improved upon communication and understanding, there might be a difference in the experience of the child at the very end of life.[22]

Within the PDIA Social Work Leadership Development Program (see chapter 7), a program directed by Barbara Jones at the Albany Medical Center was specifically geared toward social work education for psychosocial providers to children with cancer. The project described the current training of social workers in end-of-life care for children with cancer, examined the end-of-life experiences of families who have suffered the death of a child to cancer, and defined crucial family support services.[23]

In addition to the consideration of the end-of-life needs of children, PDIA scholars and grantees were active in seeking out experiences of death, dying, and bereavement in a variety of settings and contexts and in relation to numerous relatively unexplored problems. While much early hospice and palliative care practice had been focused on patients with malignant conditions, several of these PDIA projects moved beyond cancer to explore a wide range of other life-limiting conditions, situations, and diseases.

Kendra Peterson, a neurologist at Stanford University Medical Center, addressed the little known area of the experiences and needs of patients dying with malignant brain tumors and their caregivers. Randall Curtis, of Harborview Medical Center in Seattle, Washington, developed a program of work on the quality of communication about end-of-life care that focused on effective patient–doctor communication to improve the quality of the dying experience in the context of HIV/AIDS. The main goals included the validation of a measure of the quality of the dying experience among persons with AIDS and the assessment of the relationship between the quality of patient–doctor communication about end-of-life care and the quality of the dying experience. In one study, patients or physicians identified twenty-nine barriers and facilitators to communication about end-of-life care. Many patients and physicians expressed discomfort talking about death and dying, and some felt that discussing end-of-life care could cause harm or even hasten death. Several patients expressed the view that a living will obviated the need for discussion with their physician. Previous experience of discrimination from the health-care system was a strong barrier to end-of-

22. Joanne Wolfe, interview by David Clark, July 15, 2004.

23. Joanne Wolfe also developed further work on pediatric palliative care in a PDIA-funded project described in chapter 4.

life communication for some patients with AIDS. Some patients hesitated to bring up end-of-life issues because they wanted to protect their physicians from uncomfortable discussions. Many patients identified the quality of communication as an important facilitator to these difficult discussions.[24]

The special needs of people with amyotrophic lateral sclerosis (ALS, also known as Lou Gehrig's disease) were attended to by Dr. Lewis P. Rowland, professor of neurology at Columbia University, chairman of neurology (1973–1998) and director of the neurology service at the New York–Presbyterian Hospital. He undertook studies, with support from PDIA, to understand the palliative care choices made by people with ALS, and this was done by following a group of recently diagnosed patients and recording when they reached well-defined palliative care milestones. The patients were assessed every four months to determine their experience with ameliorative and palliative care. Domains included adjuvant therapies (e.g., speech therapy), adaptive aids (e.g., wheelchair use, augmentative communication), home health care, PEG placement, pulmonary support, health-care directives, psychosocial care (e.g., participation in support groups, pastoral counseling), and hospitalization. Many patients did not take advantage of palliative care options before death, though 36.6 percent used hospice, 48 percent had signed a power of attorney form, and 18 percent had "do not resuscitate" orders in their medical charts. Examining time to such end points captured important features of patient and family experience with the disease.[25]

A notable program of work, with many publications and widespread interest resulting, was undertaken by faculty scholar Nicholas Christakis, on the theme of prognostication. Trained in medicine and sociology, he set out to explain prognosis from the perspective of doctors: examining why physicians are reluctant to make predictions to their patients, how prognosis is used, and the symbolism and emotional difficulties it contains. He found that doctors were hugely inclined to optimism in predicting how long their patients would live, with average forecasts some 5.3 times greater than actual survival. He argued that this has detrimental consequences for end-of-life care, delaying access to hospice programs and forestalling endeavors aimed at end-of-life care planning. In particular, it can lead to drawn out attention to aggressive but futile medical treatment, not enough pain control, unnecessary expense, and less patient and family satisfaction. There seemed to be few clues about which doctors are good at judging when a patient is ready to enter hospice and, surprisingly, the better the physician knew the patient, the more likely he or she was to err in prognostication. The work of Christakis showed that in modern American medicine,

24. See J. R. Curtis and D. L. Patrick, "Barriers to Communication about End-of-Life Care in AIDS Patients," *Journal of General Internal Medicine* 12 (1997): 736–741; and also C. M. Pierson, J. Curtis, and D. L. Patrick, "A Good Death: A Qualitative Study of Patients with Advanced AIDS," *AIDS Care* 14 (2002): 587–598.

25. S. M. Albert et al., "Prospective Study of Palliative Care in ALS: Choice, Timing, Outcomes," *Journal of Neurological Sciences* 169, no. 1–2 (1999): 108–113.

prognosis is not merely neglected, it is actively avoided—and to the detriment of care received at the end of life.[26]

In another substantial program of studies, Lewis M. Cohen and colleagues at Baystate Medical Center in Massachusetts focused their work on the end-of-life care experiences of patients undergoing renal dialysis. Faculty scholar Cohen was supported by PDIA to conduct a bioethical, psychiatric, and clinical study of the decision by patients to terminate life-sustaining kidney dialysis treatment. Several key papers emerged from this work and showed encouraging results: only 15 percent of subjects who died after the discontinuation of dialysis were deemed to have had "bad deaths"; when measured in relation to psychosocial dimensions, those experiencing a "good death" were more likely to die at home or with hospice care, when compared to those in hospital or nursing home.[27] The definition of a good death used here was consistent with Weisman's aphorism, as being "the type of death one would chose if there were a choice"—to whit, brief in duration, purposeful, relatively devoid of suffering, consistent with ego ideals, and allowing for resolution and reconciliation.[28] As the authors noted, very good deaths need to be recognized and valued as goals for palliative medicine.[29]

This work also highlighted the increasing number of deaths that are preceded by some form of treatment decision, often involving the withholding or withdrawal of life-supporting interventions. These can be enormously complex decisions, though as Cohen and colleagues noted, "The great majority of patients referred to us for requests to terminate life-support have been neither depressed nor clinically suicidal."[30] The work was important in using the rich experience of treatment cessation decisions in renal care as a vehicle for generalizing the issue of death-hastening requests. Physician-assisted dying could be placed within this category of request, though Cohen and colleagues reported no clinical experience of the issue and were careful to see it as both the least common and the most controversial of such requests. They noted: "As our society heatedly examines the care provided to the terminally ill, psychiatry also needs to reconsider whether actions that foreshorten life can be normative and permissible"[31]—a challenging point for the original definition of palliative care from the World Health

26. N. Christakis, "Death Foretold: Prophecy and Prognosis in Medical Care" (Chicago: University of Chicago Press, 1999).

27. L. M. Cohen et al., "Dying Well after Discontinuing the Life-Support Treatment of Dialysis," Archives of Internal Medicine 160 (2000): 2513–2518.

28. A. D. Weisman and T. P. Hackett, "Predilection to Death: Death and Dying as a Psychiatric Problem," Psychosomatic Medicine 23 (1961): 232–256.

29. L. M. Cohen et al., "A Very Good Death: Measuring Quality of Dying in End Stage Renal Disease," Journal of Palliative Medicine 4, no. 2 (2001): 167–172.

30. L. M. Cohen et al., "Psychiatric Evaluation of Death-Hastening Requests: Lessons from Dialysis Discontinuation," Psychosomatics 41, no. 3 (2000): 195–203.

31. L. M. Cohen et al., "Psychiatric Evaluation of Death-Hastening Requests,"195.

Organization, which emphasized that palliative care "neither hastens death nor prolongs life."[32]

Of the two million and more deaths that occur in the United States each year, one in five follows treatment in the intensive care unit (ICU), and treatment *decisions* occur in almost half the deaths that occur in American ICUs. PDIA supported work to elucidate the practice of end-of-life care in ICU and also to promote good practice, and several grantees and scholars combined their efforts on this work, taking it forward with additional funding leveraged from elsewhere. The group included Judith Nelson, working with her colleagues Diane Meier and Sean Morrison at Mount Sinai School of Medicine, as well as Kathleen Puntillo, at UCSF School of Nursing, James Tulsky at Duke University, and Thomas Prendergast at Dartmouth.

Judith Nelson joined the Faculty Scholars Program in 1999 with a project that started from the recognition that between 15 percent and 20 percent of adult patients admitted to ICUs in the United States do not survive hospital discharge. The project aimed to characterize and improve the intensive care experience and satisfaction of critically ill cancer patients and their families. Predicated on the notion that palliative care is not simply a sequel to intensive care but an essential component of comprehensive intensive care, Nelson's work demonstrated that it should be provided in a concurrent and coordinated manner to all patients in that setting. In her study of one hundred cancer patients treated in the ICU, hospital mortality was 56 percent. Half of the patients had the capacity to complete the Edmonton Symptom Assessment Scale (ESAS)[33], and between 55 percent and 75 percent of these reported experiencing pain, discomfort, anxiety, sleep disturbance, or unsatisfied hunger or thirst that they rated as moderate or severe. Depression and dyspnea at these levels were reported by 40 percent and 33 percent of responders, respectively. The study concluded that among critically ill cancer patients, multiple distressing symptoms were common in the ICU and suggested that systematic assessment of symptoms may help to direct decisions about the appropriate use of ICU therapies.[34]

In 2000, faculty scholar Kathleen Puntillo, embarked on a related project with the goal of describing symptom assessment and management practices for dying patients in ICUs, in order to use this information to design, implement, and evaluate an academic course in intensive care symptom assessment and management. A key focus of this work was on the assessment of pain in the ICU, and in addressing this, she built on an extensive portfolio of related work. In a major retrospective of her research, published in 2003, she made special mention of the support received from PDIA:

---

32. World Health Organization, *Cancer Pain Relief and Palliative Care*, WHO Technical Report Series 804 (Geneva: WHO, 1990).

33. This tool helps identify and measure the severity of common symptoms in patients receiving palliative care.

34. J. E. Nelson et al., "Self-Reported Symptom Experience of Critically Ill Cancer Patients Receiving Intensive Care," *Critical Care Medicine* 29, no. 2 (2001): 277–282.

My selection as a Soros faculty scholar with [the] Project on Death in America has provided support to my research team to investigate the particular challenges of assessing pain and other symptoms as well as providing palliative care for ICU patients at high risk of dying. And, as a side road, emergency department colleagues and I continue a series of studies on pain assessment and management in emergency departments, where similar challenges exist in providing patients comfort.[35]

Complementing such work, Thomas Prendergast, who took up a faculty scholarship in 1999, developed a curriculum for teaching the principles of palliative care to health-care professionals who work in the ICU, with a particular emphasis on negotiation and conflict resolution. In a widely cited *JAMA* article that he co-wrote with Puntillo, the two authors noted:

The technology and expertise of critical care practice support patients through life-threatening illnesses. Most recover; some die quickly; others, however, linger—neither improving nor acutely dying, alive but with a dwindling capacity to recover from their injury or illness. Management of these patients is often dominated by the question: Is it appropriate to continue life-sustaining therapy? Patients rarely participate in these pivotal discussions because they are either too sick or too heavily sedated. As a result, the decision often falls to the family or the surrogate decision maker, in consultation with the medical team. Decisions of such import are emotionally stressful and are often a source of disagreement. Failure to resolve such disagreements may create conflict that compromises patient care, engenders guilt among family members, and creates dissatisfaction for health-care professionals. However, the potential for strained communications is mitigated if clinicians provide timely clinical and prognostic information and support the patient and family with aggressive symptom control, a comfortable setting, and continuous psychosocial support. Effective communication includes sharing the burden of decision making with family members. This shift from individual responsibility to patient-focused consensus often permits the family to understand, perhaps reluctantly and with great sadness, that intensive caring may involve letting go of life-sustaining interventions.[36]

A major piece on end-of-life care in the ICU appeared from faculty scholar Randall Curtis in the form of his edited book, with Gordon D. Rubenfeld, *Managing Death in the Intensive Care Unit*. With contributions from several PDIA grantees as well as board members Kathy Foley and Susan Block, the book

---

35. K. Puntillo, "Pain Assessment and Management in the Critically Ill: Wizardry or Science?" *American Journal of Critical Care* 12 (2003): 310–316.

36. T. J. Prendergast and K. A. Puntillo, "Withdrawal of Life Support: Intensive Caring at the End of Life," *Journal of the American Medical Association*" 288 (2002): 2732–2740.

is a comprehensive appraisal of the social, ethical, clinical, and legal aspects of death in the ICU.[37] In addition, Lewis Cohen wrote a thoughtful article relating to death in the ICU, based upon interviews with some of his PDIA colleagues at the faculty scholars retreat held in Granlibaaken, California, in 2003. He notes the following:

> Two intensivists speak about how comfortable it is to withdraw or withhold life support when a team of medical professionals and the family have reached a consensus that treatment is death prolonging rather than life sustaining. Dr. Nelson comments that "almost no one that I know would want their life prolonged if they could never leave the hospital." According to Dr. Prendergast, "Continued treatment of people against their will and in situations where no one thinks there is any clinical benefit seems absurd. In these cases, it is intuitively obvious that withdrawal is an appropriate clinical act." He concludes that "it is almost always possible to maintain comfort through the process of withdrawal. The clinical team can describe to families what to expect, and everyone can be offered an opportunity for a private leave-taking."[38]

Also notable in this body of PDIA-funded work on experiences of giving and receiving care is that of the Canadian psychiatrist and faculty scholar Harvey Chochinov. He built on earlier studies relating to the desire for death and the prevalence of depression in the terminally ill to develop a rich seam of inquiry relating to the preservation of dignity at the end of life.

> Although the literature on dignity is sparse, it shows that "how patients perceive themselves to be seen" is a powerful mediator of their dignity. In a study of patients with end stage cancer, perceptions of dignity were most strongly associated with "feeling a burden to others" and "sense of being treated with respect." As such, the more that healthcare providers are able to affirm the patient's value—that is, seeing the person they are or were, rather than just the illness they have—the more likely that the patient's sense of dignity will be upheld. This finding, and the intimate connection between care provider's affirmation and patient's self-perception, underscores the basis of dignity-conserving care.[39]

In a key article reporting this work, Chochinov and colleagues note that despite widespread use of the term *dignity* in arguments for and against a patient's self-governance in matters pertaining to death, there is little empirical research

---

37. J. R. Curtis and G. D. Rubenfeld, *Managing Death in the ICU: The Transition from Cure to Comfort* (New York and Oxford, UK: Oxford University Press, 2000).

38. L. Cohen, "Pulling the Plug," *Palliative and Supportive Care* 1 (2003): 279–283.

39. H. Chochinov, "Dignity and the Essence of Medicine: The A, B, C, and D of Dignity Conserving Care," *British Medical Journal* 335, no. 7612 (28 July 2007): 184–187.

on how the term has been used by patients at the end of life. The objective of their study was therefore to determine how dying patients understand and define the term *dignity*, in order to inform the development of a model of dignity in the terminally ill. A semi-structured interview was designed to explore how patients cope with their advanced cancer and to detail their perceptions of dignity. Interviews were audiotaped and transcribed verbatim. A consecutive sample of fifty consenting patients with advanced terminal cancer was recruited over a fifteen-month period from an urban extended-care hospital housing a specialized unit for palliative care. Three major categories emerged from the qualitative analysis, including illness-related concerns; dignity conserving repertoire; and social dignity inventory. The authors suggest that these broad categories and their carefully defined themes and subthemes form the foundation for an emerging model of dignity among the dying. The concept of dignity and the dignity model offer a way of understanding how patients face advancing terminal illness, serving to promote dignity and the quality of life of patients nearing death. The authors observe the following:

> Patients in the study had no trouble identifying issues that might impinge upon or enhance their sense of dignity. The term *dignity* evoked stories and anecdotes, and was described as meaningful to them. Patients provided countless examples of times when the behaviors of family, friends, and health providers served to enhance or diminish their dignity. Patients also shared descriptions about those things that gave their life meaning in the face of impending death, and named the essential life activities, attitudes, and self-philosophies that fostered their feelings of personal dignity. For many patients, particularly those in the hospital and those with more debility, life without dignity was described as a life no longer worthy of living. For those patients less encumbered by illness, a personal sense of dignity was inseparable from life itself. Thus, the concept of dignity and the dignity model may offer a way of understanding how patients navigate the wish to go on living—or the wish to die—in the face of an advancing terminal illness.[40]

This approach highlighted how palliative care has continued to struggle with the extent to which it can address suffering beyond the realm of physical symptoms. The work, which was widely disseminated, did much to highlight the dignity concerns of patients near the end of life and raise sensitivity to important aspects of human pain, providing the groundwork required to develop effective management strategies. The rallying call of Chochinov's work is for dignity-conserving care to become part of the palliative care lexicon and an overarching therapeutic aim and standard of care for all patients close to death.[41]

---

40. H. M. Chochinov et al., "Dignity in the Terminally Ill: A Developing Empirical Model," *Social Science and Medicine* 54, no. 3 (2002): 433–443.

41. H. M. Chochinov et al., "Dignity in the Terminally Ill: A Cross-Sectional, Cohort Study," *The Lancet* 360, no. 9350 (2002): 12022–12028.

PDIA work on the experiences of giving and receiving care seems, therefore, to have been wide-ranging in character and, in some cases, of outstanding quality when judged internationally. Among some board members, however, there was still a sense, in retrospect, that few grantees had gotten close to the direct experience of what it is to face death, as Robert Butler notes:

And that leads me to the one and only kind of disappointment I've had about this and that is that I think so much energy, understandably, has been devoted to helping transform physicians, hospitals, institutions...pain and symptom relief, that we did not get as many proposals as I was hoping on the inner life...What do people really go through at the end of life? What are the more personal, even existential, aspects? We just didn't get a lot of good proposals along that line. This afternoon there's going to be a presentation by Harvey Chochinov...I think his work is maybe the closest to what I was hoping we'd see more of. Plus it's quite amazing to me that, despite the fact that clearly millions of people have died from the beginning of time, we have very little in the way of insights as to what people really do experience at the end of life—what goes on inside people's heads? And part of my hope had been that, as we began to be more effective in relieving pain and the other terrible physical discomforts, that [we] would open the door to more opportunity for relationships to family to be dealt with—reviewing one's own life and coming to terms with it...Maybe it's just the historic sequence that first we have to be assured that people have a reasonably decent quality of life at the end of life before they can even have the energy and time to address these more, I think, profound issues.[42]

Such a reflection is understandable, but there were nevertheless a large number of PDIA grantees who directly and indirectly did a huge amount to illuminate individual experiences of giving and receiving end-of-life care, and in so doing identified ways in which it could be improved.

COMMUNITY AND MEDIA REPRESENTATIONS

In addition to these clinical and individual perspectives on the experience of care at the end of life, PDIA also promoted the exploration of issues at the community level, seeing here an opportunity to engage in situated debates about care that reflected the concerns and views of people as citizens as well as consumers of services. This work was attentive to the complexities of culturally appropriate and competent care of dying people and raised many issues about how individuals and communities prioritize the care they wish to receive, which aspects they hold as most important, and how they can communicate their views to professional care givers.[43]

---

42. Robert Butler, interview by David Clark, 23 July 2003.

43. A. Back, "Culturally Clueless: Does It Have to Be Terminal?" *Journal of Palliative Medicine* 2, no. 4 (1999): 433–434.

An early illustration came in the Coalition for Dialogue on Death and Dying that was established by the Hospice of Midcoast Maine under the project co-ordination of John A. Norton.[44] The purpose here was to create a coalition of community organizations in the region to improve the culture of dying; to deliver services more effectively to dying persons and their families during the period of illness and bereavement; and to serve as a catalyst for systemic change by "bringing to the table" hospitals and other providers of medical care, insurance companies, and major employers in the region. This group was formed in 1995 to explore the culture, issues, barriers, and organizational capabilities that surround death and dying in the Mid Coast region of Maine, with a view toward positive change. A grant of $45,000 from PDIA was crucial in moving from planning to action and created a process of dialogue with a wide cross-section of community associations in health care, education, and also including local faith groups and churches. Members of the coalition published articles about its work in the local media, gave presentations at meetings, and established a website. Interviews, focus groups, and organizational analyses were conducted to uncover local experiences and concerns. Those involved took the view that the coalition had emerged as major force in the area–community, with over one hundred individuals actively involved and at least fifteen hundred reached in a direct way by its activities. By January 1997, the group could conclude: "In short, community consciousness has been raised, issues are being examined, data is persuasive, and systematic change has commenced."[45] More significantly this demonstration project proved influential to thinking at the Robert Wood Johnson Foundation, which from 1997 to 2003 funded an $11.25 million national program called Community-State Partnerships to Improve End-of-Life Care.[46]

Around the same period, in 1994, the Poynter Center for the Study of Ethics and American Institutions, led by director David H. Smith at Indiana University, was funded by PDIA to produce an ethnographic study of residents of four diverse Indiana communities. The purpose was to better understand the meaning that ordinary people attach to death. The context of the report was the

---

44. "Maine Coalition Explores Ways to Improve End of Life Care," *PDIA Newsletter*, no. 2 (September 1998), 7.

45. "Closed Grants 95," Box GR# 3244, Final Progress Report, 20 January 1997 (PDIA files).

46. The program supported the work of state-based commissions and task forces to identify and implement changes in policy and practice to improve care for terminally ill patients and their families. Groups that received funding formed state and local coalitions with other organizations interested in working on end-of-life care policies, and secured matching funding equal to one-third of their Robert Wood Johnson Foundation grant. A total of twenty-four applicants received grants. In furthering statewide projects, site staff worked with hospitals and nursing homes to improve the care of dying patients. Seven sites (California, Hawaii, Kansas, Kentucky, Michigan, North Carolina, and Rhode Island) provided some form of training for hospital staff and administrators in addressing the needs of dying patients and improving the quality of their treatment. Site staff also worked with project partners to provide or improve education about palliative care to professionals in training and practice. See Robert Wood Johnson Foundation, "Community–State Partnerships to Improve End-of-Life Care," http://www.rwjf.org/pr/product.jsp?id=17981 (accessed April 26, 2012).

assertion that many Americans die badly, often alone in hospitals after intrusive and futile treatment options have been exhausted. The study attempted to listen to the voices of people confronting the deaths of family members and friends. Respondents described death as "a part of life" and stressed the importance of spiritual preparation. It was common to distinguish between the (absent) fear of death and the (present) fear of dying. For many the greatest fear was a long, lingering death in a state of dementia. But the report, entitled *The Social Face of Death*, was also useful in emphasizing communal sources of support in the face of death and bereavement—referring to the role of religion and church, and the efforts of funeral directors and health-care staff.[47]

A notable example of this type of community-based approach was *Vermont Voices on Care of the Dying*, which was part of the *Journey's End Project* of the Vermont Ethics Network. PDIA gave funding in 1997 for the coordination and facilitation of community discussions about death and dying. Again, the report highlighted growing North American concerns about care at the end of life. Based on interviews with 382 Vermonters in 42 different focus groups, in which participants were asked to reflect on their experiences of the end-of-life care of someone they knew intimately, the full details of the report were condensed into nine elegantly crafted statements covering the following four broad areas.[48]

On communication, education, and decision making

- When we are ourselves approaching the condition of being dying persons, we want to hear about it sooner and more clearly than people do now— but we want to be told in a way that is sensitive to our varying abilities to absorb the bad news. And then we want to learn whatever we need to know in order to steer our course through unknown waters.
- We want to have adequate opportunity to understand the various care options that are available, and then to choose what fits us best.
- We want, while still relatively well, to have the help of doctors and nurses in preparing advance directives that will really work to bring us the kind of care we would want when we can no longer speak for ourselves.
- We hope all our caregivers will keep in mind that we need time and energy and opportunity for living our remaining lives, as well as for pursuing medical possibilities.

On relationships

- We want someone we can rely on (perhaps a doctor, or perhaps a nurse or social worker) to travel with us as coach or pilot, much as a midwife goes with a woman through pregnancy, labor, and delivery.

---

47. K. D. Pimple, J. A. Granbois, and D. H. Smith, *The Social Face of Death: Confronting Mortality in Paoli, Indiana* (Bloomington, IN: Poynter Center, 1998).

48. *Vermont Voices on Care of the Dying* (Vermont: Vermont Ethics Network, 1997).

- We know we will need many kinds of help from various different people; we hope they will work together in genuine teamwork so that we will not be confused and can worry less about errors.
- Crucially, we hope our caregivers never forget that we are all unique individuals; that no generality applies easily to any of us; and that we need a unique partnership with those that are helping us.

On suffering

- We need assurance that the best modern means of controlling pain and other forms of suffering will be available and provided as we need them

On the place of dying

- Most of us prefer to die at home, if our families can be helped to help us; but if circumstances demand that our last days be in an institution, we hope the environment will be made as homelike as possible, guarding our privacy and dignity as much as possible.

These results were widely debated, the report attracted considerable interest in the professional literature, and the method was adopted in at least two other projects.[49,50] *Vermont Voices on Care of the Dying* is a thoughtfully produced and attractively designed report that combines the virtues of brevity and depth. The *citizen forum* approach to a major public issue yielded important and well expressed concerns, still being explored in the same state over a decade later.[51] By such means, PDIA showed itself capable of tapping into and supporting endeavors at the community level, in which the wider public issue of end-of-life care could be explored from the perspective of lay people and concerned individuals, as well as from the viewpoint of health and social care professionals.

This kind of approach was absolutely central to the Missoula Demonstration Project, led by end-of-life expert physician Dr. Ira Byock in Montana. Although the Missoula Project was substantially and primarily supported by the Robert Wood Johnson Foundation, PDIA also gave encouragement to a work that centered on a long-term, community-based organization that came together to study and transform the culture and experience of dying in one locality, Missoula County, Montana. The results of early inquiries were then used to provide the platform for future interventions and research focused on bringing quality to life's end.[52]

---

49. S. Hwang et al., "Knowledge and Attitudes toward End-of-Life Care in Veterans with Symptomatic Metastatic Cancer," *Palliative and Supportive Care* 1, no. 3 (2004): 221–230.

50. S. McSkimming et al., "The Experience of Life-Threatening Illness: Patients' and Their Loved Ones' Perspectives," *Journal of Palliative Medicine* 2, no. 2 (1999): 173–184.

51. See, for example, the report of a citizen forum on *Improving Care for Life's Last* Chapter, led by Dr. Ira Byock and described in *Health Decisions* 12, no. 3 (April 2006), a publication of the Vermont Ethics Network.

52. Life's End Institute, Missoula Demonstration Project, http://www.dyingwell.org/MDP. htm, accessed September 25, 2012.

Working with gerontologist Dr. Barbara K. Spring, Byock set out to engage an entire Montana town in examining the dying process and making it better. Modeled after a famous long-term heart disease study which collected data on an entire community, the Missoula Project aimed not only to improve the quality of life's end in Missoula, but to stimulate other efforts throughout the country. Organized in 1996 and overseen by an international advisory committee, the project engaged in several studies to understand people's experiences, attitudes, values, customs, and concerns about death. By looking at 250 families that experienced a death within a one-year period, for instance, and by gathering data in all health-care settings that treat or care for dying people—focusing on the length of the dying process, pain, isolation, and similar important issues—researchers hoped to create a picture of dying, death, and bereavement in Missoula that could not easily be ignored. Because this area had been so neglected in American life, most dying people and their families expect very little palliative care, and as a result, make few demands for better treatment. So a specific goal of the project was to raise public expectations for improved end-of-life care.

At the University of Oklahoma Health Sciences Center, Betty Pfefferbaum and colleagues undertook a project to examine the nature and course of traumatic bereavement in children who lost a family member in the April 1995 bombing of the Alfred P. Murrah Federal Building in Oklahoma City, in which 167 people were killed. The effects of traumatic loss on children who reported a friend or acquaintance killed in the bombing were examined. Twenty-seven children who lost a friend or acquaintance and twenty-seven demographically matched controls were assessed eight to ten months after the bombing. All but three of the children continued to experience posttraumatic stress symptoms. Those who lost a friend watched significantly more bombing-related television coverage than those without losses. They also had significantly more posttraumatic stress symptoms at the time of the assessment than those who lost an acquaintance. The authors concluded that parents and those working with children should be alert to the impact of loss even when it involves non-relatives.[53] In a further paper the team noted a strong association between posttraumatic stress, grief, and difficulty functioning.[54]

Stanford University medical anthropologist and trained nurse Barbara Koenig had two separate PDIA grants. The first was a study of the African American community in Oakland, a project in which she went on to collaborate with the black physician LaVera Crawley. On completion of that piece of work, the two then applied jointly for positions as PDIA faculty scholars. In their first project they set out to examine the apparent underutilization of hospice care by African Americans and also that community's limited utilization of advanced directives. The study used ethnographic methods to examine death and the dying processes

53. B. Pfefferbaum et al., "Post-Traumatic Stress among Young Children after the Death of a Friend or Acquaintance in a Terrorist Bombing," *Psychiatric Services* 51, no. 3 (2000): 386–388.

54. B. Pfefferbaum et al., "Traumatic Grief in a Convenience Sample of Victims Seeking Support Services after a Terrorist Incident," *Annals of Clinical Psychiatry* 13, no. 1 (2001): 19–24.

across the life cycle in one African American community in Oakland, California. The research formed part of Koenig's wider portfolio of work on the relevance of culture to end-of-life issues, particularly end-of-life decision making. The study found that poor African Americans were denied effective end-of-life care, in part resulting from communication problems linked to the use of African American vernacular English, but also due to a lack of trust of health-care workers.[55] As faculty scholars, Koenig and Crawley sought to apply insights from their earlier study through a project focused on improving end-of-life care for the underserved through targeted continuing education of African American physicians. The starting point here was that patients from culturally diverse backgrounds benefit from the provision of culturally competent and sensitive care. The project sought to increase the network of physicians capable of providing comprehensive end-of-life care to undeserved communities and to provide wider opportunities for further education and training. Koenig and Crawley enabled other faculty scholars to recognize that cultural sensitivity can become codified within medical protocols, and they were eager to warn against creating stereotypes by assuming that every member of a minority group carries particular traits and beliefs about their care:

> It's a big problem in all of biomedicine…The whole issue of ethnicity as a predictive variable is useful when you are talking about trends within a population, but then making that kind of knowledge relevant in a clinical setting with an individual becomes very problematic. Would you like your doctor to imagine that you wanted X because of the color of your skin or because of your national origin?[56]

LaVera Crawley went on to work with Dr. Richard Payne in the Initiative to Improve Palliative Care for African Americans, which is described later in chapter 5.

Women on average live seven years longer than men in the United States and women make up 70 percent of the nursing home population. The National Family Caregivers Association estimated that there are eighteen million Americans providing care to a relative or friend with a long-term illness, 80 percent of whom are women. In April 1998, the PDIA-supported association Grantmakers Concerned with Care at the End of Life held a symposium to explore the issue of *Women at the End of Life: The Hidden Cost.* Among the speakers were former First Lady Rosalynn Carter, chair of the Rosalynn Carter Institute, and PDIA board member Robert Butler. The symposium raised awareness of the gendered nature of care and also of the need for better partnerships between family caregivers and the medical profession, which, it was argued, should be based on the needs of the

55. B. A. Koenig and L. V. Crawley, "*Dying In an African American Community: An Ethnographic Study of Death throughout the Life Cycle*," Final Report to PDIA, 20 June 1999.

56. "Diversity in Dying: Improving Palliative Care in a Multicultural Society," *PDIA Newsletter*, no. 6 (December 1999), 4.

caregivers and a willingness on the part of the medical profession to set limits on what families can reasonably be expected to provide. The following year, 1999, PDIA also provided funds for the Alliance for Aging Research to produce the report *One Final Gift: Humanizing the End of Life for Women in America,* which concluded that society can provide and afford much better care at the end of life that respects women's preferences, provides emotional and physical comfort, fosters family peace, and meets spiritual needs.[57]

On 8 June 1998, the PDIA received a funding application for support to enable the leading journalist Bill Moyers to make a series of television broadcasts on end-of-life care. Moyers's reputation went before him as one who had made several documentary films on key social issues and as a person unafraid to tackle challenging questions. His proposal was for a four-part series. Mary Callaway recalls the path that proposal traveled:

> He spent a lot of time talking with Kathy Foley and trying to determine exactly what should be covered...I think pretty much Kathy laid out what the entire agenda was going to be, what topics were going to be covered, and who they might interview for those topics. There was a point during the conversation when he was still looking for funding for the project...but it had become apparent that 90 percent of the people he was going to interview on the project were PDIA grantees [and] that it wouldn't be appropriate for our project to fund his initiative, because it would look too self-serving. So we in fact went outside and got other funding...the folks at Robert Wood Johnson put a huge amount of money into an outreach campaign following that presentation and we've mailed the videos all over the world for advocacy purposes.[58]

The project was two years in the making and finally aired on PBS on 10–13 September 2000 to an estimated nineteen million people (58 percent above the PBS prime-time average). It consisted of a six-hour series in four parts, entitled: *Living with Dying; A Different Kind of Care; A Death of One's Own;* and *A Time to Change.* The series title—*On Our Own Terms*—was a deliberate nod in the direction of the baby boomers and unashamedly consumerist in its orientation. The series brought together well chosen examples of end-of-life care in a variety of settings across the United States. It revealed the profound dysfunctionality of the American care system in the face of death, yet it also presented shining beacons of good practice. As one reviewer noted: "My own favorite segment was the discussion of the symptoms at the end of life, as Dr. Sean Morrison sat with a family around the kitchen table in their home preparing them for their mother's last hours."[59] In addition to Sean Morrison, several other PDIA faculty scholars and

57. "Women at the End of Life: First as Caregivers, Last as Patients," *PDIA Newsletter,* no. 4 (February 1999), 10.

58. Mary Callaway, interview by David Clark, October 29, 2004.

59. J. F. O'Donnell, media review, *On Our Own Terms: Moyers on Dying.* Presented on PBS by Thirteen/WNET New York, September 10–13, 2000. *Journal of Palliative Medicine* 4, no. 2 (2001): 233–234.

grantees were featured in the film, including William Breitbart, Carlos Gomez, Greg Gramelspacher, Diane Meier, Jane Morris, Amos Bailey, Frank Ostaseski, Richard Payne, and Deborah Witt Sherman. There was also an impassioned plea from one-time board member Joanne Lynn on the need for system change in order to achieve better end-of-life care.[60]

But the key to the success of the series was not just in the impact of the shows themselves. In addition to the production budget of $2.6 million, a further $2.5 million was spent on outreach through a coordinated set of related activities.[61,62] Seventy national organizations, along with companion programming by sixty-three local public television stations and a high quality website,[63] led to a coordinated public debate on the issues raised by the broadcasts and a massive level of print media coverage, including an extended piece and cover story in *Time*[64] and other articles in *Good Housekeeping, Modern Maturity,* and *Money.* Major newspapers across the country, including the *Washington Post, Los Angeles Times, Chicago Tribune, Houston Chronicle,* and *Orlando Sentinel* all ran stories. Barnes and Noble booksellers featured the program on its website and had special selections of books on end-of-life care in nine hundred stores. Over three hundred local coalitions held town hall meetings and public discussions. In the months that followed, dozens of stations re-ran the broadcasts. PDIA derived huge benefit from the entire venture. The *Time* article mentioned or quoted six individuals involved with PDIA and the cover and story photographs came from Arts and Humanities Program grantee Eugene Richards. The *PDIA Newsletter* of March 2001 reported the whole event in detail, drawing an ecstatic conclusion:

> Transforming people's attitudes about dying and galvanizing communities for action, the impact of the PBS series has gone beyond the broadcast to start a new national conversation.[65]

Exactly one year after the Moyers broadcasts first took place, America confronted death in an unprecedented way. On 11 September 2001, the attacks on

---

60. Joanne Lynn observed much later that it was she who had persuaded Bill and Judith Moyers to name the series *On Our Own Terms,* instead of *On My Own Terms,* which had been the original idea. She noted: "I think the title ended up being much better for its tendency to pull us together." Joanne Lynne, personal communication, 4 July 2010.

61. http://www.current.org/outreach/out020dying.html (accessed February 7, 2007).

62. The funders of *On Our Own Terms* included The Robert Wood Johnson Foundation, the Fetzer Institute, the Nathan Cummings Foundation, the Kohlberg Foundation, Inc., the Laurence S. Rockefeller Fund, the John D. and Catherine T. MacArthur Foundation, and Mutual of America Life Insurance Company.

63. PBS.org, Resources, "On Our Own Terms: Moyers on Dying," http://www.pbs.org/wnet/onourownterms/resources/vidmus.html (accessed February 7, 2007).

64. A kinder, gentler death, *Time,* 60–73.

65. "PBS series: On Our Own Terms—Moyers on Dying Attracts High Ratings and Fosters National Dialogue," *PDIA Newsletter,* no. 8 (March 2001), 17–18.

the World Trade Center in New York City and the events in Pennsylvania and at the Pentagon shook the world. Within hours, friends and family members in New York began posting descriptions of missing loved ones in hospitals. Others added their own offerings, surrounding the pictures with poems, candles, and prayers. Spontaneous shrines appeared in parks, in front of firehouses, and on street corners as public spaces were transformed into sites of collective mourning. Afterwards millions of Americans were left struggling with the experience of death and bereavement at a national level and in relation to a complex and poorly understood set of motivations on the part of the perpetrators. A PDIA editorial of December 2001 raised a penetrating question:

> As we think about this tragedy, will we find new ways to discuss dying in America? Not just these sudden, violent deaths, but also expected death after long illnesses—the kinds of death that most Americans experience. Will people think about the care they want to receive at the end of their life? Will they want a chance to say goodbye? [66]

By some strange quirk of fate, the final years of the Project on Death in America coincided with a period of massive post-9/11 collective mourning and remembrance that brought issues of loss and bereavement into the public consciousness perhaps as never before. Such a watershed adds complexity to the question of making sense of the PDIA contribution and should always be kept in mind.

In a guest editorial published in 2005, David Wendell Moller of the Medical Humanities Program at the University of Missouri–Kansas City School of Medicine noted the previous decade's outpouring of interest in palliative care: "Through an impressive array of scholarly research, ethnographic description, and ethical dialogue, the experience of dying persons was made visible–finally."[67] Some of this effect must undoubtedly be attributed to the efforts of PDIA grantees whose work has been described in this chapter. And as Wendell Moller observes, there were disturbing aspects to the things revealed. The resulting picture showed unrelieved suffering and indignities on a wide scale. Attempts to *take control* of dying had resulted in unrealistic expectations of the benefits of technology and a growing tendency to avoid and postpone the inevitable. The outcomes were high financial costs, emotional distress, and physical suffering. Many of the projects undertaken by PDIA grantees and scholars and described in this chapter made

---

66. "A Community of Grievers," *PDIA Newsletter*, no. 9 (December 2001), 2. The same issue also included a photographic essay on the New York response to the attacks in an article by Steve Zeitlin and Ilana Harlow entitled "Giving a Voice to Sorrow: Commemorative Art, Ritual, and Story in New York City," 7–11.

67. D. Wendell Moller, "None Left Behind: Urban Poverty, Social Experience, and Rethinking Palliative Care," *Journal of Palliative Medicine* 8, no. 1 (2005): 17–19.

a contribution to the understanding of these issues. They fulfilled the call made by Kathy Foley in 1996 when she observed: "We need broad public discussions to address what Americans value, to address what kind of society we are, and how we care for our dying."[68] The initiatives provided a rich ethnographic platform of description from which a program of action could be launched. For in the matter of America's culture of dying, the PDIA goal was not simply to *understand* the world, but also to *transform* it.

---

68. Excerpted from testimony before the House Judiciary Committee on the Constitution, 29 April 1996, and quoted in *PDIA Newsletter*, no. 2 (September 1996), 1.

4

Service Innovation and Practice Developments

During the mid-1990s, as PDIA rolled out its programs and grants, clear evidence was accumulating about problems in the delivery of end-of-life care in the American health-care system—especially in hospitals. In particular, a solid platform of information was being provided by the SUPPORT study in a series of important publications that was having a wide impact.[1] In the initial two-year observational phase of this study, investigators at the five participating institutions documented serious shortcomings in the care of critically ill patients. In general the SUPPORT study patients, all of whom had a prognosis of six months or less and half of whom lived for less than six months, were likely to die after prolonged stays in intensive care, on mechanical ventilation, in a coma, or in moderate to severe pain. About half the patients could not express a preference for cardiopulmonary resuscitation (CPR). Yet more disturbing was the second phase of the study, in which investigators sought to improve the process of care. Specially trained nurses provided physicians with detailed prognostic information about individual patients and the treatment preferences they had elicited from them and from family members. The attempt to improve communication and decision making was a failure. Unchanged were the median number of days until a *Do Not Resuscitate* (DNR) order was written, physician understanding of patient preferences, the number of days spent in intensive care, in a coma, or under mechanical ventilation, the incidence of pain, and the costs of care—were

---

1. See, for example, The SUPPORT Principal Investigators, "A Controlled trial to Improve Care for Seriously Ill Hospitalized Patients: The Study to Understand Prognoses and Preferences for Outcomes and Risks of Treatments (SUPPORT)," *Journal of the American Medical Association* 274 (1995): 1591–1598.

all unaltered. It was a wake-up call for everyone interested in improving end-of-life care in the American context. Through its grants program and scholarships, PDIA was ideally placed to respond to some of the issues arising—and these were indeed complex. Seventy percent of patients or their surrogates in SUPPORT had rated their care as excellent or very good, suggesting that the observed results were as much a product of user demand as provider insistence. PDIA grantee Betty Ferrell suggested the following:

> It is probably time to quit funding descriptive studies documenting inadequacies in care. We know it's bad. Time to get on with solutions.[2]

This chapter explores the PDIA-funded solutions to such problems and looks at a variety of service innovations across inpatient and domiciliary settings, as well as new developments in clinical practice relating to people with advanced disease in the face of death. Undertaken by numerous PDIA grantees and scholars, these were the testing grounds for new ideas, some of which would prove worthy of wider dissemination and "roll out"—moving beyond the status of demonstration projects to have a wider influence on the entire American health-care system.

SERVICES

A body of PDIA work focused around service development and innovation. This took the form of some large, institutionally oriented grants, as well as the endeavors of numerous individuals, including faculty scholars and members of the Social Work Leadership Program. The settings covered were diverse: from hospitals and nursing homes to community programs of various kinds, including hospices. Attention was given to the needs of children and adolescents as well as adults and older people. Perhaps inevitably, given the PDIA focus on medicine through the Faculty Scholars Program, hospitals were a major focus of activity, especially those large and complex settings where specialist care is delivered alongside teaching and academic research—in the very heartlands of American medical practice.

Hospitals

> One of the major problems identified was in medicine itself and in the fact that hospitals were places where most people died and physicians...engaged in their care had...lost their way and that our focus of change should be at a very elite level of engaging the health-care professionals.[3]

---

2. Betty Ferrell, e-mail to Mary Callaway, November 22, 1999, in response to a request for suggestions about future funding for end-of-life care issues.

3. Kathy Foley, interview by David Clark, July 22, 2003.

This observation from PDIA board chair Kathy Foley draws attention to the importance of the hospital environment, the place where, as a British medical commentator once observed, "the serious dying takes place."[4] It was in the hospital context that many PDIA faculty scholars sought to tackle the reform of end-of-life care, often by engaging boldly with the powerful vested interests of the institutional culture and in the face of the particular value systems of academic medicine. This work recognized that hospitals remain the places where most Americans die and where so many physicians learn to practice, and it acknowledged that for many health-care workers, death in the hospital is regarded as a personal and professional failure rather than an inevitable occurrence to be attended with skill and compassion. At a time when palliative medicine was still not formally established as a specialty in the United States,[5] when dedicated revenue streams for palliative care within health-care institutions were of limited availability, and when sources of research support from within the medical science mainstream were still few in number, a focus on hospital palliative care was of enormous significance. Moreover, experience quickly showed that patients and families were overwhelmingly appreciative when a skilled and sensitive interdisciplinary palliative care team could offer comfort and dignity to those facing their last days in hospital.

Faculty scholar Sharon Weinstein undertook the first systematic effort to investigate patient death at the University of Texas MD Anderson Cancer Center in Houston. In a highly resourced and prestigious setting such as this, she found that PDIA funding gave her work a certain kind of legitimacy:

> I suddenly had a credibility that I hadn't had before and I started to ask questions like: "How many people die here in this building as a 400–500 bed cancer hospital?" And nobody collected those statistics for the institution. So I was the first person to actually ask the questions about death, give the first talk on euthanasia and assisted suicide in the building, and…work with the Ethics Committee and some different clinical groups to start doing studies on advanced directives and things like that. But that was a time when the oncology culture was changing, and this was just a way to accelerate it.[6]

In a period when the hospital was moving toward disease-management pathways, Weinstein was delegated to write all of the palliative interventions that would go with each surgical procedure, making pain and symptom management part of the care plan. Over the next eighteen months, she and her colleagues wrote 125 care plans that were implemented. The result was that during a two-year period, more than five thousand patients were treated according to these standardized

---

4. C. Douglas, "For All the Saints," *British Medical Journal* 304, no. 6826 (1992): 479.

5. See chapter 7.

6. Sharon Weinstein, interview by David Clark, July 22, 2003.

care plans, and all of them had their pain and symptom management, their psychosocial needs, and their aftercare built into the plans. Even as PDIA was closing, another faculty scholar, Anthony N. Galanos at Duke University in North Carolina, was making a cogent case for why hospitals should respond to the need for improved palliative care, arguing that the pressure from the public opinion polls and the press are incontestable and that palliative care should be seen as a positive response and not a reduction in options, as he notes in the following:

> It is the patient and family who have come to the hospital for answers to their conundrum. In response, the hospital-based palliative care team does not emphasize what will be taken away, but what will be done *for* the patient and family despite a life-threatening illness.[7]

Several PDIA grantees and faculty scholars used their supported time to develop specific hospital-based palliative care programs. Andrew Billings had been nurturing his interest in palliative care outside the hospital and medical school environment through his work at Trinity Hospice, Boston, and this brought him into contact with many oncologists at Massachusetts General Hospital. His PDIA faculty scholarship allowed him to cut back on his community health work and shift full time into developing a "palliative care presence" in the hospital. Well known to his colleagues there and with a number of allies, he set about developing a hospital palliative care service with a consult program, along with outpatient provision and home care. The emphasis was strongly interdisciplinary—"very much on a hospice model in the hospital."[8,9] Susan McGarrity developed a similar approach on a regional basis at Pennsylvania State University Hospital, where she sought to integrate with community services.[10]

Peter Selwyn, at the Montefiore Medical Center in New York, focused on the care of patients with late-stage AIDS in "Leeway" a 30-bed skilled nursing facility. It undertook clinical, palliative and end-of-life care, teaching, and research with the goal of improving clinical outcomes for patients and their families and creating a greater understanding among care providers about the end-of-life issues faced by people with AIDS in the locality and elsewhere. This early work at

---

7. A. N. Galanos, "Hospital-Based Palliative Care Units: Answering a Growing Need," *North Carolina Medical Journal* 65, no. 4 (2004): 217–220.

8. Andrew Billings, interview by David Clark, July 23, 2003.

9. In 2006, Andrew Billings was honored with an American Academy of Hospice and Palliative Medicine Project on Death in America (PDIA) Palliative Medicine National Leadership Award, recognizing a physician leader who has advanced the field of palliative care by the education of the next generation of palliative care leaders. The award program promotes the visibility and prestige of physicians in both academic and clinical settings who are committed to mentoring future leaders and serving as role models for other health professionals engaged in improving the care of the dying.

10. McGarrity noted in her first annual report to PDIA that "the enthusiasm for the palliative care service among the nurses, social workers, chaplains, residents, students and, most importantly, the patients, has been tremendous. The physician support has been much slower in coming." (Susan McGarrity, PDIA Year-End Report, April 29, 1997).

Montefiore led to a major demonstration project, one of six funded by the Health Resources and Services Administration, on the integration of HIV and palliative care. The results suggested an important and ongoing need for palliative care services for patients with advanced HIV/AIDS, even in the era of antiretroviral treatment and in a context where AIDS evolves into a form of chronic disease. Patients were readily referred from predominantly inpatient settings with very advanced disease and with problems that included a mix of medical and psychosocial issues, which the consultation team then sought to resolve. Death was predicted only by baseline functional status, not by traditional HIV disease markers. Mortality reflected both AIDS-related and non-AIDS-specific causes.[11]

Such developments presupposed how *measures* of their effectiveness might be developed, and this theme was taken up by faculty scholar Neil Wenger at UCLA. He acknowledged the low quality of death in American hospitals and the need to reduce expensive care that had little therapeutic benefit, and he attempted to address this through the development of objective measures for quality end-of-life care.[12]

Some PDIA scholars and grantees focused on the palliative and end-of-life care needs of trauma patients, taking the "hospice" approach deep into the acute medicine setting and pushing the philosophy of palliative care to the limits of its existing range. Physician Anne C. Mosenthal and nurse Patricia Murphy, joint faculty scholars based at the University of Medicine and Dentistry of New Jersey and University Hospital, worked to improve end-of-life care within an inner-city trauma center. They began by reviewing case notes in ICU and found this raised more questions than answers. Was the uncertainty of the prognosis of these patients a barrier to trauma surgeons making the transition to palliative care? They turned to an approach that sought to promote palliative care principles and values regardless of the likelihood of survival. As they noted: "The phrase 'palliative care in trauma' might seem an oxymoron," but if palliative care and curative care are viewed as two parallel therapies that are not mutually exclusive, then there is the potential to bring new support to the patient and to avoid futile treatments when death is imminent.[13] Faculty scholars Michelle Ervin of the Howard University Health Sciences Center in Washington, DC, and Tammie Quest of the Emory University School of Medicine in Georgia, approached similar issues from their practice in emergency medicine and, moreover, saw this as a portal to delivering good end-of-life care to the poorest members of society. Michelle Ervin explains:

> What PDIA did was validate a feeling that I had. Working in the emergency department, seeing patients presenting with newly-diagnosed cancers, unknown lesions on their X-rays, end-stage renal disease...this really

11. P. A. Selwyn et al., "Palliative Care for AIDS at a Large Urban Teaching Hospital: Program Description and Preliminary Outcomes," *Journal of Palliative Medicine.* 6, no. 3 (2003): 461–474.

12. K. Rosenfeld and N. Wenger, "Measuring Quality in End-of-Life Care," *Clinics in Geriatric Medicine* 16, no. 2 (2000): 387–400.

13. A. C. Mosenthal and P. A. Murphy, "Trauma Care and Palliative Care: Time to Integrate the Two?" *Journal of the American College of Surgeons* 197, no. 3 (2003): 509–516.

helped focus me and my work in emergency medicine. I *love* emergency medicine, I *love* working shifts. But if you can imagine the broad spectrum of diseases that present in the emergency department, it really helped focus *my* interest, and I'm not just interested in the ethical issues of patients that present in emergency departments, but really patients that are presenting with death and dying issues. Ethics is part of that, but it's also not giving up on those patients. It's also respecting what their wishes are, what their family's wishes are. It's helping to design a curriculum that says, yes, this patient is going to die from their cancer or they're going to die from their congestive heart failure, but at this point in time, it's not acceptable to give up on them and say they're going to die. You aggressively treat the symptom that they're presenting with, not because they're going to be cured, but because it's going to make them feel better at this time.[14]

One hospital-based program deserving special mention is that at Mount Sinai School of Medicine in New York.[15] Developed by a four-strong team of PDIA faculty scholars (Diane Meier, Judith Ahronheim, Jane Morris, and Sean Morrison) it proved a platform from which several major developments would be launched, some of which proved to be enduring and extensive.[16] Diane Meier explains the origins:

We applied as a group of four actually; we were the only team that was funded in that first cohort—one nurse, three physicians, all in geriatrics, applied together as a team in order to do a faculty education intervention at Mount Sinai School of Medicine. [We were] appealing to the audience with what they're accustomed to and what they care about, which is legitimized external expertise: legitimized, published, funded, and the best in the field, able to present the best evidence in the field, competent speakers and presenters. And, while I and my colleagues taught a few of these seminars, the vast majority were taught by outside experts. I thought that it did a great deal to elevate the profile of palliative medicine as a legitimate specialty, one with a body of knowledge behind it, one that was intellectually and scientifically compelling, as well as one that was important for the care of patients and families. I think it made it *dramatically* easier for us to subsequently launch a clinical program, because some of the key opinion leaders in our institution had been through the seminar series and, therefore, were supportive and [became] advocates at the sticky places.[17]

---

14. Michelle Ervin, interview by David Clark, July 24, 2003.

15. D. E. Meier, R. S. Morrison, and C. K. Cassel, "Improving Palliative Care," *Annals of Internal Medicine* 127 (2007): 225–230.

16. For an early example of the team's work, see J. C. Ahronheim et al., "Treatment of the Dying in the Acute Care Hospital: Advanced Dementia and Metastatic Cancer," *Archives of Internal Medicine* 156 (1996): 2094–2100.

17. Diane Meier, interview by David Clark, July 22, 2003.

Interestingly, the Mount Sinai approach was not confined to a small number of specialties traditionally associated with hospice and the care of the dying, but involved the whole spectrum of medicine. This was in recognition of the fact that seriously ill persons, those living with life-threatening illness and multiple chronic comorbid illnesses, as well as those who are dying, are found in every walk of medicine and that cancer accounts for only a quarter of deaths in the United States, with a far greater proportion due to chronic degenerative illnesses like dementia, congestive heart failure, chronic lung disease, end-stage renal disease, and liver disease. So as Diane Meier put it: "if we ignore those physicians we are as good as ignoring those patients."[18] From here the group was able to move toward the creation of a clinical service which also had success in securing monies from the National Hospital Fund (more on this later in the chapter) under its Hospital Palliative Care Initiative. The new program, which began in 1997, just two years after the faculty scholars' work was underway, had three key components: a strong clinical service; an educational strand primarily directed at Mount Sinai medical residents and fellows; and the beginnings of a research infrastructure and research program. The initiative flourished, but was for a while entirely dependent on external funding: this brought a measure of autonomy but did not secure long-term viability; to achieve this, it was important, as Meier put it, to be on the hospital's "have to have" list. Simple appeals to altruism seemed doomed to failure in tackling this problem. Meier explains their approach:

What was a starter with hospital administrators was pointing to the extremely long ICU and hospital lengths of stay of persons with serious and terminal illness. No one knew how to have conversations about goals of care, and the *reason* for this growing number of persons and the enormous cost that they represented to the hospital. [Yet it] was ameliorable, was soluble. The solution was an expert team with the skill set and the time reserved to have the two-hour family meetings three times a week with the family who won't take Grandpa off the ventilator... So palliative care can kind of come in late in the course of events, establish a new therapeutic liaison, try to get on the same side of the table with the family—it's usually the family at this stage—and help them achieve what in their view is the best outcome. If it means going to a long-term vent facility in a nursing home, because in their culture and in their family discontinuing a ventilator is unacceptable, then that is success in our view. But it gets them off the dime. It means we have a plan. We can move towards discharge.[19]

This combination of visionary and practical thinking enabled the Mount Sinai team to achieve even greater successes. By the year 2000, Meier was working with the Robert Wood Johnson Foundation to establish the Center to Advance

18. Diane Meier, interview by David Clark, July 22, 2003.

19. Diane Meier, interview by David Clark, July 22, 2003.

Palliative Care[20]—a national organization devoted to increasing the number and quality of palliative care programs in the United States. She had also been part of a team that conducted a study of the prevalence of hospital-based palliative care services in the United States.[21] [22] Now, as one of the leading American figures in the field of palliative medicine, Meier was appearing in numerous publications, including the *New York Times*, the *Los Angeles Times*, *Newsday*, and *The New Yorker*, and had figured prominently in the Bill Moyers television series, *On Our Own Terms*, described in chapter 3.[23]

Throughout this, she worked closely with Sean Morrison. He explains some of the successes achieved in the research program, in which he concentrated efforts on studies that could be used to build a case for hospital service improvement:

> We've three major areas: one obviously is federal funding, that we've been very successful in securing—investigator funding for both career development and for leadership, and also project funding, funding for research projects...We have a portfolio of federal grants in related areas, which means that we can hire a number of different people and have them working on separate grants and create an infrastructure. We've used foundation support to fund our research projects...bringing our research to the foundations and tying into what they see as opportune...And we've also used philanthropic support, approaching families of patients who might want to fund ongoing evaluation and research in palliative care. So we targeted three major areas to keep that going.[24]

Building on this, Morrison also went on to found his own major initiative, the National Palliative Care Research Center.[25] Working in close partnership with the Center to Advance Palliative Care (see more on this in chapter 9), Morrison's group aims to improve care for patients with serious illness and care for their families by promoting palliative care research. Specifically, the center provides a mechanism to establish priorities for palliative care research, to develop a new generation of researchers in palliative care, and to coordinate and support stud-

---

20. Center to Advance Palliative Care, http://www.capc.org/ (accessed March 27, 2008).

21. C. X. Pan et al., "How Prevalent Are Hospital-Based Palliative Care Programs? Status Report and Future Directions," *Journal of Palliative Medicine.* 4, no. 3 (2001): 315–324.

22. R. S. Morrison et al., "The Growth of Palliative Care Programs in United States Hospitals," *Journal of Palliative Medicine* 8, no. 6 (2005): 1127–1134.

23. She was honored with an American Academy of Hospice and Palliative Medicine Project on Death in America (PDIA) Palliative Medicine National Leadership Award in 2007, which recognized a physician leader who has advanced the field of palliative care by the education of the next generation of palliative care leaders.

24. Sean Morrison, interview by David Clark, July 24, 2003.

25. National Palliative Care Center, http://www.npcrc.org/ (accessed March 27, 2008).

ies focused on improving care for patients living with serious illness and for their families. Morrison writes:

> The field of palliative care has experienced substantial growth and development over the past 10 years... one in four hospitals in the United States has a palliative care program, including 100% of hospitals in the Veterans Health Administration. Palliative care is becoming an integral part of long-term care facilities. At the National Palliative Care Research Center, we are committed to developing the knowledge and skills that will further promote and advance the field of palliative care and thus improve care for persons living with advanced illness. The vision and support of our philanthropic partners and the Mount Sinai School of Medicine has allowed us to develop a truly unique national research center whose mission is to foster groundbreaking research, support the development of a new generation of investigators, provide an administrative home for researchers, and address the major issues facing both patients with advanced illness and their families. Finally, we will aim to take our research findings and rapidly translate them into effective clinical practice.[26]

There can be little doubt that the funding made available to the team at Mount Sinai as part of cohort one of the PDIA Faculty Scholars Program was hugely repaid by the successes of the grantees and their many activities, both within and far beyond their own hospital.[27] Morrison, in turn, is unequivocal in his praise for the support received from PDIA, as in this excerpt from an interview at a faculty scholars retreat in 2003:

> You know, when I think back I learned media training here; I learned how to move my research from the academic world into the public world because of skills that I developed here. I learned leadership skills here. I learned to think about a broader perspective rather than an individual research perspective: how do I fit my career goals within the broader framework of the movement? That was something that was taught both by people I interacted with and also through Susan [Block] and Kathy [Foley] and other members of the Board bringing people in to really establish that skill set. I've been part of two other career development programs, very similar scholarships in aging research, *none* of them did what PDIA did.[28]

In addition to the work of individual enthusiasts interested in the improvement of palliative care in the hospital, PDIA also supported a major coordinated

26. National Palliative Care Center—Message from the Director, http://www.npcrc.org/about/about_show.htm?doc_id=385728 (accessed March 27, 2008).

27. D. E. Meier, "Palliative Care Programs: What, Why and How?" *Physician Executive* 27, no. 6 (2001): 43–47.

28. Sean Morrison, interview by David Clark, July 24, 2003.

initiative in New York City in partnership with the United Hospital Fund. The Fund is a public charity created in 1879 to advance the work of New York City hospitals. It has evolved over the years into an organization that works with the full breadth of the health-care system, with a commitment to creating positive change in health care in New York City, and with a particular eye toward the special needs of the most vulnerable New Yorkers, especially those who are uninsured. David A. Gould, senior vice president at the Fund and the principal staff person responsible for program development and grant-making activities, explains the background:

> I knew of the Project on Death in America, because I'd probably read about it in the newspaper or something, but I also knew one of the board members, who was chortling with me one day that he was at long last writing an RFP as opposed to responding to one, and when I saw him in the spring of, I guess, '96, and [I] said, "So what did you find?" The answer was "Gee, we got all these wonderful scholars who stepped forward," and I said "Well, what did you get from health-care provider organizations?" And the answer was basically not a lot, and not very much that was good. And I thought, well, that's really regrettable, because you need those organizations. And I said, "What if I put together a consortium of New York City hospitals that would really think seriously about making significant changes in how they deal with persons that are near the end of life?" "Well, that's very interesting," [was the response]. So I did a quick exchange of memos and he introduced me to Kathy Foley.[29]

The response from PDIA was rapid and positive:

> And so what PDIA did was—first of all, it was not very intrusive at the point of process—they looked at it and they said this seems to make sense. You guys know the universe in which you work and have worked for a 100+ years. Our bet is on you and this is the extent of our bet, and you can use our commitment to leverage a lot of other support starting with your own board, which is exactly what happened.[30]

PDIA invested $300,000 to support the Fund in building a consortium of twelve New York hospitals to design and implement a palliative care initiative for assessing and changing the way hospitals provide care to persons at the end of life.[31] The focus was firmly on palliative care. While some thought it was simply a matter of bringing hospice into the hospital, the emphasis here was on a larger

---

29. David Gould, interview by David Clark, October 27, 2004. The PDIA board member being referred to here was David Rothman.

30. David Gould, interview by David Clark, October 27, 2004.

31. *Project on Death in America, July 1994–September 1997, Report of Activities* (New York: Open Society Institute, 1998), 35.

universe of care, and the ultimate goal was to integrate hospice with inpatient care and outpatient services and home-care services. As Gould observed:

> Our saying that palliative care was an important issue to the hospital community, to the institutional community, certainly complemented in some respects and built off of the work that the Project on Death in America was doing—"say, end-of-life care is a serious issue and we can deal with it, you can't keep averting your eyes from it."[32]

The Fund launched its Hospital Palliative Care Initiative in 1996.[33] In the first phase of the project, grants of $20,000 each were awarded to twelve hospitals for data gathering and planning over a six-month period.[34] In the second phase, two-year grants of $225,000 were awarded to five of the hospitals to implement demonstration projects for promoting palliative care.[35] Phase one identified three sets of lessons: (1) the need for professional training and clinical competency to assess palliative care needs and deliver palliative care services, (2) the existence of institutional barriers that limit the ability of the acute care hospital to expand its mission to incorporate palliative care, and (3) a lack of institutional resources to promote palliative care within the hospitals. As the project report noted: "These themes are hardly revelatory. Their significance lies in the fact that they were articulated in each hospital by its physicians, nurses, administrators, and other staff, as well as by family members and patients."[36]

The five hospitals chosen to take forward these lessons in phase two of the program were Beth Israel Medical Center, Brooklyn Hospital Center, Montefiore Medical Center, Mount Sinai Medical Center, and St Vincent's Hospital and Medical Center. Each adopted a slightly different model and set of priorities. No definitive approach that could guarantee success was identified, and it was concluded that each hospital must develop a strategy reflecting its unique culture and resources. Nevertheless, the development of a clinical service that can provide leadership and demonstrate the benefits of palliative care seemed more effective than efforts to alter directly the practices of health-care staff. Initiating palliative care services was found to be very demanding of staff time and other

---

32. David Gould, interview by David Clark, October 27, 2004.

33. The Hospital Palliative Care Initiative had gained additional support from other foundations, including the Emily Davie and Joseph S. Kornfeld Foundation, the Greenwall Foundation, and the JM Foundation.

34. C. Zuckerman and A. Mackinnon, *The Challenge of Caring for Patients Near the End of Life: Findings from the Hospital Palliative Care Initiative* (New York: United Hospital Fund of New York, 1998).

35. S. S. Hopper, *Building Hospital Palliative Care Programs: Lessons from the Field* (New York: United Hospital Fund of New York, 2001).

36. C. Zuckerman and A. Mackinnon, *The Challenge of Caring for Patients Near the End of Life: Findings from the Hospital Palliative Care Initiative* (New York: United Hospital Fund of New York, 1998), 11.

resources, and initial resistance on the part of primary physicians could not be underestimated, along with the need to engage the support of key departments and directors. A lack of overarching funding for palliative care services was a major challenge, and there was continuing concern about the reliance on foundation and project-based support, with a clear need to position new services in relationship to the broader hospital environment. Over the course of the project, an understanding grew of the potential of palliative care to benefit a wide range of patients and families affected by progressive, life-threatening illness. The key question emerging was how initial pilot projects could be sustained?

In the year 2000, the Robert Wood Johnson Foundation supported The Milbank Trust in the publication of a monograph concerned with the development of palliative care programs in hospitals.[37] It highlighted nine case studies, and no less than eight of these had been supported by PDIA or were closely associated with it.[38] The introduction was written by Christine K. Cassel, Professor and Chair of the Henry L. Schwartz Department of Geriatrics and Adult Development at Mount Sinai School of Medicine, who had helped to initiate and lead the process that produced the report. She had first encouraged Diane Meier and colleagues to apply for PDIA faculty scholar funding.[39] The case studies were written by innovative clinicians who saw the need for palliative care at their hospitals and devoted themselves to creating programs to meet that need. Committed to helping patients live and die without unnecessary suffering, these leaders sought to provide comprehensive care based on respect for patients' goals, preferences, and choices. Cassel observes the following:

> Whether they were senior or junior faculty members, all the leaders overcame significant barriers to the development of palliative care within their hospitals. They found varied routes to success, reflecting diverse institutional cultures and differing levels of financial resources... These pioneers differ, as well, in clinical philosophies, personal styles, and methods of work. Sometimes their subspecialty or research prompted them to act; others were motivated by clinical work... The narratives exemplify the current debate

---

37. *Pioneer Programs in Palliative Care: Nine Case Studies* (New York: Milbank Memorial Fund and Robert Wood Johnson Foundation, 2000).

38. These eight were Balm of Gilead Center, Cooper Green Hospital (F. Amos Bailey); Palliative Care Program, Beth Israel Deaconess Medical Center/CareGroup (Lachlan Forrow); Massachusetts General Hospital Palliative Care Service (J. Andrew Billings); Palliative Care Program, Medical College of Virginia Campus of Virginia Commonwealth University (Laurel J. Lyckholm, Patrick Coyne, and Thomas J. Smith); Pain and Palliative Care Service, Memorial Sloan-Kettering Cancer Center (Richard Payne and Kathleen M. Foley); The Lilian and Benjamin Hertzberg Palliative Care Institute, Mount Sinai School of Medicine (Diane E. Meier, Jane Morris, and R. Sean Morrison); Palliative Care and Home Hospice Program, Northwestern Memorial Hospital (Charles F. von Gunten); Comprehensive Palliative Care Service, University of Pittsburgh–UPMC (Robert Arnold).

39. Diane Meier, interview by David Clark, July 22, 2003.

that exists about the definition of "palliative care." Is it end-of-life care? Or is it broad and integrated physical, psychological, social, and spiritual care for patients with serious diseases that may be life-threatening? Most of the authors of these studies believe they should care for patients with advanced, incurable illnesses when aggressive treatment of pain and other symptoms may be needed. Several believe that palliation and cure are not mutually exclusive and that palliative care should be practiced during all stages of serious illness, even while aggressive curative treatment continues... The authors' programs serve different groups of people and employ diverse clinical models appropriate for particular patient populations. Certain authors developed post-acute care linked with hospice and home care. Others created palliative care units or consultation services within their hospitals or have combined both models to provide a continuum of care throughout serious illnesses...there is considerable variation in the financing of hospital-based palliative care programs and in institutions' methods of collecting and reporting data. Programs may be supported almost entirely by their clinical revenue or may rely heavily on philanthropy and foundation grants... There is no consensus about how to measure the quality of palliative care. But essential characteristics of hospital-based programs do emerge.[40]

These characteristics, according to Cassel, have four dimensions. First, palliative care programs in hospitals should be constructed around an interdisciplinary team, including at least a doctor, nurse, social worker, pharmacist, and chaplain. Second, patients, families, and physicians should discuss goals and preferences and should plan the care together. Third, palliative care should reach patients throughout the hospital, encourage collaboration across clinical and administrative boundaries, and foster respect for the wishes of patients and families. Finally, such programs should provide bereavement services for families and for staff members. The case studies highlighted the situation beyond their immediate locale and drew attention to the concern that acute care settings, especially tertiary teaching hospitals, may need the most improvement when it comes to palliative care—and it is here that the most barriers to its development may exist.

The case studies, drawing heavily on PDIA experience, were a source of information and advocacy for service improvement and policy change. Combined together, all the efforts described here—many of them the work of PDIA grantees—had a significant impact on the hospital health-care system. In just five years, between 2000–2005, the number of palliative care programs in American hospitals increased by 96 percent from 632 (15 percent of hospitals) to 1,240 (30 percent of hospitals).[41] Further progress was reported subsequently. By 2008,

40. C. Cassel, "Introduction." In *Pioneer Programs in Palliative Care: Nine Case Studies* (New York: Robert Milbank Memorial Fund and Robert Wood Johnson Foundation, 2000).

41. S. Connor, "Hospice and Palliative Care in the United States," *Omega* 56, no. 1 (2007–8): 89–99.

a team of authors, including Sean Morrison, found that 52.8 percent of the hospitals surveyed offered services aimed at alleviating pain and suffering. More than half of the fifty-bed or larger hospitals in the United States were offering palliative care services, though the availability of these varied widely across geographic regions. The number of large hospitals (>249 beds) with palliative care programs had increased to 72.2 percent, though fewer small hospitals (>50 beds) reported offering these services. Growth in palliative care had occurred mainly in not-for-profit hospitals and has been most notable in the Midwestern and Western regions of the United States. Importantly, the study found that 84 percent of medical schools were now associated with at least one hospital that had a palliative care program, implying access to training in palliative care for future doctors and facilitating its incorporation into their daily patient care routines. Additionally, the authors observed that the availability of palliative care services was inversely related to Medicare expenditures, suggesting that when appropriate care is applied to the right patient at the right time, overall costs go down because futile or ineffective approaches are abandoned in favor of the effective new intervention.[42]

Hospices, Nursing Homes, and Community Services

Despite the heavy emphasis on PDIA support for service development in major academic medical centers, the board did not overlook services located in other settings, particularly in the wider community. There was a limited amount of PDIA support for existing hospice programs, such as Joseph's House in Washington DC, founded in 1990 and which cared for homeless men (and later women) with AIDS, describing itself as "primarily a community as opposed to a hospice."[43] PDIA also supported the Jacob Perlow Hospice to become the first major US hospice program for deaf people and those with hearing difficulties; its aim was to provide a culturally sensitive and linguistically appropriate service by supporting staff and volunteers. There was also a PDIA-funded study on the decision to enter hospice, conducted by Ronald S. Schonwetter at the University of South Florida College of Medicine.

PDIA social work leader Mary Raymer of the National Hospice and Palliative Care Organization, and Dona Reese, assistant professor of social work at the University of Arkansas, conducted an important nationwide research study of hospice programs that showed that providing adequate social work services in conjunction with physical care significantly reduces overall hospice costs and results in fewer hospitalizations and higher client satisfaction. In the early years of the new century when hospices were appearing to cut back on nonmedical

42. B. Goldsmith et al., "Variability in Access to Hospital Palliative Care in the United States," *Journal of Palliative Medicine* 11, no. 8 (2008): 1094–1102.

43. Joseph's House Annual Report, PDIA grant number 1253, 1996.

services, the study provided good evidence to support the maintenance of multi-disciplinary care and of social work in particular. Based on a stratified random sample of 66 home hospice programs and 330 individual cases, it showed that the presence of a social worker at the patient's first interview with hospice staff contributes to lower hospice costs, lower labor costs, lower health aid costs, and improved functioning of the hospice team,[44] as Raymer noted:

> While reducing social work services may initially produce cost savings, our study strongly suggests that it is much more cost effective in the long run to preserve the role of social work, which can enhance team functioning as well as impact financial outcomes.[45]

Since the 1990s, several problems have confronted those endeavoring to introduce hospice and palliative care principles and practice into *nursing home* settings in the United States. Most patients referred to hospice programs from nursing homes do not have a cancer diagnosis, so there are problems of eligibility and duration of care, given the unpredictable trajectory of their illness. Other issues concern the differing cultures and systems of care and the possible concern of nursing home staff that they are losing long-term relationships with patients who transfer to hospice. Underlying these issues are also the problems that can occur when a nursing home resident elects for hospice MediCare and must then sign a form to give up a variety of services, including hospitalization, skilled nursing home care (if it is for the terminal condition), and home health care.[46] Yet one in four Americans reaching the age of sixty-five will die in a nursing home (some 20 percent of all deaths) and the need for improved palliative care in the sector is clearly extensive. Several PDIA grantees and scholars responded to such challenges and addressed them in a variety of research, education, and service development projects.

Early PDIA work in this field was developed by Sarah A. Wilson, associate professor of nursing in the College of Nursing at Marquette University, Wisconsin. Her project began in 1995 and was focused on identifying family, staff, and administrators' perspectives on death and dying in long-term care. A total of 155 persons participated in 22 focus groups. Evidence was found of a strong attachment of staff to residents, but educational needs were identified relating to pain and comfort, grief management, communication skills, and spiritual care.[47] As a setting for end-of-life care, nursing homes provide both challenges

44. D. J. Reese and M. Raymer, "Relationships between Social Work Involvement and Hospice Outcomes: Results of the National Hospice Social Work Survey," *Social Work* 49 (2004): 415–422, 2004.

45. "A New Study by Social Work Leader Mary Raymer: Social Work Services Save Money," *PDIA Newsletter*, no. 9 (December 2001), 13.

46. I am grateful to Susan Miller for these points (Susan Miller, interview by David Clark, 15 July 2004).

47. "Fostering Humane Care of Dying Persons in Long Term Care," PDIA Final Report Form, 31 March 1998.

and opportunities. Wilson's work went on to examine factors that impede the delivery of high-quality end-of-life care in nursing homes, such as inadequate staff and physician training, regulatory and reimbursement issues, poor symptom management, and lack of psychosocial support for staff, residents, and families. In addition to exploring hindrances to providing end-of-life care, she and her colleagues identified characteristics of nursing homes and their staff that support the care of terminally ill residents, as well as an overview of models for delivering end-of-life care in nursing homes, including the provision of hospice services, specialized palliative care units, and consultation services.[48]

Social work researcher Mercedes Bern-Klug at the University of Iowa was supported under PDIA's Social Work Leadership Development Awards to identify psychosocial issues that affect nursing home residents. Building on a doctoral study of the social construction of dying in the nursing home setting and its implications for social work, she conducted a survey of over one thousand nursing home service directors in an exercise designed to map problems and issues across the sector.

The work of the *Pilot Project to Improve End of Life Care in Nursing Homes*, based at the Midwest Bioethics Center in Kansas City, sought to bring about attitudinal and behavioral change in the staff of the selected facilities through an intervention program that included palliative care education,[49] technical assistance, case consultation, and mediation. The project aimed to measure changes in staff attitudes and knowledge, the use of advance directives, transfers to hospital at time of death, and referrals to hospice and pain management services. The strategy was to achieve this by fostering cultural change in the organizations and promoting facility ownership of the processes of change. Four facilities comprised the intervention group, with matching "controls." The project took place in 1999–2000, and at the beginning of 2001, Myra J. Christopher wrote to Mary Callaway about the evaluation results: "The day we reviewed the initial data, I said to the staff, 'Dear Lord, this is the SUPPORT Study all over again, only this time in long-term care.'"[50]

But of course, SUPPORT, despite its equivocal results, had achieved a huge leap forward in awareness of end-of-life issues in the hospital context, and those involved in the much more modest ($75,000) Kansas City project, hoped the same could be done for nursing homes. They began by rolling out a series of meetings on the subject, and involved some PDIA faculty scholars as speakers, including Amos Bailey and Laura Hanson. Picking up on the inspirational language of PDIA, the final report of the project concluded that "if a journey begins with a single step, then this project makes a meaningful contribution to improving the culture and transformation of death in America."[51]

48. M. Ersek and S. A. Wilson, "The Challenges and Opportunities in Providing End-of-Life Care in Nursing Homes," *Palliative Medicine* 6, no. 1 (2003):45–57.

49. This included an impressive seminar, Ethical Issues and Palliative Care in Long-Term Settings, held in July/August 1999 by Midwest Bioethics Center.

50. Myra J. Christopher, letter to Mary Callaway, January 6, 2001.

51. "A Project to Improve End-of-Life Care in Nursing Homes," Final report to PDIA, January 6, 2001.

North Carolina faculty scholars Laura Hanson, a geriatrician with public health training, and Martha Henderson, a nurse also educated in theology, worked with Kimberley S. Reynolds to produce an important volume and teaching aid in this area, *Improving Nursing Home Care of the Dying: A Training Manual for Nursing Home Staff.*[52] It contained chapters on recognizing the final phase of life, understanding and supporting families, advance care planning, and choices about eating and drinking, as well as pieces on pain management, emotional and spiritual care, and self-care. The book provided sage advice, case studies, and a variety of assignment tools and exercises to educate nursing home staff about the care of dying residents. Hanson and Henderson went on to contribute a number of other important journal publications on palliative care in the nursing home. They showed both the weaknesses and the strengths of nursing home provision in caring for the dying. For example, Americans who die in nursing homes differ from hospice or hospital populations, being older, more often female, widowed, and with less education. Residents are also more often impoverished and dependent on Medicaid or self-pay for health care. At the same time Americans distrust nursing homes and many do not die there by choice. Likewise recently bereaved relatives express more dissatisfaction with nursing homes than other forms of care at the end of life.

Yet continuity of care may be a real strength of nursing home provision, leading to more substantial "family-like" relationships that may prove of deep worth in the face of death.[53] In one study Hanson, Henderson, and a colleague used focus groups with experienced nursing home staff and physicians to define a good death in the nursing home context and to describe the factors that promote or prevent good care of the dying in this setting.[54] The participants highlighted a number of themes as barriers to high quality care of the dying in nursing homes—lack of training, a regulatory emphasis on rehabilitation, and a resource-poor setting—but they also affirmed the value of their experience and personal relationships with residents as a basis for good care. The good death in the nursing home was defined as comprising (1) individualized care based on a continuity of relationships with caregivers; (2) effective teamwork by staff, physicians, and family; and (3) comprehensive advance care planning that addresses prognosis, emotional preparation, and appropriate use of medical treatments. It was an important piece of work, creatively produced by a physician–nurse partnership and drawing attention to a relatively under-acknowledged aspect of end-of-life care provision.[55]

---

52. M. L. Henderson, L. C. Hanson, and K. S. Reynolds, *Improving Nursing Home Care of the Dying: A Training Manual for Nursing Home Staff* (New York: Springer, 2003).

53. L. C. Hanson, "Creating Excellent Palliative Care in Nursing Homes," *Journal of Palliative Medicine.* 6, no. 1 (2003): 7–9.

54. L. C. Hanson, M. Henderson, and M. Menon, "As Individual as Death Itself: A Focus Group Study of Terminal care in Nursing Homes," *Journal of Palliative Medicine* 5 no.1 (2002): 117–125.

55. Martha Henderson, interview by David Clark, July 24, 2003.

A solid foundation of research evidence on the delivery of end-of-life care in nursing homes was provided by faculty scholar and social scientist Susan Miller. She had a particular interest in the problem of the short length of stay in hospice programs:

> I wanted to think about how organizations contributed to short lengths of stay. What I proposed was a qualitative study where we would interview staff who took care of dying residents at the nursing home and look at residents who had hospice and had a longer stay, which we defined as over seven days, and interviewed staff and tried to identify why somebody was referred so late to hospice or why they weren't referred, and we looked at the full range, but also we're trying to identify organizational things that could be more readily changed than denial of terminal illness. I'm not the first one to identify this. Laura Hanson also has talked about this, the lack of a standardized assessment regarding terminal status... but there really were no nursing homes that had a good process for identifying whether somebody was terminal, nothing in place. There were some that seemed a little bit better than others. I did this work in Rhode Island and we had six nursing homes in our study. I have two physicians working with me; one is a geriatrician who also is a medical director in nursing homes, and one is a hospice medical director, and they helped us in reviewing the qualitative interviews. [One] administrator had no idea you could have a six-month prognosis in a hospice, because he had seen so frequently people going in so late; he thought it was much shorter.[56,57]

This formed part of a much wider corpus of work by Miller (one of the few non-clinician faculty scholars) that addressed issues such as the enrollment and hospitalization of dying nursing home patients,[58] the emergence of Medicare hospice care in US nursing homes,[59] as well as studies of the assessment of pain in nursing home residents.[60]

Nurse and research scientist Betty Ferrell was one of a smaller number of PDIA grantees that focused her work on improving end-of-life care in community settings. Already known to Kathy Foley and Mary Callaway for her extensive work on pain, she obtained funding for a project entitled Homecare Outreach for Palliative Care Education (HOPE). From a survey of 134 home care agencies

56. Susan Miller, interview by David Clark, July 15, 2004.

57. S. C. Miller, S. Weitzen, and B. Kinzbrunner, "Factors Associated with the High Prevalence of Short Hospice Stays," *Journal of Palliative Medicine* 6, no. 5 (2004): 725–736.

58. S. C. Miller, P. Gozalo, and V. Mor, "The Enrollment and Hospitalization of Dying Nursing Home Patients," *The American Journal of Medicine* 111 (2001): 38–44.

59. S. C. Miller and V. Mor, "The Emergence of Medicare Hospice Care in US Nursing Homes," *Palliative Medicine* 15 (2001): 471–480.

60. S. C. Miller, V. Mor, and J. Teno, "Hospice Enrollment and Pain Assessment and Management in Nursing Homes," *Journal of Pain and Symptom Management* 26, no. 3 (2003): 791–799.

published in 1998, only 32 percent reported the availability of specially trained nurses for care of the terminally ill patient, and only 16 percent of the agencies reported providing such training.[61] Based on earlier studies of understanding pain management at home and family perspectives on pain, the project was aimed at busy home-care nurses with the intention of strengthening their work in pain and palliative care, by integrating key concepts of palliative care into the general home-care setting.[62,63] Ferrell reflects on the project and the outcome:

> So the PDIA funding supported the first HOPE project and it was very instrumental in giving us the support to get in there and demonstrate it could be done; and that home-care agencies wanted to participate; that patients would benefit; that this could really happen. And in terms of the outcome... it was very successful, resulting in publication and in really very good outcomes in terms of working with the home-care agencies. We then went on to the National Cancer Institute and were able to get funding for a larger version of the HOPE project that involved more home-care agencies, and in the end resulted in a national conference where we brought home-care agencies from across the country to come and learn about the HOPE project. So for us the PDIA funding was very important because it was a relatively short, efficient grant process. We got the funding in a timely way, were able to carry out our project successfully, and then we were able to really use that to make our case for larger funding.[64]

In the year 2000, the United Hospital Fund of New York embarked upon a third end-of-life care initiative, concerned with moving palliative care into community services. It was a $2.5 million dollar program involving six projects over three years and built heavily on the Fund's earlier experience, which had been wholly within the hospital context.[65,66] The initiative grew out of the experience of developing palliative care programs in the acute hospital and the awareness that had emerged about the importance of continuity of care and the need for other organizations, such as home care agencies and nursing homes, to incorporate the palliative care approach. Although not directly funded by PDIA, this work is an example of a chain of activities subsequently taking on a life of its own,

---

61. B. R. Ferrell, R. Virani, and M. Grant, "HOPE: Home Care Outreach for Palliative Care Education," *Cancer Practice* 6, no. 2 (1998): 79–85.

62. Betty Ferrell, interview by Michelle Winslow, January 9, 2004.

63. B. R. Ferrell, R. Virani, and M. Grant, "Improving End-of-Life Care Education in Home Care," *Journal of Palliative Medicine* 1, no. 1 (1998): 11–19.

64. Betty Ferrell, interview by Michelle Winslow, January 9, 2004.

65. S. S. Hopper, *Crossing Organizational Boundaries in Palliative Care: The Promise and Reality of Community Partnerships* (New York: United Hospital Fund of New York, 2003).

66. S. S. Hopper, *Moving Palliative Care into the Community: New Services, New Strategies* (New York: United Hospital Fund of New York, 2004).

first catalyzed by PDIA support, which helped to leverage organizational and financial resources, and then continuing to be reported on to the PDIA board as it progressed.[67]

Pediatrics

In the United States each year approximately 50,000 children die and at any one time some 500,000 children live with life-threatening conditions that may result in death. About 12,500 children are diagnosed with cancer annually, and in 1998, 2,500 children died of cancer-related causes. Some die young of prematurity and congenital defects. Others die following trauma. Then there is a group of children who die of cancer and congenital heart disease, most of whom live with their illness for a number of years. There is not a clear pathway for those children and their parents and siblings who live their whole lives with a life-threatening condition. Such children need supportive interventions not only when they are at the end of their lives, but their situation is often heavily complicated over long periods by the developmental impact of their disease and their sense of difference from those around them. Accordingly, the children, siblings, and parents all suffer, not only from an existential and social standpoint, but also financially, because of the limited ability of the parents to continue to work while caring for a child who has extensive health-care needs.[68] Moreover, some 15 percent of American children lack health insurance entirely and the rest are covered by a multitude of private and public insurers that vary in their coverage of palliative and end-of-life care. During the period of PDIA activity, there was growing appreciation that palliative care might have some relevance to children (even when all efforts to preserve and extend life were being maintained), but this was coupled with a recognition that pediatric palliative care had failed to make some of the gains experienced in adult care and required even more of a campaigning zeal if it was to gain acknowledgment.

PDIA awarded faculty scholarships to some outstanding pediatricians and others involved in the care of children, including Joanne Hilden, Geri Frager, Marcia Levetown, Nancy Hutton, Walter M. Robinson, and Joanne Wolfe. At times these individuals might have felt that pediatrics was a little marginal to the major thrust of the PDIA initiative. They were also conscious that pediatric issues had not been covered in the Education Project in End-of-Life Care (EPEC)[69] training initiative, and it was not until considerable lobbying had taken place that pediatric palliative care became the subject of a special report in 2002

---

67. Susan Shampaine Hopper (Project Director, Palliative Care Initiative, United Hospital Fund), e-mail to Kathy Foley, February 24, 2000.

68. Marcia Levetown, interview by David Clark, July 14, 2004.

69. Education Project in End-of-Life Care, http://www.epec.net/EPEC/webpages/index.cfm (accessed May 27, 2008; site discontinued). The current website is http://epec.net/.

by the Institute of Medicine.[70] Nor was the care of dying children addressed in any way in the Bill Moyers television series, *On Our Own Terms*, first aired in 2000, which had done so much to raise public awareness about end-of-life issues in general. Nevertheless, within the broad program of PDIA, some specialists in palliative care for children were able to develop important service and practice innovations.

Joanne Wolfe, a staff physician in the Department of Pediatric Oncology in the Dana-Farber Cancer Institute and Children's Hospital, Boston, established a palliative care service for children ("The Pediatric Advance Care Team") and then went on to evaluate it. The project was initially for children with cancer and then expanded to include those with other life-threatening illnesses. Wolfe found a "normal distribution" curve of acceptance for the idea in the hospital. Some took to it in the early days, others needed more time to get on board, and others continued to resist over a period of time.[71,72] Like so many PDIA scholars working in cutting-edge hospital settings, she found there was a need for a clear rationale when introducing palliative care to colleagues. Wolfe's approach was evidence-based, but it also had other dimensions:

> I think having good relationships and mutual respect for one another enabled us to further this project without it being too challenging. There were always hurdles, but from the very beginning we recognized that there was a lot of diplomacy to promoting the concept of palliative care, and that we needed to approach it in a nonthreatening manner, in a nonconfrontational manner, and through that strategy, we were able to gradually penetrate many different areas and subspecialties involved in caring for kids with advanced illness. It was a very intentional strategy.[73]

Looking at the care of children with cancer before and after the advent of the new service, Wolfe and colleagues found parents of children who died of cancer reporting significantly less suffering from pain and dyspnea in the last month of life. These parents were also much *more* likely to report being prepared for their child's end-of-life course. There was also evidence of earlier referrals to hospice and a trend toward earlier documentation of DNR orders. Wolfe regarded the evidence as "pretty sound data" to suggest that, from the perspective of parents at least, the care of dying children at the hospital had improved since the introduction of the service. Building on this and with continuing support from PDIA and the Emily Davie and Joseph S. Kornfeld Foundation, she went on to develop

---

70. *Institute of Medicine, When Children Die: Improving Palliative and End-of-Life Care for Children and Their Families* (Washington, DC: Institute of Medicine, 2002).

71. Joanne Wolfe, interview by David Clark, July 15, 2004.

72. J. Wolfe et al., "Symptoms and Suffering at the End of Life in Children with Cancer," *New England Journal of Medicine* 342 (February 23, 2000): 326–333.

73. Joanne Wolfe, interview by David Clark, July 15, 2004.

one of the only pediatric palliative care fellowship programs in the United States at that time.

Marcia Levetown was working at the University of Texas Medical Branch in Galveston as a junior faculty member and was in the Department of Pediatrics where she was trying to implement a palliative care program. Yet after she won her faculty scholars award, she met with much less support locally than she had anticipated. She was also mindful of the poor evidence base for pediatric palliative care and, therefore, she engaged in some efforts to promote international collaboration in a context where several in the field appeared to be working in their own "silos." She began to focus her work on this latter area in an initiative known as ChIPPS (Children's International Project on Palliative and Hospice Care Services), which created a compendium of pediatric palliative care that brought together knowledge from around the world on the development of programs and the delivery of care. The compendium was distributed to thirty-one National Hospice and Palliative Care Organization member hospices in the United States and five hundred international hospices and forged a substantial network of cooperation, as well as giving rise to the creation of the National Alliance for Children Living with Life-Threatening Conditions. This work led to her practical handbook on palliative care for infants, children, and adolescents, which contained chapters from a range of international experts, including PDIA grantees, and also included a foreword by PDIA board chair Kathy Foley. Rich in case-based material, the book provides a wide-ranging resource, from epidemiological and societal contexts to special care environments and specific patient groups.[74]

PDIA faculty scholar Joanne Hilden and Grace Christ, project director of the PDIA Social Work Leadership Development Awards Program, also made substantial contributions on issues relating to children and death.

Hilden, a pediatric oncologist, and her co-author, Daniel Tobin, created a compassionate "road map" to guide families through what they may face when a child has a life-limiting illness, showing how informed choices can be made and how the child might be involved in the decision making.[75] The book sought to fill an information gap for parents with seriously ill children and was widely cited and well reviewed. Hilden also collaborated with PDIA faculty scholars Bruce Himelstein and David Weissman on an important review article about pediatric palliative care that appeared in the *New England Journal of Medicine* in 2004. The authors describe how in the previous ten years, a range of palliative care clinical programs had been developed in hospitals, hospices, home care programs, and long-term care facilities to help fill the gap between traditional hospital care and community-based hospice care. Yet the presence of a

74. B. S. Carter and M. Levetown (eds.), *Palliative Care for Infants, Children, and Adolescents* (Baltimore and London: The Johns Hopkins University Press, 2004).

75. J. M. Hilden and D. Tobin, *Shelter from the Storm: Caring for a Child with a Life-Threatening Condition* (Cambridge, Mass.: Perseus Publishing, 2003).

designated pediatric palliative care team in all health-care facilities that serve life-threatened children is generally regarded as a luxury rather than an essential service component. The key message of the paper is that pediatric palliative care should provide long-term, continuous care for children with chronic and/or life-threatening illnesses, and the goal should be to improve the quality of life for young patients and their families by advocating for patient comfort, dignity, and choice throughout treatment, regardless of the child's medical outcome.[76]

Christ's book focused not on the medical problems of dying children, but on the difficulties experienced by those children who survive the death of a parent through cancer.[77] It contains a qualitative analysis of the experiences of 88 families and 157 children who coped with the terminal illness and ultimately the death of a parent. It shows how healing occurs in bereavement through relieving painful feelings, integrating the new reality of loss, constructing a legacy created by continuous revision of the image of the dead parent, and reconstituting individual and family life following the loss. The book is a rich inventory of the inventive solutions that families and friends devise to respond knowledgeably, confidently, and effectively to children and adolescents facing the loss of a parent.

Gerri Frager of the Isaac Walton Killam-Grace Health Center in Halifax, Nova Scotia, had already developed considerable skill and interest in pediatric palliative care before she applied for a PDIA faculty scholarship to start a service for children in the Maritime Provinces of Canada, Nova Scotia, New Brunswick, and Prince Edward Island. She identified three barriers to the provision of appropriate end-of-life care for children: (1) personal distress in caring for terminally ill children; (2) the knowledge gap created by the challenge of understanding the wide-range of life-limiting illnesses affecting children; and (3) the difficulties faced by children, parents, and health-care professionals when forced to make the transition to a palliative care mode, often with little coordination in their states of readiness.[78] She describes her experience in trying to address these issues within her own area of geographically dispersed population:

> For the first three years, I was chief cook and bottle washer for pediatric palliative care at our health center. I would do the consults and see children. Not only were there clinical issues that I was engaged with but lots of opportunities to look at how pediatric palliative care could be integrated into teaching, into research, into different aspects of clinical care, so that was a big, tall order, and something that I was very enthusiastic about. But it's a real challenge to spread yourself out in so many areas that are so much in need. So a big piece of starting the service up was sitting on provincial

---

76. B. P. Himelstein et al., "Pediatric Palliative Care," *New England Journal of Medicine* 350, no. 17 (2004):1752–1762.

77. G. C. Christ, *Healing Children's Grief: Surviving a Parent's Death from Cancer* (New York: Oxford University Press, 2000).

78. Gerri Frager, "PDIA Year-End Report," July 1996.

boards and national committees looking at how to integrate pediatrics in the broader context of palliative care. For the first three years, I did that on my own and then we hired a clinical nurse specialist. The first three years, I was funded through PDIA for 60 percent of my salary, and I worked with the hematology oncology service for the other 40 percent. But then, after those three years, our provincial government Department of Health took my funding on board and I'm now funded 100 percent to do pediatric palliative care.[79]

Nancy Hutton, director of pediatrics in the Intensive Primary Care Clinic at the Johns Hopkins Children's Center in Baltimore, initiated a project to make the center a pain-free institution. In her work she interviewed family members and was struck by how eager some parents were to talk about the dying of their children, and to focus on their own feelings rather than on the medical issues. Surprisingly, many families felt their children had received the best possible care, whereas some staff expressed anger and frustration at the care that had been delivered.[80] Walter Robinson examined the medical and ethical aspects of end-of-life care for chronically ill children at Harvard Medical School and Children's Hospital, Boston.

In the PDIA newsletter of April 2000, Kathy Foley noted some of the progress being made in children's palliative care. Children's Hospice International, working closely with Health Care Financing Administration (HCFA) and Congress, had recently announced a $1 million federal appropriation for Children's Hospice Demonstration Model Programs, offering an opportunity to remove roadblocks to appropriate care for children and their families and promoting a continuum of care from diagnosis through bereavement. Meanwhile support from the Robert Wood Johnson Foundation was assisting local and national initiatives in pediatric pain and palliative care, and grassroots organizations, such as Partnerships for Caring and Americans for the Better Care of the Dying, were drawing attention to the special needs of children for appropriate palliative care.[81] In addition, a working group of pediatric specialists and ethicists was convened at the National Consensus Conference on Medical Education for Care Near the End of Life, sponsored by PDIA and the Robert Wood Johnson Foundation. The charge to the working group was to consider the unique aspects of death in childhood, identify critical educational issues and effective instructional strategies, and recommend institutional changes needed to facilitate teaching about end-of-life care for children. The group concluded that, despite the challenges, the cognitive and psychologic skills needed to provide end-of-life care to children can be taught effectively through well-planned and focused learning experiences. The ultimate goals of such instruction should be to provide more humane care

79. Gerri Frager, interview by David Clark, July 15, 2004.

80. "The Dying Child: Physicians Search for the Best Ways to Relieve Pain while Providing Treatment," PDIA Newsletter, no. 7 (April 2000), 7–8.

81. K. M. Foley, "The Growing Movement for Pediatric Palliative Care," PDIA Newsletter, no. 7 (April 2000), 2.

to very sick children, enhance bereavement outcomes for their survivors, and develop more confident clinicians. Six specific principles regarding end-of-life care in the pediatric setting emerged as essential curricular elements that should be taught to all medical care providers to ensure competent patient-centered care: (1) communicating in a cognitively and developmentally appropriate manner, (2) sharing information with patients to avoid feelings of isolation and abandonment, (3) serving the needs of patients by ensuring that ethical principles of self-determination and their best interests are central to the decision-making process, (4) minimizing physical and emotional pain and other symptoms by prompt recognition, careful assessment, and comprehensive treatment, (5) developing partnerships with families to support them in their care-giving efforts, and (6) addressing the personal and professional challenges faced by providers of end-of-life care for children. These principles apply to the care of all children regardless of diagnosis and prognosis. With this in mind, the group concluded, teaching about end-of-life care for children does not require a new and separate curriculum, but rather calls for taking better advantage of the many teachable moments provided by caring for a dying patient in routine settings.[82]

Toward the end of the PDIA initiative, in 2002, a major landmark publication did much to highlight the importance of pediatric palliative care.[83] Sponsored by PDIA, the National Institutes of Health, the Greenwall Foundation, and the Robert Wood Johnson Foundation, the Institute of Medicine report *When Children Die* included contributions from several PDIA award holders and grantees (Grace Christ, Joanne Hilden, Marcia Levetown, Mildred Solomon, Cynda Rushton, Joanne Woolf, and Barbara Koenig). It outlined specific recommendations to improve care for children with life-limiting illnesses and those facing death, and their families—sparing preventable suffering over the onset of illness, its physical and emotional toll, the difficulty of making treatment decisions, the confusion of navigating complex health and financial systems, and the pain of grieving. In particular, the report recommended that the rules set by Medicaid and some private health plans that require families to choose between receiving hospice care and continuing life-prolonging therapy should be revised. It also highlighted the problems of coordinating care when a myriad of providers is involved. The report found that if few health professionals are trained in palliative care, even fewer are equipped to handle the needs of children with life-limiting illness, and there is only a weak evidence base to support best practice. Nevertheless, it was an essential document in the struggle to raise awareness of and improve practice relating to the care of seriously ill and dying children.[84] It quickly led to the formation of a National Alliance for Children

---

82. O. J. Z. Sahler et al., "Medical Education about End of Life Care in the Pediatric Setting: Principles, Challenges, and Opportunities," *Pediatrics* 105, no. 3 (2000): 575–584.

83. *Institute of Medicine, When Children Die: Improving Palliative and End-of-Life Care for Children and Their Families* (Washington, DC: Institute of Medicine, 2002).

84. "New Report from the Institute of Medicine: Improving Care for Dying Children Requires Comprehensive Approach," *PDIA Newsletter*, no. 11 (Fall 2003), 6–7.

with Life-Threatening Conditions, which set goals for reform in clinical practice, research, advocacy, and education.[85] The following year, in 2003, the New York Academy of Medicine hosted the first national symposium for health-care professionals and parents that focused on family-centered care for gravely ill children. Social scientist Mildred Solomon, PDIA grantee and principal investigator with the Initiative for Pediatric Palliative Care (one of the sponsors of the event), took part in the meeting. So too did David Browning, who was supported by PDIA through the Social Work Leadership Program.[86,87] Meanwhile Social Work Leadership awards enabled Nancy Cincotta to organize a National Initiative to Unite Social Workers and Families in the Interest of Dying Children and supported Nancy Contro in a project for Latino Families needing pediatric palliative care at the Lucile Packard Children's Hospital in Palo Alto, California.[88] From a variety of disciplines and perspectives, PDIA was helping the cause of pediatric palliative care to advance and get a hearing, and in the lifetime of PDIA grant making, the landscape of pediatric palliative care in the United States changed considerably.

CLINICAL PRACTICE

PDIA funded a large number of initiatives that aimed to transform clinical practice in end-of-life care. These ranged from major programs of work with high ambition and extensive range, to locally based interventions in specific institutions. Some are highlighted here and many others are referred to in other chapters.

Faculty scholar James Tulsky, based at Duke University Medical Center, sought to improve communication with dying patients through an educational curriculum for medical students and house staff. The project aimed to develop communication skills that would enable physicians to become more familiar with the biographies of their patients, to listen for their anxieties about death, to help explore meaning in their patients' lives, and to discuss life-sustaining treatment preferences within the context of a deeper understanding of patients' values.[89] In a study conducted in teaching hospitals in California, Tulsky had

---

85. "Institute of Medicine Report Spurs Formation of National Alliance for Children with Life-Threatening Conditions," *PDIA Newsletter*, no. 11 (Fall 2003), 7.

86. "First National Pediatric Palliative Care Symposium on Family-Centered Care or Parents and Health Professionals," *PDIA Newsletter*, no. 11 (Fall 2003), 9.

87. David Browning and others continued to work on the IPPC initiative after the conclusion of PDIA, and in 2004–2005, the initiative held a series of regional interdisciplinary team retreats across North America.

88. *Project on Death in America, January 2001–December 2003, Report of Activities* (New York: Open Society Institute, 2001), 25–33.

89. J. Tulsky, "Annual Report to PDIA Faculty Scholars Program," 31 May 1996, PDIA Closed Box 1995/GR# 3232.

found that almost a third of 101 medical house officers had never conducted a *Do Not Resuscitate* (DNR) order while being observed by a more senior clinician and 71 percent had been observed twice or less. Tulsky observed: "We have to dispel the notion that anyone can do this well after simply watching one or two discussions conducted by a more experienced physician."[90] In a study conducted with another faculty scholar, Robert Arnold, based at the University of Pittsburgh, Tulsky and colleagues explored the quality of communication that led to the completion of written advance directives in fifty-six cases in the outpatient primary care medicine context.[91] Conversations about advance directives averaged 5.6 minutes and physicians spoke for two-thirds of the time. In 91 percent of cases, physicians discussed dire scenarios in which most patients would not want to be treated and 48 percent asked patients about their preferences in reversible scenarios. Physicians often used vague language and patients' preferences were rarely explored in detail. The authors concluded that these approaches would likely be of little benefit in the future and fell short of standards proposed in the literature, as Tulsky notes in the following:

> What they ended up doing was having conversations with patients about the overall issue, but not talking about the kinds of situations where it's actually difficult to make decisions... So it really wasn't very helpful. They talked more about documents and forms, but they probably ended up with an advance directive that wouldn't be incredibly useful if a patient had a serious illness.[92]

One aspect of the daily challenge of making change in clinical practice is captured by faculty scholar Sharon Weinstein, referring to her work at the University of Utah, Huntsman Cancer Institute. She reflects sensitively about the issues involved in working *with* colleagues while, at the same time, trying to bring a reforming influence to bear:

> What we're trying to do has had to be clearer and clearer and more and more simple. I'm constantly asking people what do they mean by palliative care. We have to be able to articulate that over and over again, and [the replies are] "What's wrong with what we're doing?" or "How is that different from what we're currently doing?" and "How is it not hospice?" The challenge has been over and over to articulate the vision of what palliative care is in an integrated model. It's to say two things: (1) everybody should do a better job of it, no matter what they're doing, (2) and there is an expertise to it that one can call upon; it's almost a standard medical model. I'm saying, you know,

---

90. In B. Wells, "We Need to Talk...Conversations about End of Life Care," *Duke Medical Perspectives* 17, no. 1 (1997), 29.

91. J. Tulsky et al., "Opening the Black Box: How Do Physicians Communicate about Advance Directives?" *Annals of Internal Medicine* 129 (1998): 441–449.

92. In Wells, "We need to talk...," 30.

"Every primary care doctor needs to know when somebody might be having a heart attack, but they don't need to be an invasive cardiologist." So we want to raise the bar throughout all of medicine to what integrated palliative care looks like, and then we want people to recognize this as a special skill that they can acquire.[93]

A traditional view in oncology has been that speaking of poor prognosis and death is too burdensome for patients and families. This view is compounded by oncologists' lack of preparation to deliver palliative care, leading to common statements such as "There is no more hope," "There is nothing more to be done," and "It's time to give up." I repeatedly point out the implications of these statements and offer alternative language for oncologists to use when it is accepted that there is no realistic possibility of cure. This "new" language emphasizes compassion and continued care. Another way I have contributed to the changing culture is to support my colleagues in oncology as they wrestle with these difficult issues.[94]

Another physician project with a specific focus on practice was Eduardo Bruera's work at Edmonton General Hospital in Canada, which involved the creation of a multidimensional "toolkit" for the assessment of terminally ill cancer patients and their families. Key components included an assessment tool for patients to describe their physical and psychological symptoms, cognitive function, spiritual needs, and family support.

As Bruera noted: "If we are going to treat patients properly when they are dying, we need to know their main problems—not from our perspective but from theirs." He observed that a physician or nurse can leaf through a cancer patient's medical chart and find measurements of blood chemistry, temperature, heart rate, progression of tumor, and so on "but what we can't see in the chart is her suffering... and if it's not measured, it's easy to ignore. What we are attempting to do is make this suffering very visible so that it becomes one of our priorities,"[95] Bruera and his colleagues at the University of Alberta's division of palliative care medicine devised a unique assessment tool which they named the *Integrated Multidimensional Tool Kit*. It was designed to be simple, efficient, and versatile and useable at home, in a hospital, or in hospice. "What kills good ideas is bureaucratic inertia," Bruera points out. "So you need a system that measures things reliably, audits how things are going, and allows everyone to do their work."[96] It was a simple and replicable approach to assessing what thirty years earlier, Cicely Saunders had designated "total pain."[97]

93. Sharon Weinstein, interview by David Clark, July 22, 2003.

94. S. Weinstein, "Year-End Report to PDIA Faculty Scholars Program," April 30, 1997.

95. See www.soros.org/initiatives/pdia/articles_publications/publications/memo/research (accessed 2 May 2008; site discontinued).

96. Ibid.

97. C. Saunders, "The Symptomatic Treatment of Incurable Malignant Disease," *Prescribers' Journal* 4, no. 4 (1964): 68–73.

Theresa (Terry) Altilio, of the Department of Pain Medicine and Palliative Care at Beth Israel Medical Center and holder of a PDIA Social Work Leadership Development Award, was able devise a two-year social work fellowship with the primary focus of creating advocacy for the inclusion of multidimensional pain and symptom management in the curriculum for social workers. The project included the development of a list-serv for social workers, as well as considerable education and development activity. The work on pain was interesting in that it tried to focus on the unique aspects of the social work contribution, without rejecting the "medical model," and in the context of a close team working with medical and nursing staff and the recognition of the impact of pain on family caregivers. She produced some compelling case studies of complex problems in pain management and how they could be addressed through imaginative multidisciplinary working.[98] She explains her approach:

> Pain and symptom management is a category that's very appropriate for social work because...the way you look at pain and symptom management is really the way social workers are trained to look at human experience and problem solving. We're really trained always to start where the patient is. We're trained to look at the person in their environment, to look at all aspects of a person's life and, really, if you think about pain and some of the basic pain principles, you accept the patient's report of pain, and if you're expert, that's where you start but it's not where you finish. You expand beyond the patient's report to different areas of [his or her life] that are impacted by the pain experience and by the experience of having pain on a day-to-day basis. Whether that pain is chronic pain or pain of life-threatening illness doesn't matter; a lot of the approach is really the same.[99]

An early social work project funded by PDIA was that of Matthew J. Loscalzo, at the Johns Hopkins Oncology Center, who undertook a piece of work to develop a problem-solving approach to helping families care for dying persons with cancer.[100,101] The initiative encountered a number of barriers and it proved difficult to recruit participants, though those who did take part were quite positive about their experience. A similar theme was later picked up by Aloen L. Townsend, associate professor of social work at the Mandel School in Cleveland, Ohio. She and her colleagues conducted research to understand the needs of family caregivers and discovered, among other things, that "dispositional optimism"

98. T. Altilio, "Pain and Symptom Management: An Essential Role for Social Work." In J. Berzoff and Phyllis R. Silverman, *Living with Dying: A Handbook for End-of-Life Healthcare Practitioners* (New York: Columbia University Press, 2004).

99. Theresa (Terry) Altilio, interview by David Clark, July 12, 2004.

100. Final Progress Report to PDIA, "A Problem-Solving Approach to Helping Families Care for Dying Persons with Cancer," 1997.

101. "Lectures by Experts on Terminal Illness Issues," *Hopkins Medical News* (Fall 1998).

serves as a beneficial resource in caring for others.[102] Other social work projects that sought to improve clinical practice at the end of life included Elizabeth Mayfield Arnold's work on assessing unmet needs in hospice patients, and a survey of the needs of social workers doing cross-cultural practice in end-of-life care by Margo Okazawa-Rey and Norma del Rio. There was also a project by Judith Dobrof on a structured support program for caregivers, and an initiative by Shirley Otis-Green to enhance bereavement and end-of-life care for Latinos within a cancer setting.[103]

Some practice development projects focused on specific patient groups, such as the work of June Simmons in Los Angeles, who developed a model for the provision of comprehensive end-stage care to patients with Alzheimer's disease; another was Susan Taylor-Brown's creation of Family Unity, a consortium to improve the ability of social workers to work with families affected by HIV/AIDS.[104] Other projects had a specifically institutional context, such as Eric Krakauer's work at Massachusetts General Hospital on clinical policy development, which aimed to reduce barriers to optimum care by developing and advocating for policies and guidelines. He illustrates how this worked:

> I felt that I needed to have a more reliable tool to assure comfort in patients who were dying, who wanted to be comfortable, who did not wish life-sustaining treatment. I felt like I needed to be able to tell people that they didn't have to suffer and feel confident that I could make sure that they didn't. I've always thought that a good analogy is knowing how to do CPR in the intensive care unit. Every day I was on call in the ICU, before I went to work I would quickly review the CPR protocols, because I needed to feel that, in the worst case scenario, I knew how to respond. If somebody arrested, I knew how to resuscitate them. And it's analogous to palliative care. If somebody, in the worst case scenario, if somebody's pain is so severe that an ocean of morphine and adjuvant pain medications does not control their pain, I need to know that I can make them comfortable.[105]

Other PDIA-funded work focused on the more personal dimensions of care at the end of life and, in particular, its impact on practitioners and caregivers. Faculty scholar Daniel Sulmasy wrote a thoughtful book which he described as "a work *of* spirituality" in health care, written from the perspective of a person

102. See, for example, A. A. Atlenza, M. A. P. Stephens, and A. L. Townsend, "Dispositional Optimism, Role-Specific Stress, and the Well-Being of Adult Daughter Caregivers," *Research on Aging* 24, no. 2 (2002): 193–217.

103. *Project on Death in America, January 2001–December 2003, Report of Activities* (New York: Open Society Institute, 2001), 25–33.

104. *Project on Death in America, January 1998–December 2000, Report of Activities* (New York: Open Society Institute, 2001), 29–35.

105. Erik Krakauer, interview by David Clark, July 14, 2004.

of faith working as a physician.[106] Meier, Back, and Morrison, in a typical faculty scholar collaboration, addressed ways in which physicians respond to patients' problems and experiences with emotions of their own, which, they argue, may reflect a need to rescue the patient, a sense of failure and frustration when the patient's illness progresses, feelings of powerlessness against illness and its associated losses, grief, fear of becoming ill oneself, or a desire to separate from and avoid patients to escape their own feelings. Such emotions can affect both the quality of medical care and the physician's own sense of well-being, since unexamined emotions may also lead to distress, disengagement, burnout, and poor judgment. The authors devised a model for increasing physician self-awareness, which includes identifying and working with emotions that may affect patient care. The approach was based on the standard medical model of risk factors, signs and symptoms, differential diagnosis, and intervention. They took the view that while "it is normal to have feelings arising from the care of patients, physicians should take an active role in identifying and controlling those emotions."[107]

This chapter has highlighted a huge range of service development and clinical practice innovations promoted by PDIA to improve end-of-life care across many settings. It gives an insight into the breadth and depth of the board's grant making in these areas. Some initiatives, on subsequent inquiry, appear not to have been sustained. In some cases it was hard to see resulting changes, publications that documented results, or evidence of long-term and sustainable outcomes. But in many of the projects described here this was not the case, and clear evidence existed that PDIA funds had catalyzed significant innovation and change with long-term effect. The United Hospitals Fund grant transformed the development of palliative care in New York City, developing teams in multiple hospitals and creating a cadre of enduring programs and initiatives, some of which were supported later by others. PDIA-funded work on communication issues led to a major transformation in medical education. James Tulsky, Bob Arnold, and Anthony Back published an influential volume *Mastering Communication with Seriously Ill Patients*[108] and went on to receive National Cancer Institute funding for a communications skills training initiative called OncoTalk.[109] Most importantly, the work described here was aimed directly at the health-care system and in many instances related to actual service innovations and improvements, examples that could be used elsewhere to leverage interest and resources for end-of-

106. D. P. Sulmasy, *The Healer's Calling: A Spirituality for Physicians and Other Healthcare Professionals* (New York/Mahwah, NJ: Paulist Press, 1997).

107. D. E. Meier, A. L. Back, and R. S. Morrison, "The Inner Life of Physicians and Care of the Seriously Ill," *Journal of the American Medical Association* 286 (2001): 3007–3014.

108. A. Back, R. Arnold, J., and Tulsky, *Mastering Communication with Seriously Ill Patients: Balancing Honesty with Empathy and Hope* (New York: Cambridge University Press, 2009).

109. University of Washington: OncoTalk—Teach, About the Faculty, http://depts.washington.edu/oncotalk/faculty_tch.html (accessed May 2012).

life-care improvement. The hospital-based projects, the work in nursing homes and in pediatrics, were all of crucial importance in this regard. As Kathy Foley put it: "In short we planted the seeds of the issues, supported the pilot studies or papers, and then the newly emerging leaders ran with it."[110] Such successful grant making in the recognized centers of health-care delivery would, in turn, give the PDIA board the courage and motivation to extend its reach to a wide range of underserved communities, where end-of-life care could not only be shaped as an issue of service improvement, but also as a matter of social justice.

---

110. Kathy Foley, personal communication, April 18, 2010.

5

Opportunities, Barriers, and Underserved Communities

The early PDIA board could be considered light on policy-oriented personnel. Velvet Miller had a background in Medicare and Medicaid, but pressures of work ended her involvement within a year of PDIA being formed.[1] Other board members were clinicians, academics, and community activists who, like Bob Butler, Joanne Lynn, and Kathy Foley, had some experience of the larger landscape of macro policy making, but in the main were coming to it rather new. Nevertheless, there was an interest in supporting work that had policy implications. The initial years saw PDIA mainly in a "responsive mode." As Bo Burt described it, "Clearly there was policy analysis, policy advocacy to be done, and there were legal things that could be done, so let's open the field to anybody who wants to come in, and let things happen."[2] This was the board's approach in the first three years; thereafter, a more targeted orientation was adopted involving specific programs identified by the board where PDIA could make its own particular contribution, at a time when other funders, and especially the Robert Wood Johnson Foundation, were becoming more active in the field. There was never a major policy initiative within PDIA in the sense of a single issue around which significant resources could be oriented, but as this chapter (and the one following) will show, the board did support a range of policy work and showed growing commitment over time to highlighting the needs of disadvantaged and dispossessed individuals, groups, and communities. These areas of activity should be kept in mind when considering some of the more service- and clinically-oriented activities described in the previous two chapters.

---

1. Kathy Foley, interview by David Clark, July 22, 2003.

2. Bo Burt, interview by David Clark, July 23, 2003.

POLICY MATTERS

In the initial PDIA RFA "the shaping of government and institutional policy" did feature as one of seven areas of interest. Early forays into the policy domain embraced the challenge of evaluating and advocating for change relating to dying and bereavement—at federal, state, and local levels. They also acknowledged the role of large health-care delivery systems (such as the work described in chapter 4 with the New York Hospital Fund), plus government reimbursement for services, as well as workforce development issues. Some interventions were focused on the production of standards and guidelines for end-of-life care. Later some strategic grants were awarded to major palliative care organizations, for capacity building purposes.

The first PDIA triennial review contained a small number of items of major policy significance that had been given PDIA support in the early years.[3] Chief among these was undoubtedly the Institute of Medicine report entitled *Approaching Death: Improving Care at the End of Life*,[4] published in 1997. Here PDIA invested heavily with a $200,000 grant that was instrumental in the production of a major report that had wide-ranging significance. PDIA colleagues were well represented in the work that led to the production of the report. Two board members, Joanne Lynn and Bo Burt, served on the committee, as did grantee Richard Payne, at that time chief of the pain and symptom management section and professor of medicine at MD Anderson Cancer Center at the University of Texas. They formed part of a group of leading clinicians and other authorities on end-of-life issues that took responsibility for the report. Kathy Foley had an important role in providing technical advice and background guidance, while several other PDIA funded experts—William Breitbart, Carlos Gomez, David Joranson, Barbara Koenig, Susan Block, Andrew Billings, Daniel Sulmasy, Diane Meier, and Mary Callaway—contributed in various ways.

Approaching Death represents a comprehensive assessment of end-of-life care issues in late 1990s America, and its provenance, the prestigious Institute of Medicine, did much to enhance its credibility and impact. The report saw death as at once a fact of life and a profound mystery. It viewed "reliably excellent" and "respectful" care at life's end as an attainable goal of the health-care system, albeit one which would require "many changes in attitudes, policies, and actions."[5] Capturing the mood of the times and an emerging openness to addressing the issues, it sought to influence a wide constituency of health professionals,

---

3. "The Shaping of Governmental and Institutional Policy," *Project on Death in America, July 1994–December 1997* (New York: Open Society Institute, 1998), 51–54.

4. Institute of Medicine, *Approaching Death: Improving Care at the End of Life* (Washington, DC: Institute of Medicine, 1997).

5. Institute of Medicine, *Approaching Death*, 1.

managers, researchers, policy makers, funders, and the general public. It highlighted the issue of preventable suffering and pain at the end of life; it noted
the significant organizational, economic, legal, and educational impediments to
good care; and it acknowledged the need for better evidence on quality of care
and outcomes.

Approaching Death can be seen as a landmark document—the first comprehensive report on end-of-life care ever produced in the United States. It made
seven recommendations:[6]

1. People with advanced, potentially fatal illnesses and those close to
   them should be able to expect and receive reliable, skilful, and supportive care.
2. Physicians, nurses, social workers, and other health professionals must
   commit themselves to improving care for dying patients and to using
   existing knowledge effectively to prevent and relieve pain and other
   symptoms.
3. Because many problems in care stem from system problems, policy
   makers, consumer groups, and purchasers of health care should work
   with health-care practitioners, organizations, and researchers to (a)
   strengthen methods for measuring the quality of life and other outcomes of care for dying patients and those close to them; (b) develop
   better tools and strategies for improving the quality of care, and hold
   health-care organizations accountable for care at the end of life; (c)
   revise mechanisms for financing care so that they encourage rather
   than impede good end-of-life care and sustain rather than frustrate
   coordinated systems of excellent care; and (d) reform drug prescription laws, burdensome regulations, and state medical board policies
   and practices that impede effective use of opioids to relieve pain and
   suffering.
4. Educators and other health professionals should initiate changes in
   undergraduate, graduate, and continuing education to ensure that
   practitioners have relevant attitudes, knowledge, and skills to care well
   for dying patients.
5. Palliative care should become, if not a medical specialty, at least a
   defined area of expertise, education, and research.
6. The nation's research establishment should define and implement
   priorities for strengthening the knowledge base for end-of-life care.
7. A continuing public discussion is essential to develop a better
   understanding of the modern experience of dying, the options available
   to patients and families, and the obligations of communities to those
   approaching death.

---

6. Institute of Medicine, *Approaching Death*, 7–13.

The report gained good media coverage at the time of publication[7] and was much reviewed[8,9] and cited[10,11,12] in subsequent years. It might be regarded as the formal establishment statement that was subsequently converted into popular format via the Bill Moyers series, described in chapter 3, and it was seen by one international commentator as the inspiration behind the Project to Educate Physicians in End-of-Life Care.[13] It was in the committee[14] that led to its creation that Kathy Foley and Bo Burt first met.[15] Moreover, the funding partnership for *Approaching Death*, which included the Greenwall Foundation, the Culpeper Foundation, and the Robert Wood Johnson Foundation, saw PDIA in a network of excellent company. The report was also a catalyst to further work at the Institute of Medicine and led directly to the 2001 document, *Improving Palliative Care for Cancer*,[16] which was edited by Kathy Foley and Hellen Gelband, and then to *When Children Die: Improving Palliative and End-of-Life Care for Children and Their Families*,[17] appearing in 2002 and sponsored by the Institute of Medicine.

Finally, 2003 saw another Institute of Medicine report on end-of-life issues, again with Kathy Foley as one of the authors, but this time with PDIA faculty scholar Thomas Smith also on the team; *Describing Death in America* gave attention to national expenditures for medical care in the months and days preceding death. It highlighted the knowledge gaps relating to whether that money is buying good quality care or optimizing the quality of life for those dying, and whether

7. "Not Enough Is Done to Ease End of Life, Panel Says," *New York Times* (June 5, 1997).

8. T. Nadelson, review of Institute of Medicine, *Approaching Death: Improving Care at the End of Life*, in *The American Journal of Psychiatry* 156 (1999): 655.

9. L. Stepp, review of Institute of Medicine, *Approaching Death: Improving Care at the End of Life*, in *Annals of Internal Medicine* 128, no. 11 (1998): 964.

10. J. N. Lickiss, "Approaching Death in Multicultural Australia," *The Medical Journal of Australia* 179, no. 6 Suppl (2003): S14–S16.

11. R. MacLeod, "Caring for Children Who Are Dying," *The New Zealand Medical Journal* 115, no. 1163 (2002): 198.

12. K. S. Heller, "Implementing Pain Management Guidelines," *Innovations in End of Life Care* 1, no. 3 (1999), http://www2.edc.org/lastacts/archives/archivesapril99/editorial.asp (accessed July 9, 2008).

13. J. N. Lickiss, "Education for Physicians on End-of-Life Care," *The Lancet* 357, no. 9261 (2001): 1051–1052.

14. Institute of Medicine, *Summary of Committee Views and Workshop Examining the Feasibility of an Institute of Medicine Study of Dying, Decisionmaking, and Appropriate Care* (Washington, DC: Institute of Medicine, 1994).

15. Kathy Foley, interview by David Clark, July 22, 2003.

16. Institute of Medicine/National Research Council, *Improving Palliative Care for Cancer* (Washington, DC: National Academies Press, 2001).

17. Institute of Medicine, *When Children Die: Improving Palliative and End-of-Life Care for Children and Their Families* (Washington, DC: Institute of Medicine, 2002). See chapter 4 for an account of PDIA involvement in the production of this report.

the situation is getting better or worse over time. The report recommended ways to fill the information gaps by better use of existing nationally representative data, and through some new measures—in particular, an ongoing National Mortality Followback Survey. The goal of the report was to set out methods for benchmarking end-of-life care in order to monitor change in the future.[18]

In the space of five years, four major policy documents with impeccable provenance had appeared on end-of-life issues in America. PDIA personnel had played a part in each one. The resulting challenges were enormous. As Kathy Foley noted: "There are no villains in this piece but ourselves and our culture"[19]—and these of course were now being actively addressed though various PDIA programs.[20]

Other PDIA policy initiatives in the early years were wide-ranging in character. Funding was made available to the State of New York Office of the Attorney General for a commission on quality care at the end of life, reviewing state laws and regulations. The commission identified several barriers to providing quality care to dying patients: inadequate professional and public education, legal and regulatory barriers, financial barriers, and underuse of hospice.[21] At the University of Washington, Paul G. Ramsey built on long-standing interests in medical education and competence to develop a systematic method for the assessment of physician performance in end-of-life care, a work in which he also collaborated with PDIA faculty scholar Randy Curtis.[22] A small grant was also given to R. Knight Steel at the Association of Academic Health Centers in Washington, DC, to direct attention to the education of physicians in end-of-life care issues, particularly by raising this with residency review committees and by encouraging the inclusion of end-of-life topics in specialty board examinations, where the goal was to make a major impact on postgraduate training across medical

18. J. R. Lunney et al. (eds.), *Describing Death in America: What We Need to Know* (Washington, DC: Institute of Medicine, with National Cancer Policy Board and National Research Council, 2003).

19. K. Foley, Preface. In Institute of Medicine/National Research Council, *Improving Palliative Care for Cancer* (Washington, DC: National Academies Press, 2001), x.

20. A further contribution to this line of work, to which Kathy Foley and PDIA faculty scholar Thomas Smith both contributed, can be found in J. R. Lunney et al. (eds.), *Describing Death in America*. The report examines the data available to track and evaluate the quality of life and quality of care experienced by Americans in the months immediately preceding death and recommends the creation of a National Mortality Followback Survey to monitor trends and issues.

21. Attorney General Dennis C. Vacco's Commission on quality of care at the end of life. *Final Report of the Attorney General* (July 1998). This report is cited in an article by two PDIA faculty scholars: N. S. Wenger and K. Rosenfeld, "Quality Indicators for End-of-Life Care in Vulnerable Elders," *Annals of Internal Medicine* 135, no. 8 (2001): 677–685.

22. J. R. Curtis et al., "Understanding Physicians' Skills Providing End-of-Life Care: Perspectives of Patients, Families, and Health Care Workers, *Journal of General Internal Medicine* 16 (2001): 41–49; J. R. Curtis et al., "Patients' Perspectives on Physicians' Skill at End-of-Life Care: Differences between Patients with COPD, Cancer, AIDS," *Chest* 22, no. 1 (2002): 356–362.

specialities. PDIA and the Robert Wood Johnson Foundation also jointly sponsored a meeting on the topic, held 16–May 17, 1997, that attracted eighty-five
participants and from which four key recommendations emerged: (1) the Liaison
Committee on Medical Education should require that all medical students demonstrate competence in end-of-life care as a condition of medical school graduation, (2) the residency review committee in primary care specialties and in
other specialties in which there is significant contact with dying patients should
set minimum standards for faculty training in end-of-life care and for resident
experiences in caring for dying patients, (3) medical specialty boards should
integrate end-of-life care into their examinations, and (4) to meet the shortage
of faculty trained in end-of-life care, public and private funding sources should
be encouraged to (a) support programs to train faculty to teach about end-of-life
care, (b) understand physician-related barriers to the provision of excellent care,
(c) implement and evaluate new educational models for physician education, and
(d) expand the research base for palliative care.[23]

Christine Cassel at the Mount Sinai Medical Center in New York City led an
initiative, supported by PDIA, to create a Disease Related Group (DRG) for reimbursement of palliative care services delivered to hospitalized patients. This was
a crucial policy issue, for while the Medicare program had provided funding to
hospice programs since the introduction of new legislation in 1982, the emerging
field of palliative care within the hospital environment was without a reimbursement stream and heavily dependent upon fellowships and foundation funding
for the delivery of services.

In October 1996, the Health Care Financing Administration (HCFA) announced
the approval of a new diagnosis code for palliative care. The new code was to enable coders reviewing hospital charts to indicate that palliative care was delivered
to a dying patient during a hospital stay. As a result, HCFA analysts were able to
study the feasibility of creating a special DRG to allow payment for end-of-life
care for people who die in hospitals or require hospitalization for palliative care
close to the end of their lives. Cassel and Bruce Vladeck noted the following:

> It may seem ironic to many that only in 1996 are we beginning to acknowl-
> edge that some of the care delivered in hospitals is palliative, since the major-
> ity of deaths in the United States occur in the hospital and have occurred
> there for much of this century...End-of-life care should be viewed as an
> integral part of the continuum of care provided by the health-care system.
> The hospice movement was a response to the need to improve the care in
> hospitals by getting patients out of hospitals as much as possible. It is now
> necessary to focus on the patients who remain in hospitals and die there.
> HCFA's announcement of the new diagnosis code for palliative care is
> an important step, but more remains to be done...We hope that the new

---

23. See Robert Wood Johnson Foundation, "Rx: More Training Urged for Physicians Treating
Dying Patients," (July 2006), http://www.rwjf.org/reports/grr/029360s.htm (accessed July 11,
2008).

diagnosis code will legitimize and encourage the use of palliative care. As with every aspect of our complex system of health-care delivery, continuous monitoring is needed. Health care is undergoing sea changes, and there may be unexpected consequences, especially if the code is used incorrectly or not extensively enough.... When we change the financing of health care, we are aiming at a moving target. But there is no alternative.[24,25,26]

Some PDIA grants influenced policy by helping to build capacity in the field. As we saw in chapter 1, PDIA was part of a consortium, first formed in 1995, of Grantmakers Concerned with Care at the End of Life, which sought to increase support for the field and act as a resource for foundations seeking to become more involved in end-of-life issues.[27] Two separate PDIA grants awarded to the Canadian Palliative Care Association and worth a total of $200,000 supported the development of a long-term strategy for research, education, and service expansion and saw the involvement of Canadian faculty scholars Harvey Chochinov, Gerri Frager, and David Kuhl.[28] Likewise two grants totaling $310,000 made to the National Hospice and Palliative Care Organization were aimed at

---

24. C. K. Cassel and B. C. Vladeck, "ICD-9 Code for Palliative or Terminal Care," *New England Journal of Medicine* 335 (1996): 1232–1234.

25. Others, however, were less convinced that the creation of a DRG would solve the relevant problems. In response to Cassel and Vladeck, John Mahoney of the National Hospice Organization noted: "Twenty years ago, hospice care was developed outside the inpatient hospital setting not because of the lack of appropriate hospital reimbursement but because of the limits inherent in the culture of hospitals that created obstacles to providing good care at the end of life. The SUPPORT study (Study to Understand Prognoses and Preferences for Outcomes and Risks of Treatment) reinforces the view that those limits may still exist and casts doubt on the reasonableness of believing that tinkering with DRG codes will substantially alter the institutional culture that limits good care of the dying." J. J. Mahoney, "A New Diagnosis-Related Group for Palliative Care," *New England Journal of Medicine* 336 (1996):1029–1030.

26. Joanne Lynne later commented: "What Chris Cassel (and others) got Bruce Vladeck et al. to do was provide a modifier for a DRG code, which was intended to be added to the DRG to designate a palliative care patient. This is not really a diagnosis code. It was (correctly) perceived by most observers to be a dangerous modifier to use without CMS having issued any regulations or interpretations, since many people saw 'palliative care' patients as being largely inappropriate for aggressive treatment settings and generally lower cost than other patients. Thus, most coders were not instructed to use this code, and it never really had a use broadly. At least one advocate got one system to use it aggressively ... and that system was able to monitor its progress in palliative care using the modifier code. Otherwise, I don't know of any helpful use of this modifier code." (Joanne Lynne, personal communication, July 4, 2010).

27. "Meeting of Foundations Results in Commitment to Help Transform the Culture of Dying," *PDIA Newsletter*, no. 1 (March 1996), 1–2.

28. Grantee Profile: "The Canadian Hospice Palliative Care Association," *PDIA Newsletter*, no. 10 (Summer 2002), 8–9. After the grant was made to the Canadian Association, PDIA ceased to accept applications from Canada, hoping that leadership initiatives would be catalyzed locally.

developing its infrastructure and capacity to generate funding for research, communication, and information provision, as well as to encourage earlier palliative care intervention and increased access to hospice care.[29] Grants of this kind were difficult to link to specific outcomes as they often went to support a broad range of activities within particular organizations and were intended to contribute to a wider agenda of "climate" change and organizational development in end-of-life care. In the case of the Canadian Palliative Care Initiative, however, it was clear that PDIA endorsement did much to help local activists in their efforts to support palliative care research and education, as well in the creation of a Quality End-of-Life Coalition of 23 national associations.[30]

A specific area of policy attention focused on the issue of improving access to opioid medications. This issue had been of interest to the PDIA from an early stage. It was dealt with at length in the Institute of Medicine's *Approaching Death* report, and on April 8, 1996, David Joranson, an international expert on the subject, had been invited to speak to the PDIA board about it. Formerly an administrator with the Wisconsin Controlled Substances Board (CSB), Joranson had become especially interested in the problem of cancer pain relief in 1984, when a proposal to legalize diamorphine was placed before the United States Congress. Together with the chairman of the CSB at the time, June Dahl, he established the Wisconsin Cancer Pain Initiative, which became a designated WHO demonstration project. Thus began an investigation of the effects that drug regulation was having on the legitimate use of opioids for cancer pain relief among medical practitioners in Wisconsin. It was found that many feared that if they prescribed morphine, they would be liable to investigation by the CSB, and Joranson "learned firsthand that drug regulators can have a chilling effect on appropriate prescribing."[31] The team then worked closely with the state government, and medical and pharmacy boards to produce more balanced regulation under Wisconsin law, which was subsequently seen as a model for other states to follow.

In 1989 Joranson moved to the Wisconsin Pain Research Group[32] to study drug policies and promote policy evaluation. Within the United States, he and his colleagues concluded that although federal policy was "balanced," insofar as it recognized the need for opioids in the management of pain, state policies were not. Subsequently, he became increasingly interested in the Single Convention on Narcotic Drugs and the work of the International Narcotics Control Board (INCB), recognizing the potential for the INCB to empower clinicians to lobby for opioid availability in their efforts to address unrelieved cancer pain. The Pain

29. "A Selection of PDIA Grants: September 2001–June 2002," *PDIA Newsletter*, no. 10 (Summer 2002), 13.

30. Final report on PDIA Grant, "Canadian Palliative Care Initiative," May 1, 2002–April 30, 2002 (PDIA files).

31. D. E. Joranson, "Improving Availability of Opioid Pain Medications: Testing the Principle of Balance in Latin America," *Innovations in End-of-Life Care* 5, no. 1 (2003).

32. University of Wisconsin–Madison, "Pain & Policy Studies Group," D. Joranson (1996), http://www.painpolicy.wisc.edu/ (accessed October 8, 2012).

and Policy Studies Group was established by Joranson in 1996, two years into the lifetime of PDIA, and built on earlier links with Kathy Foley and colleagues at Memorial Sloan-Kettering. The group is located in the University of Wisconsin Comprehensive Cancer Center within the School of Medicine and Public Health, and its work has focused increasingly on national and international opioid policy, developing guidelines and undertaking highly focused strategic workshops to stimulate governmental policy change. It has identified significant barriers to the availability of opioid analgesics, including inadequate knowledge of pain physiology, pain management, and pharmacology; exaggerated fear of addiction; legal and regulatory restrictions; uneven health-care coverage; the high costs of some opioid medications; and a lack of research studies and related policy initiatives.

In a project co-funded with the OSI-supported Lindesmith Center,[33] PDIA aided Joranson's group with a grant of $150,000 to develop its capacity to promote policies for the increased availability of opioid analgesics and to help establish a cancer pain and palliative care initiative for Central and Eastern Europe (see later in this chapter), including a resource guide and a website. The website was launched on 8 July 1997 and was soon receiving twenty thousand hits a month.[34] PDIA then went on to award $225,000 to increase the capacity of Joranson's group in the area of evaluating public pain policy and to enable it to support others in these endeavors. Joranson's colleague, June Dahl, was also supported with a PDIA grant for institutionalizing pain management through practice change programs. This work was conducted through the American Alliance of Cancer Pain Initiatives and focused on two states, each developing work in some twenty-five health-care facilities. Joranson and his group developed a long-term and highly successful relationship with PDIA, continuing over many years and growing into some of the international initiatives later sponsored by OSI. His work, as the *PDIA Newsletter* noted, "bridges the gap between regulators who work to prevent the illegal diversion of prescription medications and clinicians who treat pain patients."[35] The recipient of many awards and prizes,[36] Joranson authored some of the world's most crucial publications[37] and reports on access to opioid medications for pain relief and is widely acknowledged in the United States and beyond as

---

33. Lindesmith Center, http://www.lindesmith.org/homepage.cfm (accessed July 14, 2008; site discontinued).

34. Final Report on PDIA Grant, "A Resource Program to Address Barriers to Availability of Opioids for Pain Relief," January 1, 1997–December 31, 1999 (PDIA files).

35. Grantee Profile: "The Pain and Policy Studies Group," *PDIA Newsletter*, no. 10 (Summer 2002), 10–11.

36. These awards and prizes include the Marie Nyswander Humanitarian Award (2002); the Vittorio Ventafridda Award of the International Association of Hospice and Palliative Care (2004); and the Legislative Policy and Advocacy Award of the American Academy of Pain Management (2005).

37. For example, D. E. Joranson et al., "Pain Management, Controlled Substances, and State Medical Board Policy: A Decade of Change," *Journal of Pain and Symptom Management* 23,

a global leader in the field. His collaboration with PDIA was undoubtedly mutually strengthening and did much to raise the level of understanding surrounding
opioid medications and their availability.[38] He was succeeded as Director of the
Pain and Policy Studies Group by PDIA Faculty Scholar, Jim Cleary.

Much of the work of Joanne Lynn can be seen in a similar light. She was among
those consulted early by Patricia Prem and a founding member of the PDIA
board, as well as the leader of the SUPPORT study itself. A self-confessed activist, she was frustrated at times by some of the board's more reflective tendencies.
When the Faculty Scholars Program and its related activities appeared to have
set the direction for PDIA, she determined to leave the board to concentrate on
more policy-related work in end-of-life care. She explains her departure thus:

> It was comfortable to leave at that point. I mean, it was pretty clear that most
> of what was going to be able to be funded from then on was the scholars, the
> various scholars programs. They were beginning to branch out to the nurses
> and social workers, and the selection of scholars…I mean so much of it is
> roulette anyway, so it was likely to be at least as good without me as with
> me. I wasn't speaking to some special insight or something, and so, it didn't
> seem like I was going to hurt the board to leave it, and to be a little more free
> to do some of the policy things that seemed important to do.[39]

Key to this was Americans for Better Care of the Dying (ABCD),[40] a grassroots
organization created by Lynn to address patients' economic and policy concerns,
supported by PDIA with a foundation grant of $400,000—one of the largest
it ever awarded. ABCD developed a series of policy initiatives, including payment for pain medications, appropriate billing codes for palliative care, and a
"Medicaring" policy for older people in need of *hi-touch* rather than *hi-tech* care.
Its work showed that Medicare was inadequately designed to meet the chronic
care needs of seriously ill and old patients for symptom control, caregiver assistance, and home care in a context where elderly people, often having outlived
their family members and spouses, have limited resources and their complex ills
commonly include cognitive failure. ABCD aimed to (1) build momentum for
reform, (2) explore new methods and systems for delivering care, and (3) shape
public policy through evidence-based understanding. There was a sense of
urgency about these goals in a demographic context where huge demands would
face the Medicare system, brought about by the aging of the baby boomer generation. ABCD also produced high-level consumer information on end-of-life

no. 2 (2002):138–147; D. E. Joranson and K. M. Ryan, "Ensuring Opioid Availability: Methods
and Resources," *Journal of Pain Symptom Management* 3, no. 5 (2007): 527–532.

38. "Regional Experts Meet in Budapest to Examine National Opioid Policies," *PDIA
Newsletter,* no. 10 (Summer 2002), 19.

39. Joanne Lynn, interview by David Clark, July 14, 2004.

40. See Americans for Better Care of the Dying, "Care Transitions Search Widget Available,"
http://www.abcd-caring.org/ (accessed August 1, 2008).

care, exemplified in the widely reviewed and cited 1999 publication *Handbook for Mortals* by Joanne Lynn and Joan Harold.[41]

As early as March 1996, issues about the development of palliative care in Eastern Europe had appeared on the PDIA board agenda. The developments that followed,[42] outlined already in chapter 1, set a direction of travel within OSI that continued long after the conclusion of PDIA itself. Here was another significant piece of work, this time on the international policy front, which grew out of PDIA and saw Mary Callaway and Kathy Foley heavily involved in issues relating to global palliative care development through what became OSI's International Palliative Care Initiative (IPCI).[43] In time, some PDIA faculty scholars, notably Frank Ferris and Eric Krakauer and grantees such as Betty Ferrell in the context of her work with the ELNEC curriculum, also gave considerable energies to this area of international work, and this continued in the years after PDIA closed. Like PDIA itself, much of the early grant making in the international context was oriented to service development, particularly in Eastern Europe where its contribution was vital in stimulating many new initiatives in the years after the collapse of communism.[44] Over time, however, its orientation was further "upstream" in the developmental process—addressing issues within the mainstream of health policy at the country level, seeking the integration of palliative care into the health-care system, and focusing on issues such as workforce training and education, opioid availability, reimbursement for services, and the documentation of standards. Though its funding base was modest, IPCI emerged as a major force in the support of international palliative care development and benefited a great deal from its origins in PDIA.[45] Indeed, it was through the activities of IPCI that PDIA and its policy-oriented work came to wider international recognition, albeit after the PDIA programs had come to an end. (see chapter nine)

UNDERSERVED COMMUNITIES

PDIA work relating to underserved communities cannot, even with the benefit of hindsight, be constructed as a coherent program of activities. At best it can be

41. J. Lynn and J. Harold, *Handbook for Mortals. Guidance for People Facing Serious Illness.* (New York and Oxford, UK: Oxford University Press, 1999).

42. See "The Open Society Institute Supports International Efforts to Improve Palliative Care: Focus on Central and Eastern Europe and South Africa," *PDIA Newsletter*, no. 11 (Fall 2003), 13–15; "The Eastern European Palliative Care Initiative," *PDIA Newsletter* no. 8 (March 2001), 19.

43. See Open Society Foundations, http://www.soros.org/initiatives/pdia/focus_areas/a_international_palliative (accessed August 1, 2008; site discontinued).

44. For a full account, see D. Clark and M. Wright, *Transitions in End of Life Care: Hospice and Related Developments in Eastern Europe and Central Asia* (Buckingham, UK: Open University Press, 2003).

45. For more details, see M. Callaway et al., "Funding for Palliative Care Programs in Developing Countries," *Journal of Pain and Symptom Management* 33, no. 5 (2007): 509–513.

viewed as a patchy and rather idiosyncratic field of endeavor populated by activists high on commitment to service delivery, but with rather less inclination for research and publication. More critically it can be seen as a rather weakly developed approach to a complex and challenging issue and a possible blind spot in the PDIA board's thinking,[46] as observed by Robert Butler in the following:

> I guess one comment I'd have is that we, despite all of our efforts—and I think they were genuine efforts—I'm not sure we've done as well with the rich diversity of America in terms of support of various minority programs. I think a lot of the people in the black community are a little uneasy about the idea of palliative care: "Does that mean get rid of you and not do everything that might in fact improve your survival?" So I don't think we've done as well as I wish we could; I'm not sure it's any of our faults. I think we made tremendous efforts, but I would have wished that [we did more] in the broader program, quite apart from the scholars, which also do not have a heavy representation of minorities—that would be my one regret. But I'm not sure what we would have done to have made it happen. Then there are certain populations that we did support that are just so horrifying and so awful, like dying in prison, and again I'm not sure I know exactly what we could do with captive populations like that, but maybe we could have done a little more.[47]

It is indeed necessary to look quite hard for grantees and initiatives that engaged with issues concerning the care of disadvantaged groups, and the work that did occur seemed often to fail to develop or to establish critical mass or lasting impact. Certainly there were few tangible outputs from this field of activity, in contrast, for example, to some of the useful material on diversity that emerged

---

46. Ana Dumois was appointed to the board to bring a perspective from community activism and on behalf of underserved communities. She observes: "Well, you see, I think that I just complemented the board because, as I said, it is a diverse board, all professionals very well accomplished in their own field, with a very common set of values, even though ... you can have a goal and different people have different ideas of the *means* to achieve that goal. So we had very heated arguments about how to go about promoting change in our society. I think that what I brought was almost like a view from the trenches. While I am also a professional like they are—I have two PhDs and [I'm] educated in Cuba at the highest level and then here—I have always been in the trenches; I have always been working in the communities, intimately with the underserved communities. So the board members who have a commitment to those communities and who have some working knowledge of those ... communities, at times did not have, had not had, the intimacy of each one of the many diverse communities I would have ... I brought a perspective ... from the other side. So quite often in the course of the discussions or in the course of analyzing a proposal, I was able to bring in a dimension of a piece of information that they did not have." Ana Dumois, interview by David Clark, July 23, 2003.

47. Robert Butler, interview by David Clark, July 23, 2003.

from the Last Acts initiative of the Robert Wood Johnson Foundation.[48] Even the monumental textbook on end-of-life care edited by Joan Berzoff and Phylilis Silverman, with its large number of contributions from PDIA-funded social workers, devotes rather few of its 896 pages to issues of social disadvantage, cultural diversity, and disadvantaged and underserved groups.[49] The following sections therefore reflect a patchwork of activity, incomplete in itself, but which reveals some tentative encounters with the end-of-life care needs of underserved populations and settings.

African Americans

African Americans have higher mortality rates from cancer, cardiovascular disease, AIDS, and other illnesses, and face a number of barriers to adequate end-of-life care. They are more likely to be undertreated for pain than whites in emergency rooms, during hospital stays, and in outpatient clinics and nursing homes. Pharmacies in nonwhite neighborhoods may not stock sufficient medications to adequately treat patients with severe pain. Moreover, there is a perceived lack of awareness in the African American community about end-of-life care, which has contributed to low rates of participation in hospice and limited use of advance care planning documents that communicate the requests of a dying person to family members and physicians.[50] The problems are captured in these remarks from PDIA faculty scholar, Lachlan Farrow:

> Well, LaVera Crawley, who's one of my cohort [and] who's African American and has done project work, she's a PDIA scholar trying to reach out to African American communities about palliative care, and in the first couple of years of trying to do that, she'd go to inner city community groups, and she said she would regularly be just *berated*. She's there as an African American physician talking to African Americans... "You have been totally co-opted by the white medical establishment—we don't have cancer screening, we don't have mammography, we've got higher rates of prostate cancer dying. You're coming in, you're now saying... 'I'm here to help you guys *die*.'" They said, "Come back when you're giving us the good things the white people

48. See, for example, *Last Acts Statement on Diversity and End-of-Life Care* (Washington, DC: Last Acts National Program Office, 2001); *Last Acts Statement Diversity and End-of- Life Care Literature Review and Annotated Bibliography.* (Washington, DC: Last Acts National Program Office, 2001.)

49. J. Berzoff and P. R. Silverman (eds.), *Living with Dying. A Handbook for End-of-Life Care Practitioners* (New York, Columbia University Press, 2004).

50. From Robert Wood Johnson Foundation, "Prevention, An Investment That Pays Off in More Ways Than One," http://www.rwjf.org/pr/product.jsp?id=21341 (accessed August 1, 2008).

are having, and then when those things fail for us after we've got them, we'll talk to you about how you can help us feel nice when we die."[51]

These themes are also echoed powerfully in the faculty scholars grant application made jointly by physicians Jean Linzau and Michelle Ervin:

> In our communities of color we have observed that years of oppression, discrimination, relegation to second class citizenship, reports of human experimentation without informed consent, lack of truth telling, and injustice have fostered an attitude among our patients of suspicion and distrust of health professionals and systems...In many situations, only evidence of necrobiosis can convince adamant family members that all has been done...Many patients have no relation with the health-care system other than occasional visits to the emergency room or the corner clinic, only to be thrown into a system that is violative, does not answer their questions in an intelligible language, and finally tells them that they have a terminal illness, that further treatment is futile, and they must go home to die.[52]

Out of the interest shown in these issues, PDIA developed the Initiative to Improve Palliative Care for African Americans (IIPCA) which took the form of an interdisciplinary working group of African American scholars, professionals, and community leaders who gathered to delineate the historical, social, cultural, ethical, economic, legal, health policy, and medical issues that appear to affect African American attitudes, acceptance, access, and utilization of palliative and hospice services. This project was championed by Dr. Richard Payne, at the time chief of the Pain and Palliative Care service at Memorial Sloan-Kettering Cancer Center, New York City. It grew out of the board's belief that there needed to be a targeted effort on care for vulnerable and marginalized populations within American society, in a context where there were questions about access to health care and the quality of care being received by minority groups. Funding began with an initial grant of just $24,204[53] to Richard Payne and Harold P. Freeman (of North General Hospital in Harlem, New York, and chair of the President's Cancer Panel), which allowed the scope of the problem to be set out and for networks to be built with such groups as the Intercultural Cancer Council, the National Medical Association, and the Congressional Black Caucus. Seventeen leading experts from across the United States were at the core of the early initiative,[54]

---

51. Lachlan Farrow, interview by David Clark, July 24, 2003.

52. Jean A. Linzau and Michelle Grant Ervin, Proposal for Project, "End of Life Care Provider Education in an Ethnically and Spiritually Diverse Community" (January 1998). See also M. G. Ervin, Editorial, "Unequal Access to Hospice and Palliative Care," *Journal of Palliative Medicine* 7, no. 2 (2004): 301–302.

53. There were also grants from the Robert Wood Johnson Foundation and the Milbank Memorial Fund.

54. Terrie Reid Payne, letter to Mary Callaway, March 9, 2000.

and a key meeting was held in February 2000 in which the participants began to identify the main barriers to palliative care for African Americans and to contrast these with other populations. Then on 14 December 2000, as the momentum around the initiative began to increase, Payne met with the PDIA board for a detailed discussion of how the initiative could be expanded from a base at North General Hospital in a predominantly black neighborhood of New York City.[55] The board was favorably disposed and IIPCA, now funded with a grant of $399,947, introduced in 2001 a program of palliative care within the hospital and a separate element of wider work within the local community. Most important, however, North General also became home to a national program office for IIPCA, tasked with stimulating broader interest and action. The office would serve as a resource center for the collection, evaluation, and dissemination of information about palliative care in the African American community and also act as a stimulus to research and a guide to policy making.[56] Its executive director became the aforementioned LaVera Crawley, a previous PDIA grantee and faculty scholar. She characterized the problems thus:

> Blacks in this country suffer disproportionately from serious, chronic, and eventually fatal diseases, often presenting late with a higher degree of symptom burden. Yet, when many minorities do seek medical care, they face race-based health disparities that further compound the problem. These disparities— ranging from fewer referrals for appropriate diagnostic and therapeutic services to inadequate treatment for pain—have been the subject of numerous studies in the last decade. The breach of trust by the health care system to meet the needs of blacks and other minorities may explain, in part, the resistance of some African-Americans toward palliative and end-of-life care.[57]

IIPCA sought to define and promote a research, education, and policy agenda for the improvement of care for African American patients facing serious illness. It had a powerful mission statement:

> We envision a society where African American patients facing serious and potentially fatal illness—along with their families, the communities in which they live, and the healthcare providers who serve them—have knowledge of and access to state-of-the-art palliative care. This vision includes elimination of racial and socioeconomic disparities that limit such knowledge and access.[58]

---

55. PDIA Board Minutes, Item 5, December 14, 2000.

56. Richard Payne, letter to Dr. Kathleen Foley, May 3, 2000.

57. LaVera Crawley quoted in "Heritage, Health, and Hope: The Initiative to Improve Palliative Care for African Americans Holds Major Summit in Harlem," *PDIA Newsletter*, no. 10 (Summer 2002), 3–4.

58. *Project on Death in America, January 2001–December 2003, Report of Activities* (New York: Open Society Institute, 2004).

A further grant of $75,000 enabled IIPCA to hold its first national forum in January 2002 in Harlem, New York, on the theme of "Heritage, Health, and Hope." The follow-up among attending organizations was good and led to workshops and focus groups in the African American community on advance care planning and hospice care, as well as outreach programs for clergy. Such work was further supported by a joint briefing meeting for the New York Regional Association of Grantmakers hosted by PDIA, the JM Foundation, and the William Randolph Hearst Foundations, and focusing on the improvement of end-of-life care for African Americans. Held in May 2002, the meeting saw Richard Payne outline the work of IIPCA, as well as the Harlem Palliative Care Network, an initiative supported by the United Hospital Fund of New York under its community program for palliative care (see chapter 4).

IIPCA was sophisticated in its analysis of the problem. Figures published by the National Hospice and Palliative Care Association in 2000 showed that only 8 percent of patients cared for in hospice programs were African Americans. IIPCA sought to unpack such data and a key article in the *Journal of the American Medical Association* by Crawley, Payne, and colleagues, published in 2000, set out a detailed exploration of the main factors.[59] This began with the historical legacy of slavery, abuses in medical experimentation, economic injustice, and racial profiling practices—all of which may have bolstered a death-denying culture among African Americans and also a potential misunderstanding of the goals of end-of-life care. Moreover, in such a context, the spiritual culture of death and dying among African Americans may also be at odds with palliative care, for example, seeing pain and suffering as things to be necessarily endured as part of a spiritual commitment, rather than a problem to "palliated." At the same time, African American patients receive less resource-intensive care than other patients at the end of life. Key to the problem, in Payne's view, was the perception of African Americans that adopting palliative care is akin to "giving up hope":

> I suspect this is so because so many African Americans fear their cultural and personal values will not be respected when they are dying. They sometimes worry that their race and socioeconomic status make them more "disposable" and that treatment decisions will reflect that attitude. They do not see palliative and hospice care as offering better care at the end of life.[60]

For Crawley, good palliative care for African Americans must be part of an equitable continuum that includes prevention practices and risk assessment, diagnosis and evidence-based curative treatment—addressing societal factors and firmly rooted in community actions and initiatives.[61] There is also a need to raise public

---

59. L. V. Crawley et al., "Palliative and End-of-Life Care in the African American Community," *Journal of the American Medical Association* 284, no. 19 (2000): 2518–2521.

60. R. Payne, "At the End of Life, Color Still Divides," *Washington Post* (15 February 2000).

61. L. V. Crawley, Editorial, "Palliative Care in African American Communities," *Innovations in End of Life Care* 3, no. 5 (2001), http://www2.edc.org/lastacts/archives/archivesSept01/editorial.asp.

awareness of end-of-life care issues among African Americans, and the initiative was successful in doing that through articles in newspapers and magazines,[62] as well as in key journal editorials.[63] IIPCA was also bolstered through the interests and efforts of other PDIA grantees and scholars (some mentioned in previous chapters and others explored in later sections of this chapter).[64] A specific example of such synergy, created at an early stage in the initiative, is the important paper by PDIA faculty scholar Sean Morrison and colleagues concerned with the failure of pharmacies in predominantly nonwhite areas of New York City to stock adequate supplies of opioid analgesics.[65] The wider impact of IIPCA is difficult to evaluate, however. After an initial burst of activity in 2000–2002, its trail seems to grow cold, though later support came from the Robert Wood Johnson Foundation, and Payne's Center at Duke University did continue with the ideas. Disappointingly, by 2006, the figure for African American patients in receipt of hospice care remained largely unchanged—at 8.8 percent.[66]

Native Americans

In 1996, there were an estimated 2.3 million Native Americans, including Alaska Natives, in the United States. The end-of-life experiences for Native Americans mirror that of the general population in that they are commonly protracted and take place away from family and community. An early PDIA grant of $150,000 was made to Bruce Williams at Ellen Stephen Hospice, Pine Ridge, South Dakota, serving a population of 23,000 Lakota Sioux with an average male life expectancy of forty-five years. Ellen Stephen House was the first tribally sanctioned hospice to serve Native Americans,[67] but it did attract some concerns about its management and governance, which were drawn to the attention of PDIA by other experts in the field and found their way into the local press. Faculty scholar Judith Kitzes also focused her work on the end-of-life care needs of Native Americans. Her work aimed to formalize collaborative efforts

---

62. C. Smith, "Dr. Richard Payne—The Defeat of Agony," *New York* (June 5, 2000), 63.

63. H. P. Freeman and R. Payne, Editorial, "Racial Injustice in Health Care," *New England Journal of Medicine* 342, no. 14 (2000): 1045–1047.

64. See, for example, "Diversity in Dying: Improving Palliative Care in Multi-Cultural Society," *PDIA Newsletter*, no. 6 (December 1999), 3–4.

65. R. S. Morrison et al., "We Don't Carry That: Failure of Pharmacies in Predominantly Nonwhite Neighborhoods to Stock Opioid Analgesics," *New England Journal of Medicine* 342, no. 14 (2000): 1023–1026.

66. National Hospice and Palliative Care Organization, http://www.nhpco.org/files/public/Statistics_Research/NHPCO_facts-and-figures_Nov2007.pdf (accessed August 4, 2008; site discontinued).

67. Ellen Stephen Hospice, *Project on Death in America, July 1994-December 1997* (New York: Open Society Institute, 1998), 29.

between the national Federal/Tribal/Urban Indian Health Care system and the University of New Mexico Health Science Center through the establishment of a Native American Collaborative Center for the Promotion of Palliative Care. The program sought to support tribal sovereignty and self-determination in palliative care services and to evaluate collaborative palliative care training in relation to the specific needs of Native American groups.[68] Judith Kitzes explains:

> I was told over and over "You can't talk about death, you can't talk about this, you can't talk about that." I have found that those assumptions that you can't talk about it are not real, because all cultures talk about death and have their own ways of talking about death—it's a matter of allowing the space for them to talk in their own vocabulary and at their time and how they wish to talk about it. So when people tell me American Indian people won't talk about death or it's a taboo, I go, "I haven't experienced that." I'm not American Indian, and I questioned whether or not I would be an appropriate spokesman in the beginning. There are 500 tribes [and] each has its own views and sense about not talking or talking about death. [I brought] an outside voice to bring up the conversation and open the conversation...and I say the death word and the dying word as we move into it—then it can create a safer environment. And hopefully another goal (and it's happening) is to create tribal and American Indian leadership so they can speak publicly. So [by] getting the money and the resources into their hands, hopefully it will give them the opportunity then to be able to put [it in] their own words. But I have not been told to go home.[69]

A later grant for this area of work was awarded to Rita Ledesma, assistant professor of social work at California State University, Los Angeles, for a project on loss and bereavement in an American Indian and Alaska Native community. The study used qualitative methods to gather data from two samples: (1) American Indians and Alaska Natives who reside in the community, and (2) health and human services providers working with this community.[70] Ledesma's work was discussed at the Healing American Indian Nations conference in Los Angeles in November 2004 and informed a developing curriculum for professionals who work with Native Americans. She makes the following observservations:

> Indian nations represent different linguistic and cultural groups, but there are similarities. They will share a belief that when people die that they are

---

68. See J. Kitzes, "Talking Circle: Palliative Care and End of Life Care for American Indian and Alaska Native Communities," *IHS Primary Care Provider* 26, no. 5 (2001), 73–74; J. Kitzes and L. Berger, "End-of-Life Issues for American Indians/Alaska Natives: Insights from One Indian Health Service Area," *Journal of Palliative Medicine* 7, no. 6 (2004): 830–838.

69. Judith Kitzes, interview by David Clark, July 24, 2003.

70. R. Ledesma, "The Urban Los Angeles American Indian Experience: Perspectives from the Field," *Journal of Ethnic & Cultural Diversity in Social Work* 16, no. 12 (2007): 27–60.

still available to you. So when you pray, you pray to the creator, and you ask for help from your relations. When you give thanks, you thank the creator and your relations. Most tribes believe that you need some time to pass, like a year. Many tribes cut their hair when they're in mourning. It's an outward sign of pain and suffering... What I'm interested in is, how do people survive and thrive? There is resilience. People do bounce back... I can't change Wounded Knee or that my mom was in boarding school or my grandma died young, and my story is typical. I'm trying to help people understand how they go on.[71]

Deprived Settings and Populations

But there *is* a balm in Gilead to make the wounded whole, there is a balm in Gilead to heal the weary soul.[72]

The Balm of Gilead palliative care initiative began at the Cooper Green Hospital in Birmingham Alabama.[73] Led by the physician (and later faculty scholar) Amos Bailey and with an initial grant from the Robert Wood Johnson Foundation, it developed a comprehensive end-of-life program for the populations served by the "safety net" public health system in Alabama's largest county. It became the first inpatient palliative care unit in the state of Alabama.

The Balm of Gilead serves terminally ill persons, predominantly of minority ethnic status, who as a group are relatively younger than the national hospice population and typically lack personal financial resources. The demonstration project addressed the holistic needs associated with terminal illness in each of its stages and each of its treatment settings for this population. It also set out to identify the needs of the bereaved in a low-income setting, to develop collaborations and/or new resources to address the identified needs, and to evaluate the effectiveness of various bereavement response strategies. Balm of Gilead professionals and volunteers provide continuity of care across a continuum that includes inpatient palliative care, home hospice services, and specialized palliative care in nursing homes and other community residential settings. Cooper Green Hospital and the Jefferson County Department of Health became principal partners in the program. Community partnerships with local foundations, colleges and universities, faith communities, civic groups, and professional groups complete the collaborative network of the Balm of Gilead Project.[74] Despite ongoing

---

71. Quoted in M. T. Jarvis, "Natives Losses," *Los Angeles Times* (Sunday, January 23, 2005).

72. African American spiritual.

73. F. A. Bailey, The Balm of Gilead Center—Cooper Green Hospital. *Pioneer Programs in Palliative Care: Nine Case Studies* (New York: Milbank Memorial Fund and Robert Wood Johnson Foundation, 2000).

74. E. A. Kvale et al., "The Balm of Gilead Project: A Demonstration Project on End-of-Life Care for Safety-Net Populations," *Journal of Palliative Medicine* 7, no. 3 (2004): 486–493.

uncertainties about its long-term viability and the extent to which it was wholly supported by its host organization, the project was heavily featured in the last broadcast of the Bill Moyers television series, *On Our Own Terms*, first aired on PBS in September 2000. In 2001, the Birmingham VA Medical Center recruited Amos Bailey as its director of palliative care, and there he went on to develop a comprehensive palliative care program, including opening the Safe Harbor Palliative Care Unit in November of 2005. On moving to the VA Medical Center, Amos Bailey took up his position as PDIA faculty scholar. He describes some of his reactions and experiences:

> After about four years [at Cooper Green], we had this project that was up and going wherein 60+ percent of people who died in the hospital were on the palliative care unit before they died; two-thirds of the people who came to the unit went home, at least for some period of time, before they came back; but the home hospice program went from ten to sixty people. Most of the people using the county's health-care system who died were using the palliative care program before they died. And the people who weren't were usually people who came and were so critically ill so quickly that they died before there was really a possibility to transfer... But if somehow somebody recognized you as being ill and dying, you got referred to the palliative care program. And almost everyone opted to use that service, and I think that the reason people were amazed about it—people from around the country came to see what we were doing—was, well, African Americans won't *use* palliative care and they won't *use* hospice, and the medical director's white, so why is it that he's white and these African Americans are trusting him, you know? And I don't really know that I know the answer to that question, but it was kind of a remarkable thing, and so a lot of people came and said, "What is happening? Why is it this working there?" And so that's when people started saying, "Well, you should apply to PDIA" and that kind of thing.[75]

He eventually became a faculty scholar in the eighth cohort (for a time he was reluctant to apply and, at first, PDIA was not inclined to take him) and developed a fellowship training program at the VA Medical Center. His commitment to underserved groups remained unaltered, but he realized that he could become more effective as an educator than as a physician alone:

> Kathy Foley said basically, "Get over this. Get this chip off your shoulder" kind of thing... "You should be a teacher. You *are* a teacher. You have a gift for that. You need to be working at the medical school and you need to be teaching other people." So I really think that she has really helped me kind of refocus my career. And she said something that I remember still. She said

---

75. F. Amos Bailey, interview by David Clark, July 24, 2003.

that: "You could go and see however many patients you can see in a day, but that's all you'll be able to do, but if you *teach* somebody to do what you do, then you'll multiply your efforts a lot." You know, it's that whole life thing: "Give somebody a fish and they eat for a day; teach them to fish and they'll eat for a lifetime." She said just...pretty much that. And I thought "You know, you're *right*. You really are very right." So I said, "Well, that means I have to join the department, I have to become a faculty member," which to me kind of sounded like joining a country club. So I said, "Well, you know, that's where you teach people, so that is what you do," so I became a faculty member. So I did, and I'm glad that she was right. She was wise about that.[76]

Gregory P. Gramelspacher received a PDIA grant to study the experiences of the dying poor served by a public hospital system in order to develop recommendations for improving end-of-life care for deprived populations. The study consisted of a series of in-depth interviews and focus groups with community members, dying patients, their families, and health-care providers. Like faculty scholar Michelle Ervin, he noted the close relationship between poor people and the emergency departments of public hospitals: "That's the front door of the health-care system...It's a chaotic, disconnected system that isn't good for any patient, and especially isn't good for people who are dying."[77]

Laurie Jean Lyckholm (a physician) and Patrick Coyne (a nurse) from the Virginia Commonwealth University School of Medicine received a joint PDIA faculty scholarship in 2001 to work on improving end-of-life care for the medically underserved. They approached this by defining barriers to access and developing a related educational curriculum. For the medically underserved, barriers to good end-of-life care are compounded by the experiences of poverty, as well as social and geographic isolation. But Lyckholm and Coyne found it was often difficult to be precise about the definition of barriers, observing that there was rarely consensus between service users and service providers about what might constitute a barrier in any given instance. They sought to promote provider and public awareness of these complexities and identify ways to address them. Coyne describes a typical patient in this context:

An older gentleman with a new diagnosis of lung cancer who lives in a rural area...probably an hour and a half away, who was diagnosed after surgery in our hospital, ends up with a tracheotomy and goes home. He's been working in the farms for the last forty years, never put any money into the insurance system. It really isn't unknown. And here he is with this new tracheotomy, unable to talk, living in a farmhouse...he may have electricity, but now that he's not working any more, it's probably going to be shut off. He has well

76. F. Amos Bailey, interview by David Clark, July 24, 2003.

77. "Diversity in Dying: Improving Palliative Care in a Multicultural Society," *PDIA Newsletter*, no. 6 (December 1999), 5.

water and he may or may not have transportation, and he clearly usually never has a phone. And so he's pretty much out there on his own, living with this diagnosis, with no insurance coverage, no way to get back and forth to his appointments, and basically no one who's going to come out and see him because they're not going to get paid. And so what would happen pretty quickly with us is our social workers would meet him and work to get him at least enrolled in some kind of insurance program; get him a code within the hospital, which means that all of his visits will be covered, so that the State will at least recognize that he has no other means of paying for things and that they need to cover his care; call the American Cancer Society, start arranging someone in his neighborhood that may be able to help; pharmacy will work to put him in a system with all the drug companies so that he can be able to get free medication or at least discounted medications; and see if the home-help companies will look after him in terms of knowing that insurance is pending and that they can get paid down the road—they're not going to get paid for the next three or four months, but when the insurance becomes active they can go back and collect, knowing that it's retroactive. And that's a gamble they take because, if the social worker did it wrong or if he didn't give all the correct information, or if he owns, you know, five hundred acres somewhere that could be sold to pay for this care, the insurance will fall through, and he'll be alone. So it's a gamble that many home-help companies will accept; some will not.

DAVID CLARK: The complexities are not so much in what we might narrowly call the clinical care—they're in the management of the overall care package?

PATRICK COYNE: Absolutely. But part of the care package you have to take into account is the treatments you may be offering, like if it's radiation, that means he has to come back from two hours away for thirty treatments of radiation. That's not realistic. He's just not going to finish it. If you're talking about a pain medication that's going to cost $600 a month, nobody's going to pay for it. So I think the providers take into mind all of those issues as they're working out a plan so that it's a plan that will work.[78]

Toward the end of the PDIA lifespan, a grant was awarded to Radio Bilingue, a nonprofit network of five public radio stations in Fresno, California, and the only Spanish-language programming distributor in public radio. The grant enabled Radio Bilingue to produce a Spanish-language national radio campaign to raise awareness among Latinos about care options in the face of terminal illness. The result was *Ultimos cuidados, Cuidados para los Desahuciados y sus*

---

78. Patrick Coyne, interview by David Clark, July 24, 2003.

Familias (Final Care, care for the dying and their families).[79] Twelve broadcasts were made over the period October 2002–September 2003, and they covered topics such as access to hospice care, pain management, the dying process, and advance directives, as well as the Day of the Dead, whether to fight or accept death, and "music and death." These were further supported by a roundtable discussion and a series of thirty- to sixty-second educational messages, as well as four short radio dramas and a musical ballad. In addition Radio Bilingue brought together an advisory group of community activists and hospice personnel who worked together on a range of initiatives to stimulate "Latino Hospice Outreach," not just in California, but nationwide. The radio broadcasts were made available to others and became much in demand from hospice professionals.[80]

Another outreach program to promote end-of-life care access and awareness to members of the Latino community, mentioned briefly in the previous chapter, was the work of PDIA social worker Shirley Otis Green in a project entitled *Proyecto de Transiciones:* Enhancing End of Life and Bereavement Support Services for Latinos within a Cancer Center Setting. The project addressed the lack of integrated, Spanish-speaking end-of-life and bereavement support services in Los Angeles County, despite the high percentage of Latinos who reside there. It developed a community partnership model appropriate for use in cancer centers nationwide, and findings from focus groups made up of the dying, family caregivers, and the bereaved were used to develop and refine the structure of a bereavement support group (*Reflexiones*) and a general cancer group (*Compartiendo Esperanza*). The applicability of a community partnership model to other cancer centers was also demonstrated.[81] Jane Linberg, another PDIA social work leader, developed a program to provide bereavement services and support for the rural poor, especially migrant Hispanic families, living in three rural central California counties (Fresno, Madera, and Merced).

In rural New Mexico, faculty scholar Walter Forman developed a project with four hospices serving a mixed population of Hispanic people and American Indians to establish a permanent regional education, training, consulting, and research service in palliative care. He found a range of problems and support needs:

> The programs were all in existence less than four years with an average daily census between 5–8, and they all had a small staff. Each had a need for education of both the medical as well as the lay community, integrating hospice with their home-care service. There were unique problems with

79. "A Selection of PDIA Grants: September 2001–June 2002," *PDIA Newsletter*, no. 10 (Summer 2002), 13.

80. Final Report from Project, "Radio Bilingue, Ultimos Cuidados"; Grant #20006425.

81. S. Otis-Green et al., "An Integrated Psychosocial-Spiritual Model for Cancer Pain Management," *Cancer Practice Supplement* 10, no. 1 (2002): S58–S65.

regard to drug acquisition, referrals, trained staff, and access to patients. They had their own learning issues (none had texts, journals, etc.); each had to acquaint the public with the role of the hospice program; and each wished to establish a network where their own issues could be addressed.[82]

Groups with Complex Needs

People with disabilities and chronic illnesses, and their families, may need support to help them navigate through a web of health-care choices and constraints occurring at the end of life. Social worker Gary Stein focused on this area of work in a project that sought to train members of the New Jersey Health Decisions' regional Disability Ethics Network to conduct community-based consultation for individuals with disabilities and chronic illnesses, with a focus on dispute resolution and mediation.[83] Another grant went to Volunteers of America for a piece of work entitled Last Passages: Transforming the Experience of Death for Individuals with Developmental Disabilities and their Families. Building on a successful New York model it sought to establish a demonstration project in Oklahoma and disseminated results through a national conference.[84]

Prisons and Jails

The United States incarcerates a lot of people: 1.83 million men and women in 1998 within 1515 prisons. In the decade after 1987, the number of people dying in prisons doubled to reach over thirty-two hundred deaths per year. At the same time there were only twenty-six prison hospice programs in the United States with the expertise to handle prisoners with HIV/AIDS, tuberculosis, and other chronic diseases. In many instances prison facilities lacked adequate health-care programs and dying inmates were suffering from a lack of appropriate pain management and psychological support. In 1994, the nation's prisons held more than fifty-five thousand inmates age fifty or more. By 2005, 16 percent of the prison population was expected to be age fifty years or more, compared to 11 percent in 1988. Moreover, longer sentences and fewer paroled inmates meant an increasing number of inmates were growing older behind bars. In addition to

---

82. Final Report for Grant, "Palliative Care in Multi-Cultural Settings," August 1, 1995–December 31, 1998.

83. "A Selection of PDIA Grants: September 2001–June 2002," *PDIA Newsletter*, no. 10 (Summer 2002), 13; See G. L. Stein and L. Esralew, "Palliative Care for People with Disabilities." In J. Berzoff and P. R. Silverman (eds.), *Living with Dying. A Handbook for End-of-Life Care Practitioners* (New York, Columbia University Press, 2004), 499–507.

84. "A Selection of PDIA Grants: September 2001–June 2002," *PDIA Newsletter*, no. 10 (Summer 2002), 13.

issues of aging, in the mid-1990s, deaths from HIV in prisons and jails were six times higher than in the general population.[85]

Responding to these issues, the PDIA, together with the OSI Center on Crime, Communities, and Culture, co-sponsored America's first national conference in 1998 at the New York Academy of Medicine on the theme, Death and Dying in Prisons and Jails: Caring for Prisoners, Families, and Caregivers. The conference included a photographic exhibition[86] on the care of dying prisoners at Angola state penitentiary, in Louisiana, where a hospice program using inmate volunteers had recently been established and a visit had been made by Mary Callaway and OSI colleagues in the summer of 1998.[87] The conference explored the needs of inmates facing death in prisons and jails and presented sessions on the epidemiology and ethnography of death in custody. The event highlighted the inadequate state of medical care for those dying in prison in the United States. Inmates needs are generally not taken seriously, conditions are frequently misdiagnosed or ignored, with treatment often slow to come or inadequate once delivered. Inmates lack any choice regarding treatment options and have little say in advance care planning, and dying inmates are often extremely isolated. Family visits are, in turn, limited by the fact that prisons are most often located in remote, rural communities, to which many family members lack the resources to travel. When prisoners die, it is not only they and their families who suffer. Correctional staff and other inmates are not exempt from the grieving process. The conference brought together a highly experienced set of delegates, served by an excellent briefing pack, and thirty-five expert speakers provided the most comprehensive overview of death and dying in prisons and jails that had ever been pulled together at that time in the United States. It was a good example of PDIA working closely with other OSI experts in a cognate field—in this case the Center on Crime, Communities, and Culture. Some of the presentations from the conference were subsequently published in the *Journal of Law, Medicine and Ethics*.[88]

Parallel to the conference, PDIA awarded a small number of grants to prison projects. Three awards were made to the National Prison Hospice Association (NHPA), which was founded in 1991 by Fleet Maull, a hospice volunteer, writer, and inmate at the US Medical Center for Federal Prisoners in Springfield, Missouri. Maull also helped to establish the first prison hospice program at the

---

85. Briefing pack: *First National Conference on Dying in Prisons and Jails* (New York, 1998).

86. The work of PDIA grantees Bastienne Schmidt and Philippe Cheng (see chapter 2).

87. W. Rideau, "Dying in prison," *PDIA Newsletter*, no. 4 (February 1999), 8–9.

88. *Journal of Law, Medicine, and Ethics*, 26, no. 2 (1998). In the Summer of 2002, a whole issue of the *Journal of Correctional Health* 9, no. 2 was devoted to end-of-life care, with the opening paper by PDIA grantee, Ira Byock. In 2000, the Robert Wood Johnson Foundation through its *Promoting Excellence in End of Life Care* initiative published a set of standards of practice for end-of-life care in correctional settings through the GRACE Project (Guiding Responsive Action for Corrections in End of Life).

Springfield facility in 1998.[89] The first of the grants to NHPA (for $10,000) was made in 1995, early in the life of PDIA. Its goals were (1) to create a national network of information on corrections facilities providing hospice care, and a network of local hospices able to undertake the care of prisoners given compassionate release; (2) to provide education in hospice care for the staff of correctional facilities, as well as for hospice staff on issues concerning end-of-life care in prisons; and (3) to develop a handbook of guidelines for end-of-life care standards in correctional facilities. The grant seemed to catalyze a wide range of networking, lobbying, and consciousness-raising and, in particular, it highlighted areas of resistance, as well as opportunities for development:

> Upon entering the correctional facilities that we have visited, we discovered that most medical professionals do not feel prepared to deal with inmates dying in their medical units. The medical staffs need education and training about death, dying, hospice, and other palliative care programs.[90]

This small award appeared to leverage a great deal of activity and led, in turn, to a second and larger PDIA grant (of $75,000) for the calendar year 1997 and then to a third award (of $46,228) for operating support of the NHPA during 1998–99. The final report noted that, in many ways, the Robert Wood Johnson Foundation–funded GRACE project had begun to take over the aims of the NHPA, with more resources to fulfil them.[91] In this context, NHPA began to move in the direction of a volunteer organization, also contributing substantially to newsletters and other gray literature, as well as to some publications in specialist journals.[92] There was a sense by October 1999 that end-of-life care in prisons had gained a measure of recognition that had been absent five years earlier, and PDIA had undoubtedly played a part in achieving this.

Working with the NHPA, hospice veteran and pioneer Florence S. Wald also received a grant of $18,000 from PDIA, co-funded with the Center on Crime, Communities, and Culture, for a study to assess the need for adapting hospice care services for terminally ill patients under prison custody in the Connecticut State Department of Correction.[93] In 1997 and 1998, six prison infirmaries serving the state's twenty-three correctional facilities took part in an evaluation of

---

89. "National Prison Hospice Association Reaches Out to Hospices," *Colorado Hospice Organization Newsletter* (April 1995), 4–5.

90. Final Report to PDIA, "National Prison Hospice Association," July 1, 1995–June 30, 1996.

91. Year-End Report to PDIA, "Operating Support for National Prison Hospice Association," July 1, 1998–June 30. 1999.

92. For specialist publications, see F. W. Maull, "Issues in Prison Hospice: Towards a Model for the Delivery of Care in a Correctional Setting," *The Hospice Journal* 13, no. 4 (1998): 57–81.

93. M. J. Friedrich, "Hospice Care in the United States: A Conversation with Florence S. Wald," *Journal of the American Medical Association* 281 (1999): 1683–1685.

their health management practices, support services, and ancillary programs, providing terminal care for dying inmates. Correctional staff members and inmates were interviewed to assess their understanding of end-of-life care, and the need for hospice in Connecticut state prisons and community resources were identified for future partnerships in developing such services.[94]

Some years later, PDIA social worker Sheila Enders developed a handbook for advance care planning to assist persons with low literacy, mild learning disabilities, and mild cognitive defects. She used prisons and jails as a microcosm of this population and as a setting to focus her attention. The issue of end-of-life care in prisons and jails became central to her PDIA-funded work[95] and led to collaboration with another PDIA social work leader, John Linder. In the introduction to a series of four in-depth articles on prison hospice programs in the United States, they noted the following:

Aging inmates experience health concerns typical of the general, free, aging population. Inmates have higher incidence of health complications associated with various circumstances, risk behaviors, and associated medical conditions. These circumstances include prison violence, incarceration-related constraints on exercise, and diet. Inmates are more likely to have a history of alcohol abuse, substance abuse or addiction, and sex industry work. Risk-behavior conditions include human immunodeficiency virus/acquired immune deficiency syndrome (HIV/AIDS), hepatitis B and C, liver disease, tuberculosis, endocarditis, and cardiomyopathy. Hospice is increasingly the preferred response to the health and care needs of terminally ill inmates. Implementing hospice behind bars has some unique challenges in addition to those inherent in hospice work.[96]

Enders's own work, at the Central California Women's Facility near Sacramento, California, addressed the special problems of female inmates:

I did a series of sixteen focus groups and I had asked the inmates to come and talk to me about issues of medical care and health care and wanting to know what it's like for them to make medical care decisions in their circumstances. I thought I would have maybe 30 or 40 people sign up and I had 167. So rather than just stay with about six or eight focus groups, I thought I'll just continue to do this until I run out of inmates, because the information

94. N. Zimmermann, F. S. Wald, and A. S. Thompson, "The Needs and Resources for Hospice Care in the Connecticut Prison System: A Feasibility Study," *Illness, Crisis, and Loss* 10, no. 3 (2002): 204–232.

95. S. R. Enders, "End-of-Life Care in the Prison System." In J. Berzoff and P. R. Silverman (eds.), *Living with Dying: A Handbook for End-of-Life Care Practitioners* (New York: Columbia University Press, 2004), 609–627.

96. J. F. Linder et al., "Hospice Care for the Incarcerated in the United States: An Introduction," *Journal of Palliative Medicine* 5, no. 4 (2002): 549–552.

is so rich. The quotations that I have from some of them are just amazing and how they have dealt with the situation of not the best of health care in the system and making their medical care decisions based on whatever information they have. I wanted to provide them with a tool that they could use to maybe help their communication level with their providers. Many of them end up with situations where they're adversarial with their physician rather than working together and there are language problems—there are certainly literacy problems—and this would be a tool they could use to better the communication process. I can't change the system of health care that they have, but I was hoping to give them a tool to use within the system to better communicate.[97]

The study highlighted issues of decision making about medical treatment, advance care planning, and end-of-life care, and how these choices are often limited or influenced by a patient's capacity to read or comprehend crucial information. Ineffective communication between patient and physician, and the complex nature of serious illness and dying, also affect these decisions. It showed how America's incarcerated have virtually no autonomy in decision making, especially with regard to medical care and treatment. For the nearly one hundred thousand incarcerated women in the United States, medical issues differ significantly from those of male prisoners. Many women enter prison with chronic illnesses or are diagnosed with such illnesses while in prison. In addition, America's prison population reflects wider literacy problems with almost two-thirds of aging inmates lacking basic literacy skills. Maintaining a balance between the Eighth Amendment rights of prisoners and their status as wards of the state is a concern for inmates and for those responsible for their care. The purpose of the study was to identify informational barriers to making medical care and treatment decisions, particularly for those with low literacy, and the findings were used in the development of a handbook to assist patients to initiate discussion and become active participants in their own care.[98] Published ten years after the original small grant to the NPHA and continuing to push forward the improvement of incarcerated individuals at the end of life, the work of Enders and colleagues demonstrated PDIA interest in these issues over the full lifetime of its grant making.

There is a sense in which the entire population of people in need of end-of-life care can be characterized as "underserved," and in the America of the mid-1990s there was a huge need for policy interventions to address its problems and ways of overcoming them. This chapter has shown the approach, at times halting, made by PDIA in addressing these issues. Through the efforts of some of its senior

---

97. Sheila Enders, interview by David Clark, July 12, 2003.

98. S. R. Enders, D. A. Paterniti, and F. J. Meyers, "An approach to develop Effective Health Care Decision Making for Women in Prison," *Journal of Palliative Medicine* 8, no. 2 (2005): 432–439.

figures, not least the board members, PDIA did engage with policy making on end-of-life care at the very highest level, and the major reports described here from the Institute of Medicine can be regarded as landmark documents of huge importance in defining the field and mapping its parameters. They took forward the national end-of-life care agenda in the most significant way since the early 1980s and the time of the National Hospice Study and the provision of Medicare for hospice services. The four key documents, especially *Approaching Death*, established an architecture of policy thinking that allowed end-of-life issues to get a hearing, to be listened to, and gradually to be acted upon. With this bridge-head captured, there was a need to think tactically about how next to proceed. The following two chapters illustrate some of the priorities that were identified. But from the material described here, it is hard to see marginalized and underserved populations as a high priority for PDIA. Certainly some of its grantees and scholars labored mightily to engage with better end-of-life care for impoverished and minority communities and, as we have seen in this chapter, some of their efforts produced inspiring work. Richard Payne went on to become the Esther Colliflower Professor and director of the Duke Institute on Care at the End of Life at the Duke Divinity School at Duke University, seeking to improve care at the end of life through interdisciplinary scholarship, teaching, and outreach. But in other instances it is difficult to identify a lasting legacy. Perhaps PDIA was just too thinly spread at times to allow a concerted initiative focused on inequality and social disadvantage. Maybe these social worlds were just too far removed from those of most board members. Or could it be that such work proved too demanding, complex, and challenging to result in obvious gains in so short a period of time and with relatively modest resources?[99] PDIA could not do everything that was needed; and the United States was fortunate over this period to have other grant makers with interests in these areas, notably the Robert Wood Johnson Foundation, with whom many PDIA grantees also engaged in their endeavors. In combination, the activists of the period set out an understanding of the major barriers to high quality end-of-life care for all in need, and that at least is an achievement of note.

---

99. Kathy Foley did not agree with this assessment, pointing to the subsequent increase in access to hospice care by African Americans, outreach through the black churches, and the continued use of the APPEAL curriculum, developed at Duke with a focus on the principles of culturally sensitive end-of-life care for African Americans, making it the only palliative care curriculum of its kind. She saw these and other initiatives as "laying the groundwork and developing the experts and giving them a voice." Kathy Foley, personal communication, April 18, 2010.

6

Ethical, Legal, and
Financial issues

This chapter deals with some of the most complex issues that PDIA had to face. As with matters of policy and social disadvantage, the board was only partially equipped to deal with them. In Bo Burt, the PDIA had a distinguished presence from academic law and one with a long-standing interest in bioethics; he became a key resource on medico-legal issues. Joanne Lynn had a master's degree in philosophy, had served as a staff member on the President's Commission on Ethical Problems in Medicine and Biomedical and Behavioral Research, was a fellow and vice president of the Hastings Center, and had authored half a dozen amicus briefs for court cases. Beyond these two board members, however, there was no specialized expertise in ethical, legal, or financial matters, and this may be evident in the manner in which PDIA attended to these areas. Nevertheless, PDIA did develop a varied portfolio of work in ethico-legal and financial issues (some of it not well recognized) and this is described in detail in this chapter.

In the late 1990s, only 18 percent of Americans received comprehensive end-of-life care, and PDIA took the view that one approach to this problem should be to address the legal and economic barriers to institutionalizing palliative and hospice care.[1] PDIA was also in operation at a crucial time in the history of legal and ethical debate on death in America—the years of legislative change in Oregon, of Jack Kevorkian, and later of Terri Schiavo. Against this background, many grantees and scholars developed work that touched on or made central to its concerns the ways in which end-of-life issues in America related to ethics, the law, and perhaps ultimately, to money.

---

1. K. Foley, "Transforming the Culture of Dying," *Project on Death in America, January 1998–December 2000, Report of Activities* (New York: Open Society Institute, 2001), 10–11.

THE QUESTION OF ASSISTED SUICIDE

In the closing moments of his speech at the College of Physicians and Surgeons of Columbia University in November 1994 (see chapter 1), George Soros had touched on the "hotly debated subject" of physician-assisted suicide. He emphasized his belief in personal autonomy and in self-determination at the end of life, but he also acknowledged the unintended consequences and abuses that could result from the legalization of physician-assisted death, noting that the issues had to be carefully weighed. He had offered help to his own mother (a member of the Hemlock Society) to end her life, but he had been glad when she refused it. He stated: "The Project on Death in America concerns itself with the vast majority of people who are not looking for physician-assisted suicide, and there is much work to be done."[2] The personal views of George Soros on this issue are difficult to determine, though they have been the object of much mass media assertion. Along the way, the aims and activities of the PDIA have been wildly misrepresented, especially in Internet-based discussions where PDIA continues to be seen as an active proponent of euthanasia and assisted suicide.[3] At least one

---

2. G. Soros, "Reflections on Death in America," *Project on Death in America, July 1994– December 1997* (New York: Open Society Institute, 1998), 6.

3. See, for example, the response by Jamison Foser to Richard Poe's *NewsMax* cover story titled "George Soros Coup" [Poe, *NewsMax* magazine (May 2004), 25]. Foser's rebuttal appeared in *Media Matters for America*—a "web-based, not-for-profit, 501(c)(3) progressive research and information center dedicated to comprehensively monitoring, analyzing, and correcting conservative misinformation in the US media," http://mediamatters.org/research/2004/06/01/oreilly-factor-guest-richard-poe-smeared-george/131201 (accessed August 18, 2008). For example, Poe wrote, "Soros founded the Project on Death in America. Its goal was to encourage people to overcome their fear of death and to embrace the inevitable. Project on Death promoted suicide and euthanasia." Foser responded: "The Project on Death in America (PDIA) does nothing of the kind. To cite just one example of how PDIA and its leadership have opposed euthanasia: PDIA program director Dr. Kathleen Foley (a world-renowned cancer specialist at Memorial Sloan-Kettering Cancer Center) edited a book titled *The Case Against Assisted Suicide: For the Right to End-of-Life Care*." In another example, Poe wrote, "In a Nov. 30, 1994 speech justifying Project on Death, Soros asked, 'Can we afford to care for the dying properly? … [But] [a]ggressive, life-prolonging interventions, which may at times go against the patient's wishes, are much more expensive than proper care for the dying.' And what did Soros mean by proper care for the dying? He wasted no time in addressing that point. 'This brings me to that hotly debated subject, physician-assisted suicide and euthanasia,' he continued in the next sentence." Foser responded: "Why didn't Poe tell us what Soros actually said about 'that hotly debated subject'? Because, while Soros indicated that he personally thinks physician-assisted suicide should be legal, he explicitly said PDIA does not take that position. By truncating Soros's remarks, Poe created the misleading impression that Soros 'justified' PDIA by speaking in favor of euthanasia—despite that Soros clearly said that PDIA has nothing to do with euthanasia." (See link for full text of Soros's remarks and other examples of distortion.)Likewise see the League Against Intoxicants, "George Soros' Agenda for Drug Legalization, Death, and Welfare," www.fmr.no/george-soros-agenda-for-drug-legalization-death-and-welfare.78404–10285.html (accessed August 18, 2008). And in 1997, the *New York Times* also claimed that Soros had given "millions of dollars" to support

commentator has also criticized the present author and this work (albeit several years before it had been published) of the same intention.[4] What is known is that, in addition to the $45 million given to PDIA by George Soros through OSI, he also used his President's Fund at the Foundation to make a series of smaller grants in the late 1990s and early 2000s to organizations promoting assisted suicide.[5] For Soros, there would be no necessary tension between supporting a major initiative to improve the broad and complex spread of end-of-life care in America, while at the same time giving resources to single-issue groups supporting changes in the law on assisted suicide or euthanasia. Indeed such a pluralistic approach might be seen as one of the hallmarks of an "open society."

In 1994, the year PDIA was founded, the state of Oregon Death with Dignity Act (Measure 16) was approved by voters to allow terminally ill Oregonians to end their lives through the voluntary self-administration of medications, expressly prescribed by a physician for that purpose.[6, 7] The immediate aftermath was filled with a high level of public and political debate. An injunction was placed by a federal court judge, following which the new legislation eventually went to the 9th Circuit Court, where it stayed for some time. Meanwhile, the Oregon legislature sent the issue back to the voters who in the Fall of 1997 supported it for a second time, after which on 27 October 1997 the 9th Circuit Court decision also came out in support of the law being enacted.

Controversies about these issues received widespread public attention at various points through the lifetime of PDIA. Interest was particularly intense in the mid-1990s as a result of two lawsuits challenging the constitutionality of both New York and Washington laws prohibiting physician-assisted suicide. During

---

the cause of assisted suicide—another misreading of the paper trail from the 1994 speech. T. Egan, "Assisted Suicide Comes Full Circle, to Oregon," *New York Times* (October 26, 1996), http://query.nytimes.com/gst/fullpage.html?res=9F00E3DE1631F935A15753C1A961958260 (accessed August 18, 2008).

4. See Karen Ward's piece for *North Country Gazette* (March 29, 2006), entitled "The Mergers, the Money, the Minds Behind Assisted Suicide," http://www.northcountrygazette.org/articles/032906AssistedSuicide.html (accessed August 18, 2008) in which she states, "David Clark, a medical sociologist, traces PDIA's history and examines how PDIA and other private donors influenced the development of palliative and hospice care in the United States, although his depiction is obviously slanted and serves one purpose: legalization of assisted suicide and euthanasia."

5. These are reported to include grants in 1998 ($150,000) and 1999 ($125,000) to the Compassion in Dying Federation, and grants in 2000 to the Death with Dignity National Center ($100,00) and to the Oregon Death with Dignity Legal Defense and Education Center ($75,000). See: N. Hrab, "George Soros' Social Agenda for America: Drug Legalization, Euthanasia, Immigrant Entitlements, and Feminism," *Foundation Watch* (April, 2003), http://www.capitalresearch.org/pubs/pdf/x3770435801.pdf (accessed October 25, 2008).

6. Oregon.gov, "Death with Dignity Act," http://www.oregon.gov/DHS/ph/pas/ (accessed August 18, 2008).

7. Earlier, in 1990 and 1992, popular referenda in California and Washington states had seen the defeat of proposals to legalize physician-assisted suicide.

early 1997, the US Supreme Court heard arguments on the cases (*Vacco v. Quill*, No. 95–1858 and *State of Washington v. Glucksberg*, No. 96–110). On June 30 1997, the Supreme Court ruled that there is no general constitutional right to physician-assisted suicide. Some of the justices however wrote statements that suggested that a narrowly defined right might be upheld in specific circumstances.

The Institute of Medicine report of 1997, *Approaching Death*,[8] contained a section on assisted suicide, but the committee had agreed that it would not take a position on its legality or morality. However, several individuals and organizations involved in producing the report, PDIA included, did file "friend of the court" or amicus briefs with the Supreme Court in its 1996–1997 session, setting out the implications that might flow from any ruling, for or against, that it might make.[9] The PDIA amicus brief was prepared by board member and academic lawyer Bo Burt. It argued that the court should not find a constitutional right to assisted suicide, until American society, and the two states in particular, had taken measures to assure that terminally ill persons who consider such a course of action are not motivated to do so by the failure of their doctors to treat pain or depression, or by economic fears.[10] PDIA welcomed the decision of the court and also its recognition, in essence, of a right to palliative care.[11] Bo Burt, writing in the *New England Journal of Medicine*, is unequivocal in his interpretation of the Supreme Court ruling; here was a mandate not for physician-assisted suicide, but for palliative care:

> A Supreme Court majority has thus provided an unexpected but strong and very welcome directive requiring states to remove the barriers that their laws and policies impose on the availability of palliative care.[12]

Within PDIA, it is hard to find evidence of a pro-euthanasia or pro-physician-assisted-suicide orientation. According to Bob Butler, George Soros made

8. Institute of Medicine, *Approaching Death: Improving Care at the End of Life* (Washington, DC: Institute of Medicine, 1997).

9. Several of these briefs were made available on the PDIA website, www.soros.org/death/brieftxt.html.

10. *Project on Death in America, July 1994–December 1997* (New York: Open Society Institute, 1998), 73.

11. K. Foley, "Improving the Care of the Dying: Law and Policy," *Project on Death in America, July 1994–December 1997* (New York: Open Society Institute, 1998), 9.

12. R. A. Burt, "The Supreme Court Speaks—Not Assisted Suicide but a Constitutional Right to Palliative Care," *New England Journal of Medicine*, 337 (1997), 1234–1236.

no attempt to force his views about assisted suicide on the PDIA board: "It became clear sometime later as the potentially inflammatory subject of…physician-assisted suicide arose, that George was much more in favor of physician-assisted suicide, but our board wasn't; but that did not result, let's say, in his coming to us and saying 'I want you do this' or 'I want to argue you out of this.'"[13,14] Certainly there were a lot of frank discussions within the board on this issue. Susan Block was thought to have a more open approach to the question. In an editorial in 2002, she and PDIA faculty scholar Linda Ganzini observed:

"Physician-assisted death may be an acceptable option of last resort for a very small number of terminally ill patients. At this point, we do not know what rates of physician-assisted death are appropriate. High rates would suggest that the procedure is not just being used as a humane approach to eliminating intractable suffering at the request of the patient. Rather, high rates could reflect deficiencies in the competence of health-care practitioners, lack of access to suitable services, devaluation of the dying, or even pressures from others to end life prematurely. Judging from our clinical and research experience with patients with ALS and cancer, the rates of physician-assisted death that Veldink et al. report—10 percent among patients with cancer and 20 percent among patients with ALS—are unacceptably high. If society values the dying and can ensure respectful medical care for all terminally ill patients, then legalized physician-assisted death should be relevant in only a small number of cases. But this means that substantial resources and cultural change are necessary. We need the resources to improve the education of health-care professionals, a commitment to ongoing societal dialogue about the care of the dying, and a guarantee of universal access to good care for all terminally ill persons, with monitoring of quality to ensure that such care is provided. The challenge for states and countries considering laws permitting physician-assisted death will be to tie legalization to such a pledge."[15]

13. Robert Butler, interview by David Clark, July 23, 2003.

14. Kathy Foley took the slightly different view and did not think that Soros "ever said he was for or against, but he was on the fence. He, like others, was ambivalent, but the board at the very beginning made a decision that we would not fund work on this topic as a rule and we did not." Kathy Foley, personal communication, August 11, 2012.

15. L. Ganzini and S. Block "Physician Assisted Death: A Last Resort?" *New England Journal of Medicine* 346 (2002):1663–1665.

Robert Butler was concerned about the consequences for older people and the potential for coercion. He had public debates with the ethicist Daniel Callahan, who had taken the view that, beyond a certain age, Medicare monies should not be spent on older people. Kathy Foley was strongly opposed to physician-assisted suicide and went on to edit a book on the subject. Certainly the issue was prominent on the PDIA agenda in the early days.

In November 1995, PDIA invited over twenty foundations and other organizations concerned with end-of-life issues to a meeting at OSI headquarters, co-hosted with the Nathan Cummings Foundation and the Commonwealth Fund. Among the speakers was Herbert Hendin, executive director of the American Suicide Foundation, which at that time had already identified its concern with hasty efforts to legalize euthanasia. Hendin reported on his investigations into the Dutch system where, in his view, legally sanctioned euthanasia had become a "routine way of dealing with terminal illness."[16] Following the publication of Hendin's research, Kathy Foley then teamed with him to edit a volume on *The Case Against Assisted Suicide*.[17] In the book they sought to explain why such principles as patient autonomy, compassion, and rationality—often invoked by those in favor of legalizing assisted suicide and euthanasia—fail to address the actual situations of terminally ill persons. It was an impressive volume. The editors drew on some substantial names, including Daniel Callahan, co-founder of the Hastings Center; David Kissane, writing on the Australian experience; and Cicely Saunders herself, founder of the modern hospice movement. From the PDIA stable there were contributions from Joanne Lynn and Harvey Chochinov. The book formed a crushing attack on the medicalization of death. In the conclusion, Foley and Hendin observe as follows:

> By deciding when patients die, by making death a medical decision, the physician preserves the illusion of mastery of the disease and over the feelings of helplessness that lack of control induces. The physician, not the illness, is responsible for death. Assisting suicide and performing euthanasia become ways of dealing with the frustration of being unable to cure the disease.[18]

While the work was unfunded and conducted separately from PDIA, the book did articulate a viewpoint that was also emerging in PDIA—that the care of the

---

16. "Meeting of Foundations Results in Commitment to Help Transform the Culture of Dying," *PDIA Newsletter*, no. 1 (March 1996), 1–6.

17. K. Foley and H. Hendin (eds.), *The Case Against Assisted Suicide: For the* Right *to End of Life Care* (Baltimore: Johns Hopkins University Press, 2002).

18. K. Foley and H. Hendin, "Conclusion: Changing the Culture." In K. Foley and H. Hendin (eds.), *The Case Against Assisted Suicide: For the Right to End of Life Care* (Baltimore: Johns Hopkins University Press, 2002), 316.

seriously ill and dying should be regarded as a *public health* issue and reframed within a policy context. Only by such means, the editors assert, would there be "real choices for real care at the end of life."[19]

Perhaps the most concentrated effort within PDIA to study the issue of physician-assisted suicide came in the work of faculty scholar Linda Ganzini, who gained entry to cohort four in 1998–1999. Recognizing that the nation's first state to legalize assisted suicide would be closely watched by other states, she set out to examine its practical aspects, including requests for prescriptions, the characteristics of patients making these requests, processes for assessing patients, and the impact of the experience on the physician, family, and other health-care workers.[20] She takes us back to the time when the public discussion was raging in Oregon:

> As the debate was accelerating, it was clear there were a bunch of arguments for and against that were based on moral issues. But there were also arguments for and against that were based on clinical and psychological issues where there wasn't any data. And I had the somewhat naive idea that, if I could get good data, I could settle these arguments.[21]

In the hiatus before the law was enacted she began to conduct surveys of the views and practices of Oregon physicians in relation to assisted suicide.

In 1995, they had conducted a cross-sectional survey by mail of all physicians who might be eligible to prescribe a lethal dose of medication if the Oregon law were to be upheld. Of the 3,944 eligible physicians who received the questionnaire, 2,761 (70 percent) responded. Sixty percent of the respondents thought physician-assisted suicide should be legal in some cases, and nearly half (46 percent) said they might be willing to prescribe a lethal dose of medication if it were legal to do so, while 31 percent of the respondents were unwilling to do so on moral grounds. Twenty-one percent of the respondents had previously received requests for assisted suicide—and 7 percent had complied. Half the respondents were not sure what to prescribe for this purpose, and 83 percent cited financial pressure as a possible reason for such requests. The respondents also expressed concern about complications of suicide attempts and doubts about their ability to predict survival at six months accurately. The authors took the view that Oregon physicians had a more favorable attitude toward legalized physician-assisted suicide, were more willing to participate, and at that time were already participating in greater numbers than other surveyed groups of physicians in the United States. A sizable minority of physicians in Oregon

19. Foley and Hendin, "Conclusion," 332.

20. "1998–99 PDIA Scholars," *PDIA Newsletter,* no. 3 (September 1998), 10.

21. Linda Ganzini, interview by David Clark, July 14, 2004.

objected to legalization and participation on moral grounds and, regardless of their pro or con attitudes, physicians had a number of reservations about the practical applications of the act.[22]

Building on such work, Ganzini and her colleagues set out the issues as they would relate to physicians in the event of legalization. They showed how with increasing support for the participation of physicians in the suicides of terminally ill patients, there was a need to examine the concrete effects on physician practice of such a policy change. If physician-assisted suicide were to be legalized, physicians would need to gain expertise in understanding patients' motivations for requesting it, as well as in assessing mental status, diagnosing and treating depression, maximizing palliative interventions, and evaluating the external pressures on the patient. It would also require greater skills in prognostication, not only about life expectancy but also about the onset of functional and cognitive decline. Physicians would need access to reliable information about effective medications and dosages, and their position on physician-assisted suicide must be open to discussion between practitioner and patient. Protection of the patient's right to confidentiality would have to be balanced against the needs of health-care professionals and institutions to know about the patient's choice. Insurance coverage and managed care options might also be affected. All of these issues needed further exploration through research, education, decision making by individual practitioners, and ongoing societal debate.[23] Yet despite its importance, as Ganzini points out, she was struggling to get grants to support this work:

> It was in a sense of desperation then that I actually called Kathy Foley up who I'd never met before, I don't believe, and said "Hi, my name is Linda Ganzini, and I'm from Oregon and I'm interested in doing these studies, and I can't find any money, and what can Project on Death in America do for me?" At that time the board was making a decision not to fund projects any more but to fund faculty scholars…and she says, "well, give this a chance, because I think there's lots of benefits potentially to you being a scholar," and it was true, so I went ahead and applied…I don't even think I got it in on time, but they still accepted it. Then got an interview, flew to New York, had the interview—I thought it went quite badly and so was sort of surprised then when I got the PDIA.[24]

Ganzini's position as a PDIA faculty scholar became the platform from which she launched a whole set of crucial studies that did so much to map the landscape

---

22. M. A. Lee et al., "Legalizing Assisted Suicide: Views of Physicians in Oregon," *New England Journal of Medicine* 334, no. 5 (1996): 310–315.

23. M. A. Drickamer, M. A. Lee, and M. D. Ganzini, "Practical Issues in Physician-Assisted Suicide," *Annals of Internal Medicine* 126, no. 2 (1997):146–151.

24. Linda Ganzini, interview by David Clark, July 14, 2004.

of assisted suicide in the state of Oregon and which appeared in a series of heavily-cited papers in medical journals. It is a contribution of considerable significance. Ganzini was particularly interested in the effects of the Oregon act on clinical practice and physician perspectives. One important and much quoted study, conducted in 1999, examined the attitudes and practices of Oregon physicians regarding the care of dying patients since the passage of the Death with Dignity Act in October 1997. A self-administered questionnaire was mailed to Oregon physicians eligible to prescribe under the act. Of 3,981 eligible physicians, 2,641 (66 percent) returned the questionnaire by August 1999. The physicians reported on their efforts to improve care for dying patients, their attitudes, concerns, and sources of information about participating in the Death with Dignity Act, and their conversations with patients regarding assisted suicide. A total of 791 respondents (30 percent) reported that they had increased referrals to hospice. Of the 2,094 respondents who cared for terminally ill patients, 76 percent reported that they made efforts to improve their knowledge of the use of pain medications for the terminally ill. The number of physicians that had been asked by a patient if they were potentially willing to prescribe a lethal dose of medication was 949 (36 percent). Of all survey participants, 7 percent reported that one or more patients became upset after learning their physician's position on assisted suicide, and 2 percent reported that one or more patients left their care as a result. Of the seventy-three physicians who were willing to write a lethal prescription and who had received a request from a patient, twenty (27 percent) were not confident they could determine when a patient had less than six months to live. The authors concluded that since the legislative debate about assisted suicide began in 1994, most Oregon physicians caring for terminally ill patients had made efforts to improve their ability to care for these patients and many had conversations with patients about assisted suicide.[25]

Ganzini and her group did not confine their attention entirely to the experiences of physicians, however. Although by 2001, 78 percent of the 91 Oregonians who had died by assisted suicide were enrolled in hospice programs, there was little information about the experiences of hospice practitioners with these patients. A survey of all 545 hospice nurses and social workers in Oregon produced 397 responses (73 percent), including 71 percent of nurses and 78 percent of social workers. From November 1997, 179 of the respondents (45 percent) had cared for a patient who requested assistance with suicide. Hospice nurses reported on eighty-two patients who had received prescriptions for lethal doses of medication. Ninety-eight percent of the nurses had discussed the request with a co-worker, and 77 percent of the requests had been presented at a hospice interdisciplinary conference on patient care. A very important reason for the request was to control the circumstances of death. The least important reasons included depression, lack of social support, and fear of being a financial drain on family members. Although the patients were concerned about burdening others, only

25. L. Ganzini et al., "Oregon Physicians' Attitudes About and Experiences with End-of-Life Care Since Passage of the Oregon Death with Dignity Act," *JAMA* 285 (2001): 2363–2369.

11 percent of hospice nurses rated their family caregivers as more burdened than the family caregivers of other hospice patients.[26]

In 2004, Ganzini contributed an overview of the Oregon experience to date. From the available evidence, she concluded that the patients who had requested assisted suicide placed great value on personal control and independence of others, they has pervasively negative expectations of the future, and saw little value in the dying process. She noted that:

> The available evidence does not bear out widely voiced concerns that physician-assisted suicide will be requested by those who are socially disadvantaged or make their requests based on lack of access to palliative care, poor social support, or financial needs.[27]

Other PDIA-funded work in Oregon was carried out by colleagues of Linda Ganzini, physician Susan Tolle, and nurse Virginia Tilden at the Oregon Health Sciences University. They first received a small grant for a planning meeting on research in end-of-life care and then a larger grant (of $150,000) for work on experiences of service providers and bereaved family members relating to such issues as the prevalence of advance directives, preference for hospice, preferred place of death, family satisfaction, and barriers to compassionate care.[28]

Subsequently other PDIA scholars and grantees also contributed to the debate on physician-assisted suicide and euthanasia—usually[29] from a critical perspective and in the context of arguments that proposed better palliative care as the key alternative. Robert Pearlman and Anthony Back contributed to a volume edited by Timothy Quill and Margaret Battin and published in 2004. Pearlman and co-author Helene Starks drew on a longitudinal qualitative study of patients outside Oregon who seriously pursued assisted death. Despite their expressed intentions, and their success in obtaining the means to end their lives, these

---

26. L. Ganzini, "Experiences of Oregon Nurses and Social Workers with Hospice Patients Who Requested Assistance with Suicide," *The New England Journal of Medicine* 347, no. 8 (2002): 582–588.

27. L. Ganzini, "The Oregon Experience." In T. E. Quill and M. P. Battin (eds.), *Physician Assisted Dying: The Case for Palliative Care and Patient Choice* (Baltimore and London: The Johns Hopkins University Press, 2004), 178.

28. See S. W. Tolle, A. G. Rosenfeld, and V. P. Tilden, "Oregon's Low In-Hospital Death Rates: What Determines Where People Die and Satisfaction with Decisions on Place of Death?" *Annals of Internal Medicine* 130, no. 8 (1999): 681–685; S. W. Tolle and V. P. Tilden, "Changing End of Life Planning: The Oregon Experience," *Journal of Palliative Medicine* 5, no. 2 (2002): 311–317; V. P. Tilde et al., "Sampling Challenges in End-of-Life Research: Case-Finding for Family Informants," *Nursing Research* 51, no. 1 (2002): 66–69.

29. For a more descriptive, less value-laden approach, see C. Cskai, "Advance Directives and Assisted Suicide: Policy Implications for Social Work Practice." In J. Berzoff and P. Silverman (eds.), *Living with Dying. A Handbook for End-of-Life Healthcare Practitioners* (New York: Columbia University Press, 2004).

patients also engaged in extensive appraisal of the benefits and burdens of their situation. The study concluded that "the decision to hasten death culminated from an interaction of illness-related experiences, threats to the person's sense of self, and fears about the future."[30] Such issues were considered to be profoundly amenable to palliative care interventions. Back drew on the same study to explore the patients' interactions with clinicians. He concluded that in dealing with a request for aided dying, a therapeutic relationship between doctor and patient may be as important as a prescription for physician-assisted suicide, and he saw that relationship as "a rich meeting point" for both physicians and patients.[31]

Over time the PDIA board did take the view that as physician-assisted suicide was legalized in Oregon, then that state should be regarded as a laboratory of public policy experimentation. Between 1998 and 2005, the highest number of officially recorded assisted suicides in one year in Oregon was 42 and the total number in eight years was 246. Far more lethal prescriptions were written (390) than used.[32] Indeed ten years after the introduction of legislation in Oregon, a respected British journalist observed "remarkably few people have actually 'gone the Oregon way'"—only 431 in total, representing one death in one thousand.[33] As time passed, it appeared that the fears of some PDIA board members concerning assisted dying, so hotly debated within their early meetings, had not been realized.[34]

WIDER ETHICAL ISSUES

PDIA was concerned with a set of moral issues at the end of life that went much further than the single-issue case of physician-assisted suicide. Although it had no ethics program as such, many of its grantees and scholars had interests in ethical debates and dilemmas that went beyond the immediate and heavily debated public issue surrounding assisted dying and euthanasia. These centered

---

30. R. A. Pearlman and H. Starks, "Why Do People Seek Physician-Assisted Death?" In T. E. Quill and M. P. Battin (eds.), *Physician Assisted Dying. The Case for Palliative Care and Patient Choice* (Baltimore and London: The Johns Hopkins University Press, 2004).

31. A. L. Back, "Doctor–Patient Communication About Physician-Assisted Suicide." In T. E. Quill and M. P. Battin (eds.), *Physician Assisted Dying: The Case for Palliative Care and Patient Choice* (Baltimore and London: The Johns Hopkins University Press, 2004), 115.

32. Patient Rights Council, "Oregon Stats," http://www.patientsrightscouncil.org/site/oregon-stats-2/ (accessed October 2, 2012).

33. See K. Whitehorn, "How to Die 'the Oregon Way,'" *Guardian* (October 12, 2008), http://www.guardian.co.uk/world/2008/oct/13/usa-healthandwellbeing (accessed October 21, 2008).

34. "And I certainly think that, from what we know so far, that whatever concerns...made then about physician-assisted suicide, there certainly doesn't seem to be any suggestion that any of the fears that I had...have been justified. It seems to have been [dealt with] quite well from what I can see." Robert Butler, interview by David Clark, July 23, 2003.

on a range of clinical and organizational issues concerning how end-of-life care could be improved in line with societal expectations and patient and family preferences. But they also included the articulation of a wider ethics of palliative care itself, and this was something that many grantees took up in their work in more or less explicit ways.

A key nexus of issues in the policy and organizational arena was that of advance directives, health-care proxies, and informed consent—matters very central to those parts of American society that are oriented toward notions of autonomy and a consumerist approach to health care. Faculty scholar Barbara Koenig was eager to point out, however, that these are not universal values and that many cultures orient to a more group-focused approach to the care of sick and dependent persons.[35] A small grant from PDIA to promote the use of advance directives was made to the national organization Choice in Dying.[36] Initial evidence suggested that advance directives do not impact on medical care or result in a "good death." Joan Teno, then at George Washington University, received PDIA funds in the early years to study the use of advance care planning to improve end-of-life care in managed care settings. Her initial work had shown that advance directives did not produce an increase in the writing of *do not resuscitate* (DNR) orders, even when the patient wanted to avoid cardiopulmonary resuscitation. Physicians rarely counseled their patients about advance directives, and only four in ten patients asked their physicians about such statements. Moreover, only a third of physicians were aware of their patients' advance directive status by the second week of hospitalization.[37] Teno and her colleagues (who included PDIA-funded Joanne Lynn and Neil Wenger) argued that future work to improve decision-making should focus upon improving the pattern of practice through better communication and more comprehensive advance care planning.[38] The argument resulting from this was that advance directives should become part of the broader activity of advance care planning, designed to ensure that clinical care will be shaped by patient preferences, when the patient is no longer able to take part in decision making.

It was a theme that was taken up by other PDIA grantees and scholars. A study by Tulsky, Arnold, and colleagues (as we saw in chapter 4) showed that conversations about advance directives were brief, vague, and physician dominated.[39] Curtis and others applied the same focus to the intensive care setting

---

35. "Diversity in Dying: Improving Palliative care in a Multicultural Society," *PDIA Newsletter*, no. 6 (December 1999), 2–5.

36. *Project on Death in America, July 1994–December 1997*, 53.

37. *Project on Death in America, July 1994–December 1997*, 46.

38. J. Teno et al., "Advance Directives for Seriously Ill Hospitalized Patients: Effectiveness with the Patient Self-Determination Act and the SUPPORT Intervention," *Journal of the American Geriatrics Society* 45, no. 4 (1997): 500–507.

39. J. A. Tulsky et al., "Opening Up the Black Box: How Do Physicians Communicate About Advance Directives?" *Annals of Internal Medicine* 129, no. 6 (1998): 441–449.

where communication difficulties arise, in part, because a family may be facing an unexpected poor prognosis associated with an acute illness or exacerbation and, in part, because the ICU orientation is one of saving lives.[40] In a study conducted at The New York Hospital–Cornell Medical Center, faculty scholar Joseph Fins and colleagues found that DNR orders were in place for 77 percent of all patients considered to be dying and 46 percent had comfort care plans. The presence of a health-care proxy was significantly associated with DNR orders and comfort care plans and, on average, comfort care plans were put in place fifteen days after admission, as compared with an overall mean length of stay of seventeen days. Substantial proportions of patients with comfort care plans continued to receive antibiotics (41 percent) and blood draws (30 percent). Only 13 percent of the patients on mechanical ventilation and 19 percent of those on artificial nutrition and hydration underwent withdrawal of these interventions prior to death.[41]

Another faculty scholar, Thomas Prendergast, reviewed a decade of experience with advance directives since the Patient Self-Determination Act was signed into law in November 1990. With few exceptions, empirical studies yielded disappointing results. Advance directives were recorded by medical personnel more often but were not completed by patients more frequently. The process of recording them did not enhance patient–physician communication. When available, advance directives did not change care or reduce hospital resources. The most ambitious study of advance care planning, the Study to Understand Prognoses and Preferences for Outcomes and Risks of Treatments (SUPPORT), failed to show any change in outcomes after an extensive intervention. Later research (including clinical trials) suggested that preferences for care are not fixed but emerge in a clinical context from a process of discussion and feedback within the network of the patient's most important relationships. The approach that emphasizes communication, building trust over time, and working within the patient's most important relationships was therefore seen as the most hopeful model for clinicians working in intensive care units.[42]

One early PDIA grant focused on cross-cultural dimensions of death and mourning in relation to organ donation. Lesley A. Sharp at Barnard College noted that organ donation in the United States relies heavily upon "universalist" assumptions about death and often downplays cross-cultural differences in grief and mourning. Sharp's work showed that the donation process can alter grieving and may prolong and intensify the period of mourning. Using an anthropological

40. J. Curtis et al., "The Family Conference as a Focus to Improve Communication About End-of-Life Care in the Intensive Care Unit: Opportunities for Improvement," supplement, *Critical Care Medicine* 29, no. 2 (2001): N26–N33.

41. J. J. Fins et al., "End-of-Life Decision-Making in the Hospital Current Practice and Future Prospects," *Journal of Pain and Symptom Management* 17, no. 1 (1999): 6–1.

42. T. J. Prendergast, "Advance Care Planning: Pitfalls, Progress, Promise," supplement, *Critical Care Medicine* 29, no. 2 (2001): N34–N39.

perspective, the project investigated cross-cultural differences in Hispanics, African Americans, and Anglos in Manhattan, comparing professional atti-tudes to lay beliefs.[43] Sharp argued that a pronounced disjunction characterizes symbolic constructions of the cadaveric donor body in the United States, where procurement professionals and surviving donor kin vie with one another in their desires to "honor" this unusual category of the dead. Of special concern is the medicalized commodification of donor bodies, a process that shapes both their social worth and emotional value. Among professionals, metaphorical thinking is key: death and body fragmentation are cloaked in an "ecological imagery" that stresses renewal and rebirth. Such objectification also obscures the origins of transplantable organs, renders individual donors anonymous, and silences kin who mourn their dead. In response, donor kin have grown increasingly asser-tive, generating alternative public mortuary forms that exclude professional mediators. In so doing, they challenge the medical assumption that anonymity is central to transplantation's continued success. Sharp showed how through donor quilts and Web cemeteries, they proclaim the personal identities and concerns of donors, even long after death.[44] It was a fascinating and generally overlooked example of PDIA-supported work.

Of related interest was the PDIA Task Force on Human Experimentation on Persons Near Death. Its starting point was to examine two different models for treating research subjects. One of these was concerned with strengthening the regulatory protection of terminally ill subjects—for example, by limiting the power of surrogate decision making. The other was concerned with increasing the potential for gravely ill subjects to obtain promising experimental drugs as participants in clinical trials and as volunteers outside the bounds of formal research.[45] The task force was co-chaired by Sherry Brandt-Rauf, JD, of the College of Physicians and Surgeons at Columbia University, and Neil MacDonald, MD, director of the Center for Bioethics at the Clinical Research Institute of Montreal, and a noted palliative care leader and activist.[46]

In 1991, and long before the start of PDIA, subsequent faculty scholar Carlos Gomez had written a book about assisted suicide and euthanasia in the Dutch context in which he had a taken a critical stance.[47] His explanation of how he got interested in this and the subsequent professional journey he followed opens up a whole moral landscape of clinical ethics at the end of life that can be seen as

43. *Project on Death in America, July 1994–December 1997,* 12.

44. L. A. Sharp, "Commodified Kin: Death, Mourning, and Competing Claims on the Bodies of Organ Donors in the United States," *American Anthropologist* 103, no. 1 (2001): 112–133.

45. *Project on Death in America, July 1994–December 1997,* 73–74.

46. The task force seems not to have published a final report.

47. C. Gomez, *"Regulating Death: Euthanasia and the Case of the Netherlands"* (New York: Free Press, 1991).

central to much of what PDIA was about and which was touched on also in the work of many other grantees:

> I was a graduate student in public policy and got interested in the end-of-life decision-making debates going on in the '80s, and in particular got interested in physician-assisted suicide, did my fieldwork in the Netherlands, and came away concerned and argued against it in a book. And I was hit over the head with a critique that said in essence "I know what you're *against*, I just don't know what you're *for*." At that point I was a medical student and was about to enter my residency training and I thought I knew everything and sort of solved all the problems, and got into residency training and was just horrified at what I saw, and understood why people would want to kill themselves, why patients with advanced cancer would in fact do things or ask physicians and so on. But it also struck me that the things that we weren't doing were fairly simple and fundamental, and why we had lost them or why we weren't doing them, at least in my institution, I don't know that we were unique...was a genuine mystery to me. And it hit me very hard in my internship year when I was on the oncology service, when I was the on-call intern, and basically I could do anything I wanted to with pain medications, anxiolytics, psychiatric drugs. Nobody commented. But God forbid that I should change any antibiotic or chemotherapy order. And my best teachers in terms of symptom management as an intern were the nurses, who found a sympathetic ear in the intern, not the senior resident, not the fellow, not the attending, and they taught me how to dose morphine, what the conversions were, how to assess anxiety in a patient, how to talk to patients about their decisions, and I found that amazing that my own profession, my own teachers weren't giving me that, and I was getting it from someone else. As I went on, this became more and more apparent and I would see patients for example, when I was rotating through an ICU, where I felt bloodied by the experience and felt dirty. I felt that I was doing a violence to people, and felt morally inept...didn't feel good about what I was doing.[48]

PDIA grantee and social scientist Mildred Solomon was able to address some of these issues through a major grant ($189,951) to examine ethics, law, and pain management, with a focus on the care of terminally ill cancer patients.[49] Her starting point was the way in which innovative treatments have led to conflicts in the goals and values of cancer medicine, especially between "aggressive" treatment to cure versus attempts to relieve suffering and provide for a dignified and peaceful death. Hers was a leadership initiative designed to challenge health-care institutions to improve the care of dying cancer patients and their families by undertaking a program to educate staff in ethics, law, and pain management, foster better decision making about treatments, and stimulate action planning to improve palliative care. The team began its work by conducting interviews with

---

48. Carlos Gomez, interview by David Clark, July 23, 2003.

49. *Project on Death in America, July 1994–December 1997*, 47.

forty-one oncology specialists from a range of disciplines to determine their perceptions of the barriers to optimal palliative care in oncology. Based on these interviews, case discussions and a training agenda were developed, which were launched at a leadership retreat in Florida in January 1997 for a program that included nineteen cancer care institutions.[50]

Pamela Hinds, coordinator of nursing research at St. Jude's Children's Research Hospital in Memphis, Tennessee, highlighted the problems of end-of-life decision making in the care of children and adolescents with life-threatening illness, and their parents. In a two-year project (1995–1997) she explored the dilemma of health-care professionals who wish to include adolescent patients in the decision making but who fear the young person may lack sufficient understanding of the situation to be able to participate competently. Her study sought to define the factors that pediatric oncology patients, their parents, and health-care providers consider when deciding to end curative or life-sustaining care. It showed that seriously ill children aged ten years and above are able to understand that they are participating in decision-making about their cancer-related treatments and their lives, and they are able to appreciate the options and the likely outcomes. The team was able to produce a set of fifteen guidelines for assisting parents in end-of-life decision making.[51]

Faculty scholar Joseph Fins, of the 1996–1997 PDIA cohort, embarked on an inquiry into reconstructing the care of the dying through the integration of clinical ethics and palliative care. He recognized that the care of the dying could be improved through the enhanced integration of the two fields and set out to develop a model educational program and collection of scholarly literature by linking the disciplines. This interdisciplinary program was based in a newly-developed hospice-like alternative care unit (ACU). The centerpiece of the program was a joint fellowship in clinical ethics and palliative care, producing professionals with an integrated knowledge of both fields.

Several grantees engaged in discussions and scholarship relating to the relief of intractable suffering and the particular intervention known as *terminal sedation*. Timothy Quill and Ira Byock argued that some patients who have witnessed harsh deaths want reassurance that they can escape if their suffering becomes intolerable. In addition, a small percentage of terminally ill patients receiving comprehensive care reach a point at which their suffering becomes severe and unacceptable, despite unrestrained palliative efforts; some of these patients request that death be hastened. They presented "terminal sedation" and voluntary refusal of hydration and nutrition as potential "last resorts" that can be used to address the needs of such patients. They argued that these two practices allow clinicians to address a much wider range of intractable end-of-life

50. Closed Box 1613 (1995): PDIA Year One Progress Report for *Decisions Near the End of Life: Focus on Cancer Care* (September 30, 1996).

51. P. S. Hinds, L. Oakes, and W. Furman, "End-of-Life Decision Making in Pediatric Oncology." In B. R. Ferrell and N. Coyle (eds.), *Textbook of Palliative Nursing* (Oxford and New York: Oxford University Press, 2005), 450–460.

suffering than physician-assisted suicide (even if it were legal) and can also provide alternatives for patients, families, and clinicians who are morally opposed to physician-assisted suicide.[52] A lengthy debate in the *Annals of Internal Medicine* letters column ensued, followed by further articles, many of them involving authors who had received PDIA support.[53]

Faculty scholar Stephen Miles offers interesting observations on the role of his PDIA peers in contributing to end-of-life ethics in the United States:

> I think PDIA's strongest players have been [working on] the question of how do we move that ethics discipline into teaching house staff, how do we assess its impact in terms of steering patient care, particularly in academic health centers? Also then how do we develop the types of platforms that are not bioethics centers but that are platforms *within* medical and nursing education that teach to the next generation of clinicians so they won't have to rely on specialized experts, but they'll be equipped with these tools within themselves to do this.[54]

He goes on to describe the components of those ethics and the broad range of issues with which PDIA was concerned:

> I think there are a couple of components. Number one, there's the application of patient choice to this set of profoundly controversial moral decisions. Number two, there's been the statement that it is equivalent to withhold[ing] or withdraw[ing] treatment, which allows for the construction of therapeutic trials: if you have a stroke and I don't know what your outcome is going to be, if there is a difference between withholding and withdrawing treatment, then I'm stuck in a Faustian choice—if I don't put a feeding tube in to sustain you for six weeks, and you *don't* recover, or you *would be* recovering, then you lose because you don't have the feeding tube, the opportunity to pursue the kind of life that you would have wanted by advance directive saying "Keep me alive so long as I can relate to my family." On the other hand, if I place the feeding tube and I can't withdraw it actually because there's a difference between withdrawing and withholding in the first place, and you come up to six weeks and you've *not* recovered, then I'm stuck with violating your living will in a different direction. And by stating that the two forms are equivalent, it opens up the space for therapeutic trials, just as we do for all other forms of medical treatment. The third element of the ethics piece is that feeding tubes are a life-sustaining treatment just like any other. And then the fourth element

---

52. T. Quill and I. Byock, "Responding to Intractable Terminal Suffering: The Role of Terminal Sedation and Voluntary Refusal of Food and Fluids," *Annals of Internal Medicine* 132, no. 5 (2000): 408–414.

53. "Sedation, Alimentation, Hydration, and Equivocation: Careful Conversation About Care at the End of Life," *Annals of Internal Medicine* 136, no. 11 (2002): 845–849.

54. Stephen Miles, interview by David Clark, July 24, 2003.

is that for persons not capable of making a decision, the decision making should be made from the patient's perspective as represented by those who have the most loving and intimate knowledge of the patient. Curiously, though, there's been a shallowness to that model that's excessively rational. It doesn't take account of the profound—what we used to call transference and counter-transference issues—in the whole discussion. It assumes that the transaction is essentially about consent and non-consent to treatment or to a technology, and so it medicalizes the problem, and it does not address the question—the paradox from the family's side—which is: "How do I remain faithful without abandoning the patient?" or "How do I let go and still remain faithful?" which are really two sides of the same coin. And from the standpoint of the clinician, it also discounts the degree to which physicians feel more uncomfortable talking with patients than they do with families, and it assumes that there's an equivalence from the word of a family member talking to a patient, whereas in fact the data show that if you defer talking to a patient to go to the family, it biases the treatment choices in a more aggressive manner. That is, if I ask the person who *you* would prefer to make choices on your behalf [to] make a choice, based on what they think you would want, and I give them a scenario like, "If you were profoundly demented and needed a feeding tube to prolong your life, would you want it?" you'd agree about two-thirds of the time with your self-designated proxy, but 80 percent of the time the proxy would be more aggressive than you would. So there's this biasing that occurs. The problem is, because we really haven't taken in, we've *assumed* that a physician is...psychologically neutral or healthily disengaged from this discussion to the point where they are managing it properly, [but] the ethics winds up not working the way that the philosophers and the academic ethicists say it is.[55]

LEGAL AND FINANCIAL MATTERS IN END-OF-LIFE CARE

PDIA took the view that the provision of palliative care to ameliorate the pain and suffering of terminally ill individuals is "infused at every level with legal issues and concerns."[56] In Bo Burt as a board member, it had a champion for such issues. It was also clear that the law and finance were often closely related in end-of-life matters in the United States, so PDIA made a number of forays into the convoluted world of American health-care financing. A PDIA memorandum on the economic barriers to palliative care noted that the United States stands alone among industrialized countries in its lack of a tax-supported, universal

---

55. Stephen Miles, interview by David Clark, July 24, 2003.

56. "Legal Initiative": *Project on Death in America, January 1998–December 2000, Report of Activities* (New York: Open Society Institute, 2001), 71.

health-care system, its patchwork assemblage of palliative care/hospice benefits, and its treatment of essential health-care services as "entitlements."[57] There was much to tackle.

In January 1998 a group of lawyers was invited to an exploratory meeting to assess the desirability and feasibility of litigation to address state and federal legal barriers to adequate care at the end of life. The Center to Improve Care for the Dying was centrally involved in the organization, and the meeting took place in Washington, DC, on 23 September. Typically for PDIA, there was a detailed agenda and an extensive briefing pack that included materials on Medicare funding for hospice, physician-assisted suicide, and barriers to pain management. Around 30 participants were involved, including PDIA board members, and the attendees comprised a judicious mix of end-of-life activists and legal experts from a broad spectrum of right-to-life, right-to-die, disability, and civil liberties advocacy groups.

The stated goal of the meeting was to pursue litigation in this arena, centered around three major topics: (1) Medicare hospice benefit, (2) the role of the Department of Health and Human Services, and (3) Medicare entitlements beyond hospice.[58] The problem of the "six-month" prognosis rule as a determinant for access to funded hospice care was discussed, and the argument was made that a person should be hospice-eligible if given a "better chance than not" of dying within six months; Joanne Lynn suggested that this would enable thousands more to qualify under a more expansive interpretation. Could litigation be pursued around this issue? The interstate variation in the implementation of Medicare hospice benefit was also noted, despite the fact that it is based on federal statute. The "terrible choice" between Medicare and Medicare hospice benefit was highlighted, which allowed "no middle ground" between life-prolonging care and hospice. Ira Byock pointed out that this dichotomy did not exist in Canada or the United Kingdom. The group discussed the possibility of suing to include palliative care as a legitimate use of hospital funds. This all seemed fertile ground for development and, following the meeting, the PDIA board decided to fund a position for a palliative care lawyer at the Bazelon Center for Mental Health Law in Washington, DC.

The Judge David L. Bazelon Center for Mental Health Law was funded with an initial grant of $239,272 by PDIA to undertake an examination of how litigation might be used to secure the rights of terminally ill people to receive adequate palliative care. It addressed the "six-month rule," as well as regulatory restrictions on the prescription of opioids. It acknowledged that while litigation is no

---

57. Open Society Foundations, "Economic Barriers to Palliative Care," http://www.soros.org/initiatives/pdia/articles_publications/publications/memo/economics(accessed July 9, 2008; site discontinued).

58. A full report of the meeting was circulated on September 28, 1998 by Janet Heald Forlini, JD: Box 734907, Litigation Meeting, "Legislation and Policy Analyst at the Center to Improve Care of the Dying," (September 23, 1998).

panacea, properly targeted legal action can be a vehicle for overcoming practices that impede access to appropriate care at the end of life. A second grant of
$233,866 was made to the center in PDIA's second trimester. The Palliative Care
Law Project sought to use legal advocacy to bridge the gap between recognized
standards for high quality end-of-life care and the actual experiences of terminally ill people and their families.[59] In the same period, PDIA gave a grant of
$81,576 to establish the *Pain and Palliative Care Reporter* on the Internet, which,
linked to the Bazelon Project, served to collect and disseminate legal materials
and links to assist attorneys and patients.[60]

But Bo Burt's judgment on the outcome of the Bazelon Project was harsh:

> We tried something in the legal area which failed: that was in my view one
> of the worst failures, and I felt a particular chagrin for that because it was
> my field, but it just had to do with the funding recipient that we chose. We'd
> looked at the field, we identified what we thought needed to be done, we
> looked at the possible grantees out there, and we actually chose a grantee,
> and it was complicated. I was the chair of the board of that organization [the
> Bazelon Center], and it had done great work in the mental health field, but
> for a variety of complicated reasons it just did not succeed anywhere near
> what we had hoped...So that was a big chunk of money...and nothing to
> show for it.[61]

By the late 1990s. it was also clear from legislation and court decisions in the
United States that although most people die in hospitals, often with considerable high-technology involvement, patients did have the right to decide whether
to receive medical treatments, even when the refusal of such treatment could
lead to death. Translating such a legal right into daily clinical and organizational
practice was however a challenging task. *End-of-Life Care and Hospital Legal
Counsel: Current Involvement and Opportunities for the Future* was a report produced jointly by the Milbank Memorial Fund and the United Hospital Fund—
two good allies of PDIA. With an introduction by PDIA board member Bo Burt
and grantee Christine K. Cassel, it described the role of hospital counsel in the
day-to-day practices affecting terminally ill patients and made recommendations for improvement. It highlighted the considerable legal challenges faced by
clinicians, and many of those interviewed for the report were uncertain about
legal issues and anxious about liability. At the same time, hospital legal counsel
reported that only a small percentage of their work time was devoted to decisions

---

59. "Shaping Public and Legal Policy to Improve End-of-Life Care," *Project on Death in
America, January 2001–December 2003, Report of Activities* (New York: Open Society
Institute, 2004), 45.

60. "Pain and Palliative Care Law Reporter on the Internet," *Project on Death in America,
January 1998–December 2000, Report of Activities* (New York: Open Society Institute,
2001), 72.

61. Bo Burt, interview by David Clark, July 23, 2003.

about patient care, and even less time to end-of-life care. Indeed their participation in end-of-life issues was usually in response to a crisis that had worked its way up through the ranks of clinicians; hospital counsel were found rarely to initiate educational outreach to assist clinicians on the legal aspects of care at the end of life. The report made three key recommendations: (1) calling for hospital counsel to become better educated about the attitudes and practices of clinicians providing end-of-life care, (2) encouraging more advance care planning to clarify patients' wishes, and (3) urging hospital counsel to do more to inform legislators about clinical practices and pressures at the end of life, as well as helping clinicians to understand the implications of new laws.[62]

As we saw in chapter 5, in 1998 PDIA funding was made available to the State of New York Office of the Attorney General for a commission on quality care at the end of life, reviewing state laws and regulations. The commission identified several barriers to providing quality care to dying patients: inadequate professional and public education, legal and regulatory barriers, financial barriers, and underuse of hospice.[63] Of course many of the legal issues considered by PDIA had significant financial components. Indeed in his 1994 speech at the College of Physicians and Surgeons of Columbia University, George Soros had raised the question of how much it would cost to deliver appropriate care to 2.2 Americans dying annually and in a context where (he claimed) half of all medical expenses are incurred in the last year of life.[64,65]

It was appropriate therefore that just a month after the legal initiative meeting took place in 1998, a session on the economics and financing of end-of-life care also took place, again in Washington, DC, on 21 October. The goal of this meeting was to identify a research agenda and opportunities for funding; participants were from a variety of fields: economics, gerontology, health services and policy research, sociology, and anthropology. As on other occasions, the preparation was impressive and the participants formidable. A full report was prepared afterwards by Haidan Huskamp, then an assistant professor of Health Economics at Harvard Medical School.[66] The meeting acknowledged the importance of

---

62. "New Publication: End-of-Life Care and Hospital Legal Counsel," *PDIA Newsletter*, no. 5 (December 1999), 5.

63. Attorney General Dennis C Vacco's Commission on Quality of Care at the End of Life, *Final Report of the Attorney General* (July 1998). This report is cited in an article by two PDIA faculty scholars:N. S. Wenger and K. Rosenfeld, "Quality Indicators for End-of-life Care in Vulnerable Elders," *Annals of Internal Medicine* 135, no. 8 (2001): 677–685.

64. G. Soros, "Reflections on Death in America," *Project on Death in America, January 1998–December 2000, Report of Activities* (New York: Open Society Institute, 2001), 4–6.

65. Writing in 2010, Joanne Lynn pointed out that "the correct figure is that about 28 percent of MEDICARE expenses are within the last year of life. No one has actually done the work to figure out what the proportion would be if one were to include long-term care. My estimates are that half of lifetime costs are in the last tenth of life ..." Joanne Lynne, personal communication, July 4, 2010.

66. Box 734907, Economics Meeting (September 23, 1998): H. Huskamp, "The Economics and Financing of End-of-Life Care," Meeting report (Washington, DC, October 21, 1998).

location of care in the financing model and asked whether financial incentives under Medicare should be redesigned to encourage death in one setting or another. It acknowledged the need for more flexibility in financing and recognized the Medicare demonstration project of the day, known as "Medicaring," as a possible way forward. It also drew attention to the "non-permeable membrane" between acute and long-term care and the need for a better interface between health and social services. Insurance coverage for pain medications was difficult to access for some patients. This was part of a wider problem of finding a Medicare payment code for palliative care provided by physicians in a context where physicians received no reimbursement for consulting with patients about their end-of-life preferences. A number of possible research areas were indentified, including the factors that influence treatment choice at the end of life, the need for a better definition of quality dying, the socioeconomic determinants of a "good death," and a randomized controlled trial of hospice care. It seemed a good "ventilation" meeting, but the next steps were much less clear, and PDIA never gained a sustained and strategic grasp on economic issues, despite the professional interests of its funder.

PDIA was able to work on financial issues in collaboration with other foundations. One of these was the Milbank Memorial Fund. Its president, Daniel Fox, had attended the October 1998 financing meeting as well as the 1995 meeting of foundations. At the latter, he had spelled out the Fund's interest in "policies for appropriate care at the end of life," which included a task force on financing that developed a proposition for the Health Care Financing Administration and the Center for Health Statistics to initiate a code for hospital reimbursement related to a DRG for palliative care.[67]

Another example of this kind of collaboration across foundations was the creation of Grantmakers Concerned with Care at the End of Life, described in chapter 1. In 1998 Grantmakers Concerned with Care at the End of Life produced *Paying for Care at the End of Life: Implications for Individuals and Families, Health-care Providers, and Society*, a report presenting the views of five experts in the field.[68] Likewise, in 2002, and with some involvement from PDIA grantees, the Robert Wood Johnson Foundation produced a detailed and closely argued statement on *Financial Implications of Promoting Excellence in End-of-Life Care*.[69]

Throughout the lifetime of PDIA there was a range of smaller grants that focused on cost issues. Some work was done in Bailey-Boushay House, Seattle, on the costs of care in a hospice for people with AIDS.[70] Lawrence J. Schneiderman in the Department of Family and Preventive Medicine at the University of

67. "Meeting of Foundations Results in Commitment to Help Transform the Culture of Dying," *PDIA Newsletter*, no. 1 (March 1996), 1–6.

68. *PDIA Newsletter*, no. 3 (September 1998), 11.

69. L. Beresford et al., *Financial Implications of Promoting Excellence in End-of-Life Care* (Missoula: University of Montana, 2002).

70. *Project on Death in America, July 1994–December 1997*, 28.

California, San Diego, conducted a cost comparison of treatments provided to Medicare beneficiaries during their last year of life in managed care and fee-for-service settings.[71,72]

Faculty scholar Thomas J. Smith also focused his attention on cost effectiveness in end-of-life care. Starting from the premise that cancer care is costly and will become more so, he examined how the aging population, new technologies, and the switch to managed care will make attempts to control costs more important. Before they switch to hospice care, patients use many more health-care dollars during the active phase of treatment, yet they may be the group that needs the resources least: white, upper-middle class, well educated. Smith set up a hospice and palliative care team for an underserved population to assess their needs and costs of care.[73] Working with others, including PDIA faculty scholar and nurse Patrick Coyne, they set out to measure the impact of the dedicated eleven-bed palliative care unit inpatient staffed by a high-volume specialist team on the cost of care. They compared daily charges and costs of the days prior to palliative care unit transfer to the stay in the unit for patients who died in the first six months after the unit opened in May 2000. A case-control study was performed by matching 38 palliative care unit (PCU) patients by diagnosis and age to contemporary patients who died outside the unit, cared for by other medical or surgical teams, adjusting for potential differences in the patients or goals of care. The unit admitted 237 patients from May to December 2000, and 52 percent had cancer followed by vascular events, immunodeficiency, or organ failure. For the 123 patients with both non-PCU and PCU days, daily charges and costs were reduced by 66 percent overall, and by 74 percent in medications and diagnostics after transfer to the PCU. Comparing the thirty-eight contemporary control patients who died outside the PCU to similar patients who died in the PCU, daily charges were 59 percent lower ($5,304 \pm $5,850 to $2,172 \pm $2,250, $p = 0.005$), direct costs 56 percent lower ($1,441 \pm $1,438 to $632 \pm $690, $p = 0.004$), and total costs 57 percent lower ($2,538 \pm $2,918 to $1,095 \pm $1,153). It was a strong argument for appropriate standardized care of medically complex terminally ill patients in a high-volume, specialized unit, with a demonstrable potential to reduce costs.[74]

---

71. *Project on Death in America, July 1994–December 1997*, 15.

72. This area of comparison between managed care and fee-for-service could prove a difficult subject for research. Faculty scholar Stephen Miles observed: "And so they gave me a green light to study the trajectories of the dying and the costs in managed care systems…with access to their data. And that was so death in managed care was actually a focus of the PDIA grant. Almost immediately after I got the grant, the firm merged with another firm, and then with another firm, and then went into a financial tailspin from which it emerged but, in the process of that, the administrative continuity to support the PDIA project essentially completely got blown away. So I was never able to secure access to the data systems or the process to analyze the data that were originally part of the [PDIA] grant." Stephen Miles, interview by David Clark, July 24, 2003.

73. *Project on Death in America, July 1994–December 1997*, 62.

74. T. A. Smith et al., "A High-Volume Specialist Palliative Care Unit and Team May Reduce In-Hospital End-of-Life Care Costs," *Journal of Palliative Medicine* 6, no. 5 (2003): 699–705.

A PDIA grant of $150,000 was made to the Medicare Rights Center to support the education of consumers and clinicians about Medicare hospice and home health benefits for the terminally ill in fee-for-service and health maintenance organizations,[75] and this was extended in the second trimester of PDIA with a further grant of $100,000 to promote this service on the Internet.[76] At the same time, a grant was made to New York State Hospice Association to develop a data matrix of hospice services and costs.[77] Another grant was made to Christine Cassel at the Mount Sinai Medical Center, New York, to conduct a mail survey to identify existing hospital-based programs of palliative care, the services provided, and the funding mechanisms.[78] This study was the first to examine the prevalence and characteristics of hospital-based palliative care programs in the United States and served as a baseline and benchmark against which future development could be compared. Data were obtained from the American Hospital Association's 1998 Annual Survey on the existence of end-of-life care and pain management services in U.S. hospitals: 1,751 hospitals (36 percent) reported having a pain management service and 719 (15 percent) had an end-of-life care service, for a total of 2,015 unique hospitals that had one or both. In total 1,120 (56 percent) responded to a follow-up survey and, of these, 337 hospitals (30 percent) reported having a hospital-based program for palliative care, and another 228 (20.4 percent) had plans to establish one. Hospital-based programs of palliative care were most commonly structured as inpatient consultation services and hospital-based hospice. They tended to be established in oncology, general medicine, and geriatrics.[79]

These were important studies that laid a foundation of understanding on the provision of palliative care within the core of the hospital system. PDIA grantees and scholars maintained an interest in cost issues across a wide range of projects, but no clear message emerged from this, and there was never a well developed randomized control trial of the cost effectiveness of palliative care. With the exception of a few individuals, the field remained relatively unattractive to health economists and the tendency was for appropriately minded clinicians to engage in costing issues where they felt able, and, in general, without major PDIA-supported economic analytical power.[80]

75. *Project on Death in America, July 1994–December 1997,* 40.

76. *Project on Death in America, January 1998- December 2000, Report of Activities* (New York: Open Society Institute, 2001), 66.

77. *Project on Death in America, January 1998–December 2000,* 66.

78. *Project on Death in America, January 1998–December 2000,* 76.

79. C. X. Pan et al., "How Prevalent are Hospital-Based Palliative Care Programs? Status Report and Future Directions," *Journal of Palliative Medicine* 4, no. 3 (2001): 315–324.

80. As Kathy Foley put it: We were thwarted by the lack of [economic] data available, but Haiden Hauskamp, who was at the first meeting, went on to develop a career in studying economic issues, as did Susan Miller and Joan Teno, who contributed to the debate, as well as Diane Meier, Tom Smith, and others. So, the seed was planted." Kathy Foley, personal communication, August 11, 2012.

Some important PDIA work was supported in relation to ethics, legal issues, and costs. Although physician-assisted suicide held center stage in the early days of PDIA development, it was not the most important or complex ethical issue. Excellent work was done on physician-assisted suicide in Oregon with PDIA support, but also important was the way in which the emergent cohorts of PDIA leaders helped forge *the ethics of palliative care* as they grappled with the complex and challenging issue of transforming the culture of dying in American society. Some of this had to be done in the context of a better understanding of legal frameworks. Ultimately it ran up against the barriers of health-care financing in the American system, and this presented a challenge that would not quickly be overcome: how to identify, draw on, and make sustainable a source of funding for end-of-life care that would meet the needs of all Americans, regardless of social class, ethnicity, or disease status. PDIA-funded work nevertheless mapped out and defined the ethical, legal, and financial questions, many of which continue to reverberate.

7

Developing the Field

Underlying all the wider goals and programs of PDIA, there emerged a gradual and strengthening commitment to one particular issue. This took shape around the compelling need to build evidence, expertise, and professional capacity to promote end-of-life care in different settings, and it was articulated in the simple phrase: "developing the field." Used repeatedly by PDIA cognoscenti and increasingly by others working in palliative care, the phrase was accompanied by a tacit set of assumptions about what it meant and that it was a desirable and realistic target at which to aim. In this chapter, "developing the field" is addressed in relation to three core areas: research, education, and professional recognition. An examination of PDIA involvement in each of these realms and the level of progress made then brings us to some core aspects of how PDIA sought to make a long-term impact on the culture of dying in American society and the particular role of the caring professions within that.

A SCIENCE OF CARE

Before PDIA got underway, two landmark studies had drawn attention to end-of-life issues in the United States and had captured attention well beyond the narrow confines of specialist interest. The National Hospice Demonstration Project was a research study funded by the US federal government that commenced in 1979. Twenty-six hospice demonstration sites participated along with fourteen control programs, and 13,374 patients were enrolled. The results showed that patients who chose hospice care did not suffer any deprivation of care. Often (although not always) they required a lower level of expenditure, and usually they were able to spend more time at home.[1] Even before the study was complete, it had informed the enactment by the US Congress of legislation to authorize a hospice care benefit. It was an indication of the power of research, when combined with effective advocacy, to shape policy. Fifteen years later, the SUPPORT study brought to the wider field of end-of-life care some of the benefits yielded by the National Hospice Demonstration Project, but this time they came not in a reimbursement stream, but in a much broader debate about how American society should organize the care of those facing death and life-limiting illness.

SUPPORT was often seen as a benchmark that set the agenda for some aspects of the PDIA program. As stated in the final PDIA triennial report, "The SUPPORT data left no doubt that George Soros established PDIA at just the right time."[2] SUPPORT also did a great deal to set the agenda for research thinking within PDIA. For example, on July 11, 1996, a meeting of major figures in the pain and palliative care field was convened jointly with the Robert Wood Johnson Foundation at OSI headquarters in New York to explore the data on pain and pain relief emerging from SUPPORT.[3] There was wider encouragement too for more research in these areas, as in the piece written with PDIA funding by the bio-ethicist Daniel Callahan, in which he notes:

> Modern medicine, at least in its research aspirations, seems to have made death public enemy number one. It is not—at least not any longer in developed countries, with the average life expectancy approaching eighty years. The enemies now are serious chronic illness and an inability to function well. Death will always be with us, pushed around a bit to be sure, with one fatal disease superseded by another. For every birth, someone long ago happened to notice, there is one death. We cannot and will not change that fact. But we can change the way people are cared for at the end of life, and we can substantially reduce the burden of illness. It is not, after all, death that people seem to fear the most, and certainly not in old age, but a life poorly lived. Something can be done about that.[4]

When PDIA began, research to support that "something" was taking place in a small number of centers, notably those doing work on pain and symptom management. Yet there were very few university chairs in the field in North

---

1. V. Mor, D. S. Greer, and R. Kastenbaum, "The Hospice Experiment: An Alternative in Terminal Care." In V. Mor, D. S. Greer, and R. Kastenbaum (eds.), *The Hospice Experiment* (Baltimore: Johns Hopkins University Press, 1988).

2. *Transforming the Culture of Dying: The Project on Death in America, October 1994 to December 2003* (New York: Open Society Institute, 2004), 16.

3. Box 734891: Pain Meeting, June 11, 1996.

4. D. Callahan, "Death and the Research Imperative," *New England Journal of Medicine* 342 (2 March 2000): 654–656.

America[5] and very little evidence of active research groups with external funding, research students, fellows, and postdoctoral investigators. There was a huge need to strengthen capacity in these areas and to support the isolated individuals working in them. The profile and impact of the relevant journals needed to increase, and palliative care research needed to find its way into the high-impact generic medical journals where it would attract the interest of other specialists and provide an evidence base to support practice and service development. What we must ask in relation to this, however, is the extent to which PDIA assistance served in a wider sense to *build capacity* in the world of palliative care research, rather than simply to fund individuals with their own particular research interests and preoccupations.

The first PDIA newsletter highlighted some of the important end-of-life care research being conducted in the United States in the mid-1990s and hammered home the message of SUPPORT: "Every facet of medical culture, from the training of doctors to reimbursement systems to over-reliance on high-tech treatments conspired to cause doctors to ignore patients' last wishes."[6,7] One year later, the Institute of Medicine report *Approaching Death*, which as we have seen had considerable input from PDIA personnel (see chapter 5), set out some directions for research to improve care at the end of life. In particular, it looked to the nation's key research organizations to show leadership. The National Institutes of Health (NIH) were urged to take the lead by organizing workshops and consensus conferences focused on an agenda for research improvement,[8] and PDIA board members Kathy Foley and Robert Butler did some early lobbying of Institute directors to raise awareness of the research needs of palliative care.[9] Bo Burt took the view that *Approaching Death* had been a work of major importance:

> The [Institute of Medicine] committee didn't do any independent research, or hardly any independent research, but it brought together the field. It had enormous impact in medical schools in raising the visibility; it had impact that I think is continuing to evolve in terms of shaming the National Institutes of Health about their funding for research. I mean the IOM [Institute of Medicine] committee held hearings...we asked everybody from the National Institutes, institute by institute, to come and tell us what

---

5. Kathy Foley at Columbia University in New York, and Balfour Mount at McGill University in Montreal, were notable exceptions.

6. "An Impressive Range of Innovative Programs in Culture and Care of Dying," *PDIA Newsletter*, no. 1 (March 1996), 3.

7. Joanne Lynn pointed out that SUPPORT showed "doctors were not AGAINST patients' wishes, just not helping to develop them or to solicit them." Joanne Lynn, personal communication, July 4, 2010.

8. Institute of Medicine, *Approaching Death: Improving Care at the End of Life* (Washington, DC: Institute of Medicine, 1997).

9. Robert Butler, interview by David Clark, July 23, 2003.

they were doing in end-of-life care, what research...So they would come in one after another and they would tell us they're doing nothing. It turned out in pain research—this was astounding to me—that there was only one of the National Institutes of Health that was putting any money at all into pain research, and when I tell this story I often ask people to guess, and they never can guess: it was the Institute of Dentistry, and the dentistry group wasn't doing any end-of-life research.[10]

In 1998, PDIA supported a key meeting, organized under the auspices of NIH and the US Cancer Pain Relief Committee. Led by Drs. Russell Portenoy[11] and Eduardo Bruera,[12] the First International Conference on Research in Palliative Care was held in Bethesda, Maryland. It took up the challenge to strengthen palliative care research and was attended by 268 experts from 22 countries. Two-thirds of the participants were physicians, more than a quarter of those attending were nurses, and 40 percent were from outside the United States.[13] The plenary lectures struck a familiar pose for palliative care meetings of the day, covering pain, pediatrics, anorexia and gastro-intestinal disorders, quality of life, neuropsychiatric and psychosocial issues, bereavement, ethical decision making, respiratory symptoms, practice change, and fatigue.[14]

Portenoy observed: "There is increasing recognition that both the ultimate acceptance of palliative care as a model of good clinical practice and the continued evolution of palliative care as a specialty will depend upon credible research that assesses interventions."[15]

It was a call to action that was taken up by many PDIA grantees who, in the years following, undertook a range of studies and evaluations designed to throw light on best practices in end-of-life care, many of which have already been explored here in earlier chapters. There was also a lasting legacy to the 1998 meeting. In 2003, Portenoy and Bruera published a substantial edited collection, *Issues in Palliative Care Research*, which contained updated versions of the presentations and also new material in a set of chapters that focused on palliative care research problems in some challenging clinical areas, such as anorexia and gastrointestinal disorders; respiratory symptoms; fatigue and asthenia; and

10. Bo Burt, interview by David Clark, July 23, 2003.

11. Dr. Portenoy is chair of the Department of Pain Medicine and Palliative Care at Beth Israel Medical Center in New York.

12. Dr. Bruera was then director of the Palliative Care Program at Grey Nuns Community Hospital and Health Care Centre in Edmonton, Canada.

13. "Palliative Care Research: Gains Recognition at International Conference," *PDIA Newsletter*, no. 3 (September 1998), 5.

14. Sixty-four abstracts from the meeting appeared in a special journal issue: *Journal of Pain and Symptom Management* 15, no. 4 (1998).

15. *Journal of Pain and Symptom Management* 15, no. 4.

neuropsychiatric conditions—as well as quality of life, end-of-life decision making, and practice change.[16]

Some faculty scholars and grantees directed considerable energy to the palliative care research agenda and, over time, emerged or strengthened their role as national and international leaders in the field: Sean Morrison, Nicholas Christakis, Harvey Chochinov, James Tulsky, Randall Curtis, Diane Meier, William Breitbart, and Eduardo Bruera. All became among the most highly cited researchers in the international palliative care field over the decade following the start of PDIA. Morrison was fulsome in his praise of the faculty scholar retreats as a stimulus to research innovation. Speaking at the 2003 retreat, he observed:

I think my best research ideas have come on the plane ride back from these meetings after sitting talking with people, running through my brain, and then thinking about it on the airplane back. And some of my best research projects have developed as a result of this meeting—certainly the most successful ones have come about as a result of the intellectual engagement and exchange that's happened here.[17]

PDIA also made some efforts to stimulate research within those caring professions less associated with empirical inquiry and evidence-based practice. Social work is one such example. In a review of the development of social work and end-of-life care, Cheryl Brandsen notes the important work of PDIA in supporting such research:

This was, in part, a piece of the agenda for the first national Social Work Summit on End-of-Life and Palliative Care held in March 2002...This is also, in part, what the Social Work Leadership Development Awards Program of the Project on Death in America is addressing as it moves forward. What is important in both of these initiatives, in addition to the priorities established, is the interactive processes, grounded in field representation methodologies, used to facilitate the group, gather ideas from social work leaders, and arrive at consensus about research priorities. To the extent that the social work leaders participating in these consensus activities are close to the ground with practice experience in end-of-life care, the research priorities that emerge are important for shaping practice, policy, and social work education...The research methodologies must be empirically sound and also diverse and include quantitative and qualitative methodologies that capture the full range of human experience.[18]

---

16. R. Portenoy and E. Bruera (eds.), *Issues in Palliative Care Research* (Oxford, UK: Oxford University Press, 2003).

17. Sean Morrison, interview by David Clark, July 24, 2003.

18. C. K. Brandsen, "Social Work and End-of-Life Care: Reviewing the Past and Moving Forward," *Journal of Social Work in End-of-Life & Palliative Care* 1 (2005): 45–70.

There was a price to be paid, however, for bringing social work into the PDIA research agenda. The board proposed that faculty scholars and social work leaders should meet together at the annual retreats. But it was an uneasy mix, with reported differences of professional orientation, status, research know-how, and experience. After some joint meetings, the idea was quietly abandoned and the social workers subsequently held their own retreats—at Lake Tahoe, Cape Cod, and on Long Island.[19] But the issue caused reverberations in the board and added to the divisions within it. Some board members remained only partially convinced that the social work program had achieved its goals or repaid the investment, whereas others saw its inclusion as a triumph and an unprecedented opportunity for the discipline. As we shall see, the social work contribution to PDIA was more defined in relation to education than to research, and this may have gone some way in contributing to the negative evaluation on the part of some board members who were ultimately more persuaded by the lingua franca of knowledge production rather than its distribution.

But as PDIA came to a close, there were still some rather critical observations on the state of palliative care research and its success in advancing the field. Faculty scholar David Weissman was founding editor of the *Journal of Palliative Medicine*, first published in 1998. Interviewed five years later and drawing on his editorial experience, he noted:

There are a lot of other things happening that scholars are doing; a lot of it falls under very focused research projects that may or may not be talked about ten years from now, but they do form the first basis in this country of a true science of this field. The one area we have not impacted... is virtually no work in the clinical area. There's a tremendous amount of health systems research, educational research, some psychology and bereavement issues, but virtually nothing about what dose of morphine *do* we give? How *do* we titrate morphine correctly? Those kinds of questions have *not* been part of the scholars' work, with very few exceptions. And that's an area that's

19. "There was always some uneasiness or, let's say, difference of opinion, about the interdisciplinary piece, because the doctors had been funded for five years, and ... I think they felt they were in a different sort of organizational and developmental period with themselves than [the] social workers who would be coming into the program. But nevertheless we tried it for a couple of years and it was a tremendously beneficial ... meeting together at Lake Tahoe and it was tremendously beneficial for social work ... In both helping them [the doctors] to understand where other disciplines were at, so they began to see in areas of diversity, in areas of service provision, communication, fragmentation, all those kinds of issues, we really had a lot more experience. So I think it's promoted a sense of confidence. We always say in social work it's the confidence in their competence that's sometimes lacking, because we're very broadly focused, so sometimes it's hard to get a sense of what your competence is and to gain sufficient confidence that you can build knowledge in that area and you can teach in that area. I think that's one thing that happened with them ... doing family conferencing—that's their Social Work 101, dealing with diversity and multiculturalism; that's what they do all the time." Grace Christ, interview by David Clark, October 27, 2004.

critically lacking, and I'm not sure where those people are going to come from in the next ten years... Because this group's not there: this group has done a lot of great things, but that's one area that hasn't happened. It has an impact on the field as we try to both differentiate ourselves and merge with the hospice community. This is the field, this is the group that's trying to define the *science* that hospice people have been doing all these years and trying to say what really works and what doesn't work.[20]

Even by 2009, PDIA scholar Harvey Chochinov, in an editorial in the *Journal of Palliative Medicine*, could bemoan the lack of engagement with research by palliative care clinicians and their too ready tendency to accept that research is a burden to patients at the end of life and can do little to enhance practice.[21]

Despite such comments, we have seen in earlier chapters many examples of innovative research stimulated, funded, and supported by PDIA. The rich intellectual environment of PDIA and the commitment to change that was so central to its values, gave expression to a wide range of innovative methodologies, research questions, and topics of inquiry. Although they may not have advanced significantly the medical evidence base on the mechanics of symptom control, and hence the specific point made by Weissman, other studies did a huge amount to address the question of transforming the *culture* of dying, which was central to the PDIA mission. In the first triennium, PDIA funded a wide range of evaluation projects focused on special programs in palliative and hospice care as well as efforts to integrate these principles into the delivery of services for all dying persons.[22] Many scholars and grantees conducted work to assess needs, describe the delivery of care, improve practice, and promote change—and published their results for wider dissemination and scrutiny. It is also fair to say that PDIA funding often gave the individuals concerned the confidence to work in such ways and to make a contribution to the emerging evidence base of palliative care.

PROFESSIONAL EDUCATIONAL INITIATIVES

More than half of PDIA's total grant funds were used to support professional development initiatives.[23] Educational activities and programs proliferated with PDIA support and seem to have been the central "comfort zone" of the majority

20. David Weissman, interview by David Clark, July 22, 2003.

21. H. M. Chochinov, "The Culture of Research in Palliative Care: *You Probably Think This Song Is About You*," *Journal of Palliative Medicine* 12, no. 3 (2009): 215–217.

22. "New Service Delivery Models for the Dying and Their Families," *Project on Death in America, July 1994–September 1997, Report of Activities* (New York: Open Society Institute, 1998), 27.

23. *Transforming the Culture of Dying: The Project on Death in America, October 1994–December 2003* (New York: Open Society Institute, 2004), 18.

of scholars and grantees. Lists of awards year after year throughout the duration of PDIA refer to the intention to develop, implement, and in some cases evaluate educational interventions aimed at a wide range of health and social care professionals, as well as in some cases specific groups of service users, communities, or populations. The PDIA board addressed the need for improved palliative care education through two separate columns of activity: the Faculty Scholars Program and the Social Work Leadership Program. There were also some strategic and crosscutting initiatives focused on areas such as medical and nurse education.[24]

Some important work was done to address the end-of-life care "content" of major textbooks for health professionals, with a view to highlighting deficiencies and filling gaps. Joanne Lynn and colleagues had a particular role in initiating this. The June 1999 issue of the PDIA newsletter sees Lynn sitting solemnly next to a pile of medical textbooks. From a review of four of the most widely used texts, she concluded such resources "provide little information that would help a physician to care for a dying patient."[25] The investigators had searched the textbooks for content on twelve common causes of death—AIDS, dementia, chronic lung disease, congestive heart failure, kidney failure, cirrhosis of the liver, diabetes, stroke, and four types of cancer. They found a reluctance to acknowledge death and dying, amounting to denial in some instances, where, for example, dead persons were termed "non-survivors," as well as a lack of specifics on symptom management—in particular, diseases and stages.[26]

Faculty scholar Michael Rabow and colleagues built on this work with a much more detailed analysis of textbooks from a broad range of specialties. They aimed to determine the quantity and to rate the adequacy of information on end-of-life care in textbooks from multiple medical disciplines. This involved a review in 1998 of no less than fifty top-selling textbooks from multiple specialties (cardiology, emergency medicine, family and primary care medicine, geriatrics, infectious disease and acquired immunodeficiency syndrome [AIDS], internal medicine, neurology, oncology and hematology, pediatrics, psychiatry, pulmonary medicine, and surgery). The focus of inquiry was the presence and adequacy of content in thirteen end-of-life care domains. Chapters on diseases commonly causing death and those devoted to end-of-life care were identified, read, rated, and compared by textbook specialty for the presence of helpful information in the thirteen domains. Content for each domain was rated as absent, minimally present, or helpful. Textbook indexes were also analyzed for the number of pages relevant to end-of-life care.

---

24. "PDIA Supports Professional Education," *PDIA Newsletter*, no. 9 (December 2001), 14–15.

25. "Studies Promote Improvements in Textbooks on End-of-Life Care," *PDIA Newsletter*, no. 5 (June 1999), 3–4.

26. A. T. Carron, J. Lynn, and P. Keaney, "End-of-Life Care in Medical Textbooks," *Annals of Internal Medicine* 130, no. 1 (1999), 82–86.

Overall, the investigators found that helpful information was provided in only about a quarter of the expected end-of-life content domains; in around one-fifth of entries, expected content received minimal attention; and in 56 percent, expected content was absent. As a group, the textbooks with the highest percentages of absent content were in surgery (71 percent), infectious diseases and AIDS (70 percent), and oncology and hematology (61 percent). Textbooks with the highest percentage of helpful end-of-life care content were in family medicine (34 percent), geriatrics (34 percent), and psychiatry (29 percent). In internal medicine textbooks, the content domains with the greatest amount of helpful information were epidemiology and natural history. Content domains covered least well were social, spiritual, ethical, and family issues, as well as physician after-death responsibilities. On average, textbook indexes cited just 2 percent of their total pages as pertinent to end-of-life care. The authors concluded that top-selling textbooks generally offered little helpful information on caring for patients at the end of life. Most disease-oriented chapters had minimal or no end-of-life care content. Specialty textbooks with information about particular diseases often did not contain helpful information on caring for patients dying from those diseases.[27,28]

PDIA grantee Betty Ferrell and colleagues at the City of Hope National Medical Center collaborated with Michael Rabow and colleagues in doing a parallel review of the fifty leading textbooks in nursing. Both the medical textbook and nursing textbook reviews were supported by grants from the Robert Wood Johnson Foundation. The review of nursing textbooks revealed that less than 2 percent of all content was related to any aspect of palliative care.

By 1999, four nurses had received faculty scholarships from PDIA.[29] At New York University School of Education, Deborah Witt Sherman, building on a decade of past experience, developed the first program in the United States to prepare palliative care nurse practitioners in a curriculum that focused on the philosophy and principles of palliative care, death and grief education, pain and symptom management, as well as related ethical and legal issues.[30] Marianne Matzo, professor of nursing in the Department of Health Services at New

27. M. W. Rabow et al., "End-of-Life Care Content in 50 Textbooks from Multiple Specialities," *Journal of the American Medical Association* 283 (2000): 771–778.

28. PDIA grantee Betty Ferrell led a similar exercise in the nursing texts in a project funded by the Robert Wood Johnson Foundation and others. Of the material reviewed across 45,683 pages in 50 textbooks, only 901 pages had any end-of-life content, representing 2 percent of the total content. In particular there was little information on pain and its management at the end of life. See B. R. Ferrell, M. Grant, R. Virani, "Strengthening Nurse Education to Improve End-of-Life Care," *Nursing Outlook* 47, no. 6 (1999): 252–256.

29. "Nursing the Dying: Palliative Care Reaffirms the Nurse's Mission," *PDIA Newsletter*, no. 4 (February 1999), 3–5.

30. D. W. Sherman, "Training Advance Practice Palliative Care Nurses," *Generations* 23, no. 1 (1999): 87–90.

Hampshire Community Technical College, prepared a novel curriculum for associate degree nurses and placed a heavy emphasis on dealing with students' own imaginings of death as a starting point.[31] Martha Henderson's educational work on improving the care of people dying in nursing homes has already been described in chapter 4. Jane Morris, a geriatric nurse practitioner at Mount Sinai Medical Center, worked with Diane Meier and Sean Morrison in a shared faculty scholarship and focused her energy on addressing the culture of nursing care at the end of life—mainly though education at the bedside.

Matzo and Witt Sherman, together with another PDIA grantee, Betty Ferrell,[32] collaborated closely on a major national initiative to extend palliative care education to nurses—the End-of-Life Nursing Education Consortium (ELNEC).[33] Important textbooks were also produced by these people, including *Palliative Care Nursing: Quality Care to the End of Life* and[34] the *Textbook of Palliative Nursing*,[35] both of which appeared to favorable reviews in 2001. As we shall see, further investment in ELNEC was a crucial part of the PDIA exit strategy.

One of the earlier grants awarded by PDIA, in October 1995, was used by Dr. Knight Steel, professor of geriatrics at Hackensack University in New Jersey, to organize a conference for senior figures involved in regulating the training of American physicians.[36] The conference was entitled *The Education of Physicians About Dying*. By bringing together representatives of those organizations that design and administer examinations and set standards for accreditation of training programs, it was believed that improvements in the care of the dying, particularly by the medical profession, could be achieved. This is of course a complex matter. The education of physicians is influenced by any number of factors, but among the most important are the requirements for training as detailed by the residency review committees, under the auspices of the Accreditation Council for Graduate Medical Education, with the content of examinations administered by the speciality boards. It was the specific intent of this conference and the work surrounding it to influence both the requirements for training and the content of the examinations. Following the conference, Dr. Steel was informed by the chair of the residency review committee, Dr. Daniel Duffy, that special requirements

---

31. M. L. Matzo, "Conversation on Caring: A Nursing Perspective," *Journal of Geriatric Nursing* 29, no. 1 (1996): 45–59.

32. See chapter 4 for a description of Betty Ferrell's work on the HOPE project for the education of home-care nurses.

33. D. W. Sherman et al., "Achieving Quality Care at the End of Life: A Focus of the End-of-Life Nursing Education Consortium (ELNEC) Curriculum," *Journal of Professional Nursing* 18, no. 5 (2002): 255–262.

34. M. Laporte, D. W. Sherman, M. L. Matzo (eds.), *Palliative Care Nursing: Quality Care to the End of Life* (New York: Springer, 2001; 2/e in 2006).

35. B. R. Ferrell and N. Coyle (eds.). *Textbook of Palliative Nursing* (New York and Oxford, UK: Oxford University Press, 2001).

36. Closed grants 1995, Box 3200: Year One Progress Report Form, October 15, 1996.

for "end-of-life pain management" and "hospice" had been added in the new framework.

Many PDIA-funded physicians endeavored to address the palliative care education needs of their colleagues, working across a variety of settings. Stephen Pantilat, at the University of California, San Francisco, concentrated his initial PDIA efforts on the *hospitalist*, a new breed of physician spending 25 percent of time caring for inpatients in place of the primary care provider.[37] The work of the hospitalist was also a special interest of PDIA scholars J. Cameron Muir and Robert Arnold. They argued that most US citizens die in acute care hospitals, often in physical pain, without attention to emotional and spiritual suffering in what amounts to an ethical failure of the health-care system, thereby creating a huge need for palliative care. At the same time, a new specialty of hospitalists was emerging, providing care for acutely ill patients, many of whom will die. Muir and Arnold proposed that the hospitalist may well become the primary deliverer of palliative care. Hospitalists could enhance the quality of care for the dying by emphasizing interdisciplinary communication and involvement of hospital-based health professionals to address emotional and spiritual distress and bereavement issues, as well as through specific quality-improvement efforts. When hospitalists are not selected and trained effectively around palliative care issues, however, the risks are great. Discontinuity of physicians can lead to miscommunication and misunderstanding (by professionals, patient, and family); disagreement about treatment focus (especially as it relates to a shift from curative to palliative care); inappropriate deferring of advance care planning to the hospital setting; and a lack of expertise in symptom control, communication skills, and attention to patient and family distress and the provision of emotional and spiritual support. These authors sought to promote convergence between the two fields—of palliative medicine and hospitalist medicine—and to thereby stimulate opportunities for mutual education and improved patient care.[38]

Some PDIA faculty scholars placed a special emphasis on educating physicians in particular dimensions of palliative care, and one group focused on *psychosocial* and *psychiatric issues*. They sought to broaden understanding about the emotional and social needs of terminally ill people and to improve medical education in these areas.[39] John Shuster, associate professor in the Departments of Medicine and Psychiatry at the University of Alabama, developed a model curriculum for teaching psychiatry and internal medicine residents about the dimensions and complications of terminal illness. William Breitbart, chief of the Psychiatry Service at Memorial Sloan-Kettering Cancer Center in New York,

---

37. S. Pantilat, "Palliative Care and Hospitalists: A Partnership for Hope," *Journal of Hospital Medicine* 1, no. 1 (2006): 5–6.

38. J. C. Muir and R. M. Arnold, "Palliative Care and the Hospitalist: An Opportunity for Cross-Fertilization," *American Journal of Medicine* 11, no. 9B (2001): 105–145.

39. "Shedding Light on Psychiatric Disorders among the Dying," *PDIA Newsletter*, no. 4 (February 1999), 6–8.

developed an observership program to provide continuing medical education in the psychiatric dimensions of palliative care and he evaluated it with the support of two other PDIA Scholars.[40] Another aspect of Breitbart's PDIA work was the decision to edit, with fellow faculty scholar Harvey Chochinov, a text on psychiatry and palliative medicine, which became the *Oxford Handbook of Psychiatry in Palliative Medicine*.[41] The two also collaborated in founding the international palliative care journal *Palliative and Supportive Care*, which began in 2003. Indeed for Breitbart, even though already well established in his field, the PDIA involvement led to a major career reorientation:

> I think that as a result of my involvement with the PDIA there was this fundamental shift in my identity. From being a psycho-oncologist or psychiatrist who focused on symptom management, pain, and other symptoms, I eventually changed my sense of my work and my identity to that of a palliative care practitioner. And it actually changed my goals, my sense of mission in psycho-oncology…and in palliative care, which was to essentially expand the focus of palliative medicine beyond an emphasis on pain and physical symptom control to include psychiatric and psychosocial, existential, and spiritual issues. So my involvement with PDIA really changed my identity and my goals.[42]

As Shuster, Breitbart, and Chochinov noted in an editorial, there were huge challenges to the development of education in this field:

> Educational efforts should emphasize the prevalence and morbidity of psychiatric complications in terminal illness. Target audiences should include the general public; students and trainees in all health-care professions; and health-care providers in hospice and palliative care, primary care, and medical specialties (including psychiatry). Educational and other efforts should be designed to reduce or remove barriers to excellent psychiatric end-of-life care. Educational and advocacy efforts should aim to ensure that legal or regulatory barriers do not hinder or prevent excellent psychiatric care at the end of life.[43]

Several scholars and grantees built palliative care education programs around visiting fellows and interns. Often these were institution-specific, such as a

---

40. W. Breitbart, B. Rosenfeld, and S. Passik, "The Network Project: A Multi-Disciplinary Cancer Education and Training Program in Pain Management, Rehabilitation, and Psychosocial issues," *Journal of Pain and Symptom Management* 15, no. 1 (1998): 18–26.

41. H. Chochinov and W. Breitbart (eds.), *Handbook of Psychiatry in Palliative Medicine* (Oxford, UK and New York: Oxford University Press, 2002).

42. William Breitbart, interview by David Clark, April 1, 2004.

43. J. L. Shuster, W. Breitbart, and H. M. Chochinov, Editorial: "Psychiatric Aspects of Excellent End-of-Life Care," *Psychosomatics* 40, no. 1 (1999): 1–4.

program for internal medicine residents run by faculty scholar Wayne Ury at St. Vincent's Hospital and Medical Center of New York; his evaluation showed that the palliative care curriculum was associated with a sustained improvement in medical residents' opioid prescribing practices.[44] Daniel Johnson, at the University of Colorado Health Sciences Center, developed an evidence-based symptom management educational intervention to reduce distress at the end of life.[45] James Tulsky devised a project on improving communication with the dying patient and produced a curriculum for medical students and house staff.[46] Charles von Gunten ran such a program in Northwestern University Medical School, Chicago. He observed the following:

> If I am known as a doctor who specializes in the care of the dying, then maybe a frightened, overwhelmed intern will know to call me for help rather than walk away because he mistakenly thinks there is "nothing more that can be done." There is a joy in helping other physicians—whether they be medical students, residents, fellows, or physicians in practice—learn to care for patients with advanced, incurable illness in the context of palliative care. The new skills they learn enable them to make patients and families "heal" in ways they hadn't thought possible, and to feel a new sense of competence as physicians.[47]

David Weismann's work at the Medical College of Wisconsin established a solid foundation of activity to develop a death education program for a primary care residency, and he also collaborated in this with faculty scholar Jim Cleary. Weismann went on to work with Charles von Gunten in a larger study of end-of-life education in medical residency programs. They examined patterns of education, discerned from program directors' responses to structured surveys of institutional teaching and evaluation practices, and derived information from the performance of faculty and residents on a knowledge examination with thirty-six items. The subjects of the study were program directors, faculty, and residents at thirty-two accredited US internal medicine residency programs. The authors found that while all programs cited inclusion of some end-of-life education, the expected end-of-life domains were not systematically taught or assessed. Pain assessment and treatment training was required in only 60 percent of programs. Even fewer programs required instruction on non-pain symptoms (30 percent) or hospice and nonhospital care settings (22 percent). End-of-life assessment depended primarily on the faculty's general ratings of the resident's global

---

44. W. Ury et al., "Can a Pain Management and Palliative Care Curriculum Improve the Opioid Prescribing Practices of Medical Residents?" *Journal of General Internal Medicine* 17, no. 8 (2002): 625–663.

45. "PDIA Supports Professional Education," *PDIA Newsletter*, no. 9 (December 2001), 14.

46. Closed Box 1995, Box 3232.

47. Quoted in *Project on Death in America, July 1994–September 1997, Report of Activities* (New York: Open Society Institute, 1998), 62.

competency, and few programs used knowledge examinations or structured skill assessments. Directors identified barriers and support for improving education. On the knowledge examination, the mean score of residents increased across training levels and the mean score of faculty was higher than that of residents. The authors concluded that existing internal medicine residency education lacks personnel trained in critical end-of-life care domains. Residency programs therefore needed additional training for residents and teaching faculty in end-of-life content and skills, with assessment practices that demonstrate competencies have been acquired.[48]

Building on the work around underserved communities that we saw in chapter 5, faculty scholar Jerome Kurent, working in South Carolina, was engaged in a number of educational initiatives and also edited an introduction to the multidisciplinary field of palliative care. Arranged in chapters by disease systems, the book provides clinical guidelines as well as practical advice for the management of advanced disease, including a review of the assessment of prognosis (determining when the illness is end-stage), how to communicate and face difficult decisions with patients and families, the role of hospice care and criteria for admission, and the use and limitations of advance directives.[49] He makes it clear that PDIA endorsement was a major spur to his efforts:

> The recognition that the Project on Death in America has provided to this institution and myself has greatly facilitated my ability to get out throughout the state and serve as a platform for providing education to health-care professionals about the need to improve end-of-life care—the many different facets of end-of-life care, whether it's pain management, reaching out to diverse communities, being sensitive to the needs of under-served patients, and trying to address their very unique needs...I'm proud to say that we have quite a few electives and pieces that are worked in the various parts of medical school curricula, so in a short time we made some real change. I'd like to attribute a great part of that to the Project on Death in America's support. I would say it's had a real impact.[50]

Tammie Quest, as we saw in chapter 4, worked in the area of emergency medicine and established a curriculum in palliative care for residents. Faculty scholars Richard Brumley and Kris Hillary combined physician and nurse perspectives and built on work at the Kaiser Permanente Tri-Central Service in California to provide support for others to replicate the Kaiser model elsewhere. In Colorado, Daniel Johnson focused his efforts on decreasing symptom distress at the end

---

48. P. B. Mullan et al., "End-of-Life Care Education in Internal Medicine Residency Programs: An Inter-Institutional Study," *Journal of Palliative Medicine* 5, no. 4 (2002): 487–496.

49. G. J. Taylor and J. Kurent (eds.), *A Clinician's Guide to Palliative Care* (New York: Wiley-Blackwell, 2003).

50. Jerome Kurent, interview by Thomas Lynch, April 8, 2004.

of life through evidence-based education at the University of Colorado Health Sciences Center. Joseph Weiner developed a structured communication training program for physicians and medical students to build confidence in establishing conversations with patients about advanced care planning.[51]

Several faculty scholars showed a huge capacity to work together on issues of medical education in end-of-life care. Notable among these were the efforts of Frank Ferris and Charles von Gunten, working with PDIA grantee Linda Emmanuel,[52] to promote the program entitled Education in Palliative and End of Life Care (EPEC).[53] EPEC's mission to educate all health-care professionals on the essential clinical competencies in palliative care was hugely successful, and it continued to do this and to expand its audiences over time, often involving PDIA scholars and grantees in its training courses.

In 1997, PDIA activists Susan Block, David Barnard, and Andrew Billings were involved in a national consensus conference on medical education near the end of life.[54] Led by the three, a twelve-strong steering committee of national experts, including PDIA faculty scholars and grantees, worked to develop a national consensus conference on Medical Education for Care Near the End of Life, held in Washington, DC, May 16–17, 1997, and jointly organized with the Robert Wood Johnson Foundation. The meeting involved some ninety participants representing senior elements of the world of academic medicine in the United States, as well as experts within the field of palliative medicine; nineteen of the then thirty-eight PDIA scholars attended, many in leadership roles. It sought to bring together the wide array of groups with expertise in education near the end of life; to promote collaboration between them; to share innovative methods; and to create a consensus statement on values and priorities for medical education in the field. The rationale behind the meeting was that, at that time, a number of professional groups and clinical societies had recently stepped up their efforts to develop standards of practice for care near the end of life and were engaging in educational strategies to promote enhanced care. So an opportunity was available to bring together these groups to harness collective experience, wisdom, and authority with the purpose of leveraging change in the content, structure, and culture of medical education for end-of-life care. There were also models to build on from Canada and the United Kingdom, as well as the United States. The

---

51. J. S. Weiner and S. A. Cole "Three Principles to Improve Clinician Communication for Advance Care Planning: Overcoming Emotional, Cognitive, and Skill Barriers," *Journal of Palliative Medicine* 7, no. 6 (2004): 817–829.

52. A PDIA grant of $43,775 was made to Linda Emanuel to provide for the worldwide webcasting of a training conference videotape so that each of the sixteen modules in the EPEC curriculum could be made available on the Internet.

53. Education in Palliative and End-of-Life Care, http://www.epec.net/EPEC/webpages/index. cfm, (accessed March 4, 2009; site discontinued). The current website is http://epec.net/.

54. D. E. Simpson, "Introduction to the National Consensus Conference on Medical Education for Care Near the End of Life: Executive Summary," *Journal of Palliative Medicine* 3, no. 1 (2000): 87–92.

organizers saw a major challenge in respecting the differences in clinical settings and professional orientations among the various providers of end-of-life care education, in such a way as to avoid a one-size-fits-all approach. They took the view, for example, that intensive care emergency medicine, obstetrics and peri-natal medicine, pediatrics, and the care of persons with AIDS should all be seen as particular end-of-life contexts that may or may not fit the "supportive oncol-ogy" model of palliative care that had come to dominate curricular discussion."[55] The work took place in small groups over two days, each addressing a particular clinical context, such as advance care planning, pain and symptom manage-ment, psychosocial and spiritual care, as well as matters relating to workers' own attitudes, feelings, and experiences. The groups explored barriers to improving education about end-of-life care, such as high service demands, lack of opportu-nities to see patients as "people," and lack of faculty with the relevant expertise. They worked together on a consensus statement, as well as on plans for publica-tions addressed to medical educators in the various clinical specialties.

The published summary of the conference made four recommendations to improve education in palliative care: (1) the Liaison Committee on Medical Education should include a requirement that all medical students demonstrate competence in end-of-life care as a condition of medical school graduation; (2) the residency review committees, primary care specialties, and all other special-ties in which there is significant contact with dying patients, would set minimum standards for faculty training in end-of-life care and for resident experiences in care of dying patients and, to ensure competency, program directors should require direct observation of residents while interacting with dying patients and their families; (3) medical specialty boards should integrate end-of-life care into their examinations; and (4) public and private funding sources, including the National Institutes of Health, should be encouraged to support programs that train faculty, so as to meet the shortage of faculty trained in end-of-life care.[56]

The United States has over 600,000 social workers and they comprise the larg-est single group of mental health workers in the nation. The have multiple and complex involvements with end-of-life issues. In social work, the breakthrough to becoming a priority area within PDIA came on November 13, 1997 at the United Hospital Fund in New York, when PDIA organized a roundtable dis-cussion on the Role of Social Workers in End of Life Care, with twenty partici-pants. The invitations came from Patricia Prem, PDIA's board member trained in social work, who explained that the discussions would concern "programs to support social work leaders in becoming more effective change agents in improving end-of-life care" and they would be used to inform the development

55. Proposal to Project on Death in America: "National Consensus Conference on Medical Education for Care Near the End of Life" (n.d.), Box 734892: Medical Education for Care at the End of Life, May 15–18, 1997.

56. National Consensus Conference on Medical Education for Care Near the End of Life, Executive Summary" (n.d.), Box 734892: Medical Education for Care at the End of Life, May 15–18, 1997.

of appropriate programs.[57] The goal of the meeting was to explore the place of social workers within end-of-life care and the methods whereby they could be most effective. For some time, the idea did not move forward, but then the findings of a key article by Grace Christ and Mary Sormanti, published in 1999 and later developed in a white paper for PDIA, showed that social workers did not feel adequately trained in end-of-life care issues and considered that the training did not address their needs or the range of services that they provided. It also revealed a dearth of leadership and the absence of an organization that could advocate for them in working with dying patients.[58] Now more persuaded, in the following year, 2000, the board launched the PDIA Social Work Leadership Program. It had many facets.

In California, John Linder of the UC Davis Cancer Center set out to develop a statewide coalition of schools of social work and schools of theology. He explains the aims of his project:

> To design and then teach a graduate-level course that would bring social workers and spiritual care providers together to examine both our own collective mortality and spirituality and then to look at how can we collaborate more closely as disciplines in helping patients and the people who love them to go through the dying process.[59]

Like many of the social work leaders and faculty scholars, he benefited from collaboration with and support from other's working within PDIA, in this case social work leader Iris Cohen Fineberg. She had developed a program to train social work and medical students together in teamwork and family conferencing skills,[60] so there were parallels with Linder's interdisciplinary orientation:

> I designed all kind of exercises and opportunities for the social work students and the medical students to do things together either in small groups or in the large group, and in different configurations, so that they would have to really interact with each other on a variety of topics. So the focus was very much on the interdisciplinary process and learning about each other. My thoughts behind that were that, first of all, we knew that educational systems for health-care professionals were lacking in opportunities

---

57. P. Prem, letter of invitation to meeting (n.d.), Box 734892: SW Meeting, October 30, 1997.

58. G. H. Christ and M. Sormanti, "Advancing Social Work Practice in End of Life Care," *Social Work and Health Care* 30, no. 2 (1999): 81–99.

59. John Linder, interview by David Clark, July 13, 2004.

60. Cohen Fineberg also collaborated with PDIA faculty scholars Neil Wenger and Lachlan Forrow in evaluating her program. See I. C. Fineberg, "Preparing Professionals for Family Conferences in Palliative Care: Evaluation Results of an Interdisciplinary Approach," *Journal of Palliative Medicine* 8, no. 4 (2005), 857–866; and I. C. Fineberg, N. S. Wenger, and L. Forrow, "Interdisciplinary Education: Evaluation of Palliative Care Training for Pre-Professionals," *Academic Medicine* 79, no. 8 (2004), 769–776.

to learn about end-of-life care, but we also know that end-of-life care ideally is supposed to be interdisciplinary. And one of the thoughts I had was that shouldn't we really teach people how to do that early on and certainly expose them to doing it very early on in their careers if we really want them to be comfortable and adept at it later when they become full professionals and then perfect those skills over a lifetime?[61]

Elizabeth Chaitin, at the University of Pittsburgh Medical Center, also developed an interdisciplinary educational program and collaborated with PDIA faculty scholar Robert Arnold on the ethics of consultation in the intensive care unit.[62]

Others focused specifically on the social work profession, with a number of targeted interventions and programs. Susan Blacker worked on a post-masters' training opportunity to encourage new graduates in social work to focus on palliative care and she also established a network to promote collaboration and training. Ellen Csikai and Mary Raymer developed a national survey of social workers in various practice settings to determine current preparation in end-of-life care and the perceived educational needs. Amanda Sutton used the Internet to create a forum for social work education in end-of-life care.[63] David Cherin developed a summer workshop at the University of Washington to assist participants in designing research and demonstration projects. Jane Lindberg designed a bereavement training program in Fresno, California. Bruce Paradis developed a MSW offering at Salem State College involving a year-long field placement in an end-of-life care setting. In Kentucky, Sherri Weisnfluh built a cross-state collaboration to promote culturally sensitive end-of-life care.[64]

Jim Kerustury implemented a survey of social worker involvement in end-of-life care that he had already conducted in West Virginia to establish a network of support, information, and education:

I used the results of that survey as the baseline for developing a project that would pull together a network of end-of-life social workers in West Virginia and offer them opportunities to network with each other, to share information and, quite frankly, frustrations, and everything else that goes along with that, and in addition, offering training opportunities, and also looking for ways to integrate social workers into the movement in West Virginia that was really starting to pick up a lot of momentum, and that movement was looking at ways to improve end-of-life care, and I feel that social workers needed to definitely be involved in that movement in the state.[65]

61. Iris Cohen Fineberg, interview by David Clark, July 12, 2004.

62. M. Aulisio, E. Chaitin, and R. Arnold, "Ethics and Palliative Care Consultation in the Intensive Care Unit," *Critical Care Ethics* 20, no. 3 (2004): 505–523.

63. "New 2001 Grantees: Social Work Leaders," *PDIA Newsletter*, no. 9 (December 2001), 15.

64. "Social Work Leadership Development Awards," *Project on Death in America, January 2001–December 2003, Report of Activities* (New York: Open Society Institute, 2004). 24–33.

65. James Kerustury, interview by David Clark, July 11, 2004.

David Browning was one of the small number of PDIA social workers who took a special interest in education for pediatric palliative care. His interest was in developing a curriculum in this area directed at hospital-based staff, and to bring a social work perspective to bear in looking at how staff learn and the informal and hidden aspects of the curriculum that support learning.[66] He described it as "trying to create a learning environment that challenges the way knowledge gets held inside health-care institutions and challenges the authority of whose knowledge gets to have power."[67] Others focused on the creation of Internet-based resources, such as Karen Bullock with an online Resource Enrichment Center for improving end-of-life care at the University of Connecticut School of Social Work,[68] and Terry Wolfer and Vicki Runnion, who developed an online selection of decision cases for educational purposes. Eventually published as a book in 2008, it comprised twenty-three challenging case scenarios that are left unresolved at a point when a practicing social worker would have to carefully evaluate the issues before making decisions. Written for advanced courses in social work, it was also supported by additional teaching notes on the publisher's website.[69]

A major point to come out of the social work summit of 2002 related to the absence of suitable textbook material to support social work education in end-of-life care. A project undertaken with PDIA support by Betty J. Kramer and colleagues had three goals: (1) to develop end-of-life guidelines for the social work profession, (2) to use these guidelines to conduct a critical review of fifty textbooks frequently used in social work education, and (3) to write a text that would address some of the gaps identified.[70] Betty Kramer herself co-edited a major volume, *Men as Caregivers*, that explored issues of theory, research, and service development.[71] But the key outcome of the review was a major work edited by PDIA-funded social work leader Joan Berzoff together with international end-of-life and bereavement expert Phyllis R. Silverman entitled *Living*

---

66. This theme of the "hidden curriculum" was also pursued by faculty scholar Michael Rabow in his project at the Medical Center of Mount Zion in San Francisco, entitled *Between the Blackboard and the Bedside: An Examination of the Hidden Curriculum in Palliative Care*, in which he sought to develop an intervention to address educational barriers to training in end-of-life care.

67. David Browning, interview by David Clark, July 13, 2004.

68. K. Bullock, "Resource Enrichment Center: An Internet Resource for Working with Terminally Ill Patients and Families," In E. L. Csikai and B. Jones (eds.), *Social Work in End-of-Life and Palliative Care: A Compendium of Syllabi and Teaching Resources* (Chicago: Lyceum Books, 2007).

69. T. A. Wolfer and V. M. Runnion (eds.), *Dying, Death, and Bereavement in Social Work Practice: Decision Cases for Advanced Practice* (New York: Columbia University Press, 2008).

70. B. J. Kramer, L. Pacourek, and C. Hovland-Scafe, "Analysis of End of Life Content in Social Work Textbooks," *Journal of Social Work Education* 39 (2003): 299–320.

71. B. J. Kramer and E. H. Thompson, *Men as Caregivers: Theory, Research, and Service Implications* (New York: Springer, 2002).

with Dying: A Handbook for End-of-Life Healthcare Practitioners.[72] Written by
social workers, containing 44 chapters and spanning 896 pages, the book was a
tour de force. Its breadth was seen as a reflection of the wide range of social work
involvements in palliative care, though some caviled with the notion that it was
the first book of its kind for health-care workers.[73] One reviewer noted: "It is hard
to imagine that any social worker who works with loss, chronic illness, or the
dying will not benefit by having this important resource readily accessible."[74]

Joan Berzoff herself describes at length what the book was about and how it
came into being:

> Well this truly has been a labor of love and I consider it a testament to my
> [late] sister and to her struggles and to our struggles as a family. It is a text-
> book that we hope will be used by social workers whomever they may be
> and wherever they may be who encounter end-of-life issues. So it's not only
> for the palliative and hospice care social workers...it's for a range of set-
> tings but we also hope to reach people outside of social work, occupational
> therapists, respiratory therapists, the kinds of people who are auxiliary
> to end-of-life care work who will really need to know about what it is to
> be present with a client or family, or how one conducts a family confer-
> ence, or how one runs a group, or how one makes use of telling bad news or
> informed consent, or just a range of issues that are presented in the book.
> The book begins with five narratives of practitioners, advanced practition-
> ers whose own lives were transformed by loss and how they have used those
> losses to transform their careers. I write one; there is one written that is
> magnificent by a social worker from a children's hospital whose child died
> of leukemia in that hospital and she is able to elucidate the ways in which
> she suddenly went from being a subject and a member of a department to an
> object and someone who was feared and avoided, and she talks beautifully
> from her heart about the experience and then about how that transformed
> her practice. David Browning, likewise, has an absolutely gorgeous chapter
> about the death of his mother and how that has influenced his thinking,
> his career, and his soul essentially. There are a number of chapters that are
> so moving. That was the tone we wanted to set, a very experienced "near"
> tone...the voices of real people who are social work practitioners whose
> struggles shape and inform their practice every day. Then the textbook
> moves to theoretical issues in end-of-life care, and that means psychologi-
> cal theoretical issues, spiritual theoretical issues, ethical theoretical issues,
> social theoretical issues. Many chapters are dedicated to social theories,

72. J. Berzoff and P. R. Silverman (eds.), *Living with Dying: A Handbook for End-of-Life
Healthcare Practitioners* (New York: Columbia University Press, 2004).

73. F. C. Zanger, review of J. Berzoff and P. R. Silverman (eds.), *Living with Dying.* In *American
Journal of Hospice and Palliative Care* 21 (2004): 474.

74. M. J. Loscalzo, review of J. Berzoff and P. R. Silverman (eds.), *Living with Dying.* In *Journal
of Palliative Medicine* 9, no. 2 (2006): 494–495.

psychological theories, lifespan developmental theories, postmodern theories, psychodynamic theories, as they relate to end-of-life care practice. The book then changes its lens again to talk about practice—individual, group, family, family conferencing—but also to talk about the range of settings in which this work occurs, including places like prisons and schools and low-income communities, and with multicultural populations, with people who are disadvantaged by social class or race or gender or sexual orientation. Then the book moves to policy issues, ethical policy issues, legal policy issues, and a range of other reimbursement issues... and then finally we move to research and the ongoing need for research in end-of-life care, again using so many of the fellows from PDIA.[75]

Another major contribution to the establishment of social work as a significant player in the field was the creation of the *Journal of Social Work in End-of-Life and Palliative Care*, which published its first issue in 2005 under the founding editorship of PDIA grantee Ellen Csikai. The journal quickly established itself as a platform for academic and social work practitioner research, articles, and continuing features on the state of the art of social work practice, including interdisciplinary interventions, practice innovations, practice evaluations, end-of-life decision making, grief and bereavement, and ethical and moral issues. Many PDIA grantees and social work leaders populated its pages.

Building on these successes, and as PDIA was coming to a close, the National Association of Social Work (NASW) became involved to shore up and maintain the social work legacy. Elizabeth J. Clark, NASW executive director and PDIA grantee explains:

We proposed three things from NASW. The first was that we would take the work that had been done to date and we would turn it into formal standards of practice for social workers... a lot of work had already been done by PDIA scholars and by the group and we felt if we could actually institutionalize the standards and say these are the standards of practice for palliative and end-of-life care in social work... The second thing we proposed was to try and reach practicing social workers. One of my concerns about the PDIA program is that it has a very heavy academic focus and while I think it is wonderful to be training young social workers about palliative and end-of-life care, I say it'll take a generation before we have enough people trained to make a difference, because in the United States, we turn out about thirty-four thousand social workers a year at the bachelors', masters', and doctoral level. But if you look at the number that are practicing, we estimate right now that the number is around 607,000 practicing social workers, and those are professionally trained people, not just people in social work roles but professionally trained. My concern always is how do we get those 600,000 social workers who probably are not going to go back

---

75. Joan Berzoff, interview by David Clark, July 12, 2004.

to school, how do we train them in end-of-life care? So my concern was to try and find a mechanism to do that. The idea of having a Web course, because our website is so heavily visited, seemed like a good opportunity for us, so that was the second thing we proposed. We had the standards, we had the end-of-life Web course. And then the third thing was that we also have a mechanism where every three years we set policies…surrounding palliative care and end-of-life care. So that was the third thing…we had a policy that had been done previously; we would use the scholars from the program to help us update that policy and then that would be adopted at the next delegate assembly, which is actually summer of 2005. So those were the three things we proposed. Those are the three things that we've done.[76]

It was an impressive outcome of the PDIA social workers program and did much to consolidate its aims, both outside the academy and within the grassroots of the social work profession. It was complemented by many ongoing activities by social work leadership grantees, including two other members of the program who followed up with another major textbook, this time primarily aimed at educators and students.[77]

There can be no doubt that across the disciplines of medicine, nursing, and social work, PDIA was successful in reaching its goal to stimulate and kick-start a program of activity in palliative and end-of-life care education. It was not the major funder or initiator of the largest initiatives (EPEC, ELNEC), but it complemented and enhanced these and, in particular, many of its grantees and scholars had overlapping commitments with other funders in palliative care education that proved mutually energizing and added to a wider sense of strengthening the field at a time when education initiatives were badly needed.

SPECIALIZATION, RECOGNITION, AND INTERDISCIPLINARY ISSUES

Building on this work in research and education on end-of-life issues, there was also a growing preoccupation with how best to promote endorsement of palliative care as a specialist field of activity. This meant not only the existence of research and education programs and a body of published and peer reviewed literature, but also the organizational and policy recognition of key professional organizations, as well as agreed systems of accreditation, governance, and reimbursement. As PDIA moved forward, and especially as it wound down to closure, these issues occupied a growing amount of attention on the part of the board. Bo Burt was particularly upbeat about this:

---

76. Betsy Clark, interview by David Clark, July 12, 2004.

77. E. L. Csikai and B. Jones (eds.), *Social Work in End-of-Life and Palliative Care: A Compendium of Syllabi and Teaching resources.* (Chicago: Lyceum Books, 2007).

We created a field. That's very exciting. There was no field before. We've created a field that works with the most desperate, needy people, who are people who are dying, and we have really done it in a way, particularly with the faculty scholars, in giving these young professionals an opportunity to spend their lives in this service role, but in a way that had not been imagined until then. With our first cohort, it was interesting because they were the only people in the field aside from Susan [Block]: it was a *very* small field. But after that, everybody that we brought in, [these] were people who had thought that there was something attractive to them in dealing with death and dying, but if we hadn't existed, there was no path for them to take. But they were all very unusual people in terms of the practice of medicine. They were unusual in a number of ways. They were willing to define themselves as very much outside the prized modality of medicine, which is cure. At the beginning of our work, to be sure...physicians who worked in dying were scorned amongst their kind, and they did it for their own special reasons but they knew that they were outcasts. This was particularly true in the first cohort. It was one of the powers of bringing them together—they didn't have a professional cohort of which they were a member. They were doing good stuff that they believed in, but they were very isolated, kind of scorned by their colleagues, and they had nobody else. You know, they were lonely let me put it this way, and death itself is incredibly lonely and lonely-making. But they were soldiering on. And what we gave to the first cohort was a sense that "you're not alone," that there are people here who will support you.[78]

By the close of 1999, the PDIA newsletter could point to some successes in this regard and stated: "After five years of funding programs, the Project on Death in America is seeing signs of progress resulting from its activities and the efforts of other foundations, organizations, and individuals working to improve end-of-life care."[79] The article listed five newly created chairs in palliative care, all working in hospital settings and all in the New York area, and four of them had been beneficiaries of the United Hospital Fund's Hospital Palliative Care Initiative (see chapter 4). Three were PDIA faculty scholars: Diane Meier, Peter Selwyn, and Daniel Sulmasy; and the other two were PDIA grantees: Russell Portenoy and Richard Payne. There was evidence here of the combined effect of PDIA's initiatives and support programs—and their potential to build long-term capacity at a high level. Portenoy explained the goal succinctly:

To get every practitioner in a hospital to accept the principles of palliative care and [to] practice them, and to establish in every hospital a specialized

78. Bo Burt, interview by David Clark, July 23, 2003.

79. "Signs of Progress: New Chairs Advance Palliative Care in Hospitals," *PDIA Newsletter*, no. 6 (December 1999), 6–7.

program in palliative care with a comprehensive team approach, research and training, and interaction with hospice."[80]

Part of the success of such an approach would be determined by the potential to recruit palliative care fellows to work in training posts in key departments. To this end, as we saw in chapter 1, PDIA worked in 2002 with the Emily Davie and the Joseph S. Kornfeld Foundation to provide funds for six fellowship programs designed to "help move the field forward so that palliative care becomes more widely recognized as an essential component of medical education and clinical practice" and move it toward the "ultimate goal"—that of a "fully certified subspecialty of medicine."[81] Such accreditation presented a complex challenge and one which gained increasing attention in the closing years of PDIA operations.

The development of palliative medicine in the United States has been seen in three phases:[82] (1) the period until the work of Elizabeth Kübler-Ross and Cicely Saunders became known, (2) the development of hospice programs across the country, and (3) the development of a distinct and officially recognized subspecialty of medicine. Within this scheme, the path to subspecialty recognition for palliative medicine in the United States began in 1988 with the creation of the Academy of Hospice Physicians, later the American Academy of Hospice and Palliative Medicine. Further progress was made in the 1990s when the Institute of Medicine, the American College of Physicians, and the American Board of Internal Medicine all highlighted the need for greater physician competency in the care of persons with terminal illness.

The American Board of Hospice and Palliative Medicine (ABHPM) was formed in 1995 to establish and implement standards for certification of physicians practicing hospice and palliative medicine and, ultimately, accreditation of physician training in the discipline. The ABHPM created a certification process that paralleled other member boards of the American Board of Medical Specialties (ABMS). A paper published in 2000 by PDIA faculty scholar Charles von Gunten and colleagues showed that in the first three and a half years of the existence of ABMS, and over the administration of seven examinations, 623 physicians achieved board certification in hospice and palliative medicine. Those with ABMS primary board certifications were certified by anesthesiology (4 percent), family practice (23 percent), internal medicine (55 percent), pediatrics (1 percent), radiation oncology (2 percent), and surgery (2 percent). Applicants were drawn from forty-eight American states, as well as from Canada and three other countries. The authors concluded that there was significant physician interest in seeking professional recognition of expertise in caring for terminally ill persons

---

80. "Signs of Progress" *PDIA Newsletter*, 7.

81. "PDIA Announces New Funding Initiative," *PDIA Newsletter*, no. 10 (Summer 2002), 2.

82. T. Ryndes and C. F. von Gunten, "The Development of Palliative Medicine in the USA." In E. Bruera et al. (eds.), *Textbook of Palliative Medicine* (London: Hodder Arnold, 2006), 29–35.

and their families through the creation of a specialty in hospice and palliative medicine with certification of physicians and accreditation of training programs as key elements in the process.[83]

To support these developments, PDIA made a three-year grant in 2001 to the American Board of Hospice and Palliative Medicine for an initiative that had three aims:

1. To develop a consensus within medicine on the appropriate organizational base for a subspecialty in palliative medicine
2. To seek ABMS approval for such a subspecialty within one or more existing specialties of medicine
3. To seek formation of a residency review committee within the Accreditation Council of Graduate Medical Education (ACGME) to implement accreditation guidelines for palliative medicine fellowship programs.

Modern medical specialties are built around the twin pillars of accreditation of education and certification of competency. For the subspecialty of hospice and palliative medicine to be taken seriously as a mature medical discipline, it required credible accreditation and certification processes. The grant resources from PDIA enabled ABHPM to undertake activities designed to achieve the strategic goals of (1) ABMS subspecialty certification in palliative medicine and (2) ACGME accreditation of palliative medicine fellowships. Achieving these goals was of crucial importance in giving the subspecialty of hospice and palliative medicine an institutional "seat" within the formal professional organizations of medicine. Institutionalizing the specialty (through ABMS recognition and ACGME accreditation) would help to assure that the achievements of palliative medicine to date were passed on to the next generation of physicians and that knowledge in the field continued to grow.

There were some significant accomplishments in these endeavors during the ABHPM grant period covered by PDIA. The Palliative Medicine Review Committee (PMRC) conducted initial accreditation of fellowship programs in the expectation that these would subsequently be "grandfathered" into accreditation by ACGME. To support this, voluntary accreditation standards were developed for fellowship programs, and meetings were hosted for fellowship directors. By the end of the initiative, ABHPM had engaged in increasingly cordial discussions with the leadership of several ABMS boards regarding the sponsorship of an application to ABMS for a formal subspecialty in hospice and palliative medicine. In the three-year period of the initiative, from the end of 2000 through the close of 2003, the number of diplomates almost doubled from 779 to 1,538. Another critical concern to the ABMS was whether there would be a sufficient number of graduates of fellowship training programs to sustain the field at a

83. C. von Gunten et al., "Physician Board Certification in Hospice and Palliative Medicine," *Journal of Palliative Medicine* 3, no. 4 (2000): 441–447.

steady state. In fact, the number of fellowship programs quickly expanded from just a handful to approximately forty-five, and it was anticipated that close to one hundred fellows would graduate annually in the coming years. A critical contribution of the PDIA funding was to enable ABHPM to enlarge staff resources sufficiently to carry out the complex set of activities needed to achieve full recognition of the subspecialty of palliative medicine. PDIA funding supported a portion of the CEO's time and a portion of the program administrator's time. This allowed ABHPM staff to coordinate communication with ABMS, ACGME, and ABMS boards, to lead the start-up of accreditation activities through the PMRC, and to inform the hospice/palliative medicine community about strategies for achieving recognition. As a result of the PDIA initiative, ABHPM was able to develop a sustainable staff infrastructure to allow it to continue to provide significant leadership to the palliative care field.

Throughout the period of the initiative, ABHPM staff and trustees carried out a campaign of strategic communications to educate both leaders and grassroots professionals in the palliative medicine field about the steps needed to bring about formal recognition. This included regular communication with the board of the American Academy of Hospice and Palliative Medicine, presentations at the Academy annual meeting (notably, a keynote presentation to the membership by ABHPM chairman and PDIA faculty scholar Charles von Gunten), regular communications to Academy members through the Academy newsletter, communications to the board's own diplomates, and publication of several articles in the *Journal of Palliative Medicine*. To achieve formal recognition, it was considered important to build support that would be tangible and visible to the leadership of the other specialty disciplines. It was a huge challenge.

Diane Meier, speaking in 2003, captured well some of the pressures and issues:

Well, perhaps this is as a result of my having worked my entire career in the ivory tower of academic medicine, but it is my perspective and belief that if we ignore the power structures of medicine, we do so at our peril, and that in order to have power to influence what happens to patients and families, the line is *pay to play*. We have to, in order to get fellowship support, be an American Board of Medical Specialties approved medical specialty. In order to do that there are certain ducks we have to get lined up. There has to be a certain number of fellowships; there has to be a certain number of applicants for those fellowships; those fellows, when they finish, have to be employable. They don't want to create a new medical specialty when there's "no there there." So there's been a real effort over recent years—Charles von Gunten has spearheaded this, another cohort one PDIA faculty scholar—to very logically and rationally and sequentially line up all those requirements so that when we went to them, there would be nothing we hadn't done before we got there that they would look for, and so they couldn't send us away. And we're there. It's been very strategic and very longitudinal in the planning. And the result will be that palliative medicine will be just as legitimate as critical care medicine, and have just as much a right to exist, and have trainees and have NIH funding and have publications in major journals... it's all about being in there with the big boys, being legitimate, having a place at the table.[84]

As we shall see in chapter 9, in 2006, and after PDIA had closed, the Accreditation Council for Graduate Medical Education (ACGME) and the American Board of Medical Specialties (ABMS) approved and recognized a new specialty in hospice and palliative medicine. The case of medicine provides the most concrete and tangible example of specialist status being accorded to the practice of palliative care. In the cognate fields of nursing and social work, the challenges were slightly different and the resulting processes varied accordingly.

In January 1999, PDIA embarked on a major initiative in nursing with the launch of the Nursing Leadership Consortium on End-of-Life Care. The consortium was developed to advance the nursing profession's commitment and efforts to improve palliative care and brought together key national nursing organizations with education, administration, research, practice, and policy responsibility, as well as specialty organizations with particular expertise in end-of-life care to develop a coordinated, broad-based plan within the profession. The quality of care provided to persons near the end of life was described as being of the utmost concern to nurses, individually and collectively, and it was acknowledged that nurses in all practice settings and roles face quandaries about the provision of humane and dignified end-of-life care. Moreover, care of the dying occurs across the lifespan and is rendered across all settings including hospitals, long-term care facilities, hospices, and home environments, so that attention to the specialized care of dying people should be integrated into all clinical and education contexts and should permeate the practice of all health professionals. The consortium acknowledged that throughout the decades, nurses have been the mainstay of care for dying persons and their families and have played a vital role in promoting responsible, competent, compassionate, appropriate, and ethically sound care. Now, with the convergence of significant trends in legislation, societal opinion, judicial decisions, research involvement, and media interest, a time had come to highlight nursing concern about the quality of end-of-life care.

The specific aims of the consortium were (1) to formalize a collaborative and supportive effort within the nursing profession focused on end-of-life care; (2) to examine available educational materials, clinical guidelines, conferences proceedings on end-of-life care within nursing; (3) to develop mechanisms of collaboration and resource sharing between nursing organizations; (4) to identify gaps and future needs within the policy, research, education, administration, and practice domains of nursing; (5) to recommend specific strategies; and (6) to build agreement on a plan to improve the organization, delivery, and quality of care for those who are dying.

---

84. Diane Meier, interview by David Clark, July 22, 2003.

The consortium was an attempt to provide an organized and coordinated approach to improvements in end of-life care in nursing and to make responsible plans for new initiatives. It sought to clarify and establish an end-of-life care agenda for nursing and to contribute to interdisciplinary and consumer efforts. It would also seek to be a vehicle for new strategic partnerships, to identify funding and create mechanisms for continued communications and collaboration. The consortium meeting of June 12–14, 1999 brought together thirty-four individuals representing twenty-three nursing specialty organizations, the National Institutes of Health, PDIA, the Robert Wood Johnson Foundation, and other institutions with a variety of perspectives on end-of-life care to engage in a systematic, facilitated process for developing new projects and increasing collaboration on existing relevant activities. The participating organizations represented over 600,000 nurses in combined memberships. Working together over a two-day period, using a facilitated design process known as *interactive management*, the group was able to produce an informed and thoughtful program for nursing professionals concerning end-of-life care. The agenda that resulted from the consortium was claimed to be much more than a simple collection of good ideas from qualified individuals, but rather a consensus of views on a range of key issues. The result was a strong statement from the nursing profession. While this was not the first time that an agenda for end-of-life care had been produced, it did constitute the most thorough attempt ever to examine the issue from the perspective of American nursing professionals and sought to help those concerned with nursing issues to speak with what it called a "unified and amplified voice." For the immediate future the agenda was a reliable guide for funders, researchers, practicing health-care professionals, and others concerned with end-of-life care in the nursing context.[85]

Despite the rhetoric of the report, however, and the considerable financial investment made by PDIA, this was an initiative where it was hard to trace major tangible outcomes and where obvious "products" were difficult to identify.[86] When the Nursing Academy reconvened three years later in March of 2002, some of the progress metrics looked modest: eighteen new articles in nursing journals, six national nursing conferences that had palliative and end-of-life care on the agenda, and two organizations writing core curricula on patient care at the end of life. Despite this, further PDIA funding was provided to sustain and mentor the first cohort of nurse leaders and to support a second cohort from

85. Designing an Agenda for the Nursing Profession on End-of-Life Care was funded by The Open Society Institute: Project on Death in America, and organized by the American Association of Critical-Care Nurses. Consortium Coordinators: C. H. Rushton, RN, DNSc, FAAN; C. Scanlon, RN, JD; B. Ferrell, RN, PhD, FAAN. Workshop report released November 1999, American Association of Critical-Care Nurses.

86. Subsequently there appeared to be rather poor communication between the consortium coordinators and the PDIA office, with a resulting lack of impact.

twenty-three nursing organizations.[87] Then in the PDIA exit strategy, a grant of $200,000 was made to the Hospice and Palliative Nurses Association (HPNA) to advance professional nursing education by building on the work of the End-of-Life Nursing Education Consortium (ELNEC). Having delivered national provision of nursing education to hundreds of nursing educators and to nursing specialists in geriatrics, pediatrics, oncology, and hospice and palliative care, ELNEC was thereby able to continue to benefit from PDIA support, even beyond 2003. Johns Hopkins was well positioned to do this, having supported nursing leadership development and assisted in the integration of palliative and end-of-life care into no less than forty-four nursing specialty organizations. HPNA in turn had recognized that palliative and end-of-life care issues receive little attention in nursing homes and long-term care settings and was able to use the funding to initiate ELNEC courses in these settings with a goal of recruiting 50 percent of participants from long-term settings. On completion of the course, participants became members of a newly established *Community of Practice*, designed to meet their ongoing needs for support and education in end-of-life care.[88]

In March 2002 at Duke University, the three-day summit organized by the Social Work Leaders Program addressed, among other things, the gaps in social work education on end-of-life care at undergraduate, graduate, and postgraduate levels. The summit encouraged collaborative efforts between schools of social work, practice sites, and professional groups, and served to highlight some of the innovative approaches being developed by PDIA-funded social workers involved in educational programs.[89, 90]

An article by Katherine Walshe-Burke of the School of Social Work at Springfield College, Massachusetts, examined the education programs that had been developed by PDIA social work leaders. Walshe-Burke showed that social work education at both the bachelor's and master's level lacked vital content about end-of-life care, palliative care, and bereavement. End-of-life care training opportunities through continuing education programs were also limited. These educational and training lacunae made for a significant problem in a context where social work saw itself as a discipline confronted extensively with end-of-life issues on a daily basis and in a variety of practice settings. Through the PDIA Social Work Leadership Development Awards initiative, many programs

87. C. H. Rushton, K. H. Sabatier, and K. L. Spencer, "Nursing Leadership Academy: Advancing the Agenda for Improving Care," *PDIA Newsletter*, no. 10 (Summer 2002), 6.

88. *Transforming the Culture of Dying: The Project on Death in America, October 1994 to December 2003* (New York: Open Society Institute, 2004).

89. "Social Workers Set Goals to Strengthen Care for the Dying and Bereaved," *PDIA Newsletter*, no. 10 (Summer 2002), 17–18.

90. G. Christ and S. Blacker, "Setting an Agenda for Social Work in End-of-Life and Palliative Care: An Overview of Leadership and Organizational Initiatives," *Journal of Social Work in End-of-Life and Palliative Care* 1, no. 1 (2005): 9–22.

and models for professional social work education and training in end-of-life care were developed and these were summarized in Walshe-Burke's article; they included end-of-life care courses, symposia, training manuals, certificate programs, and fellowships.[91] Grace Christ, leader of the program, elaborated on the details and decision making involved:

> Kathy Foley's idea, when we started talking about it, [was that] she wanted to include practitioners as well as academicians...And sometimes I think we would have been better off to go that way—they'll continue in the field. It's a little bit harder sometimes with practice people who have other options available to them. But at any rate, I think one of the strengths of our program has ended up being that it is...42 social workers, 50 percent are academicians or have PhDs, and 50 percent are masters' social workers who are in direct practice. So what they settled on was it would be a Social Work Leadership Development Awards program, and it would be aimed at trying to fund projects for social workers who are leaders, who would then come together and begin a dialogue, strengthen each other, support each other, and we would develop programs in research, education, and practice.[92]

As with nursing, the social work program received, within the PDIA exit strategy, a final grant of $200,000 to further promote this work. Under the leadership of Grace Christ and Susan Blacker, a second Social Work Summit on End-of-Life Care and Palliative Care was convened, taking place in Washington, DC, June 1–3, 2005. Hosted by the National Association of Social Workers with support from PDIA and the National Hospice and Palliative Care Organization, it built on the work of the first summit, with work groups focused on practice, research, policy, and education, and using "state of the field" presentations as a point of convergence for setting priorities and developing action plans.[93] Summit planners set out to continue momentum within the profession to make end-of-life and palliative care an important strategic area of focus. They sought to further develop a network of organizations and leaders, create a mechanism for collaborative efforts, and further the profession's evolution in a key area of policy/advocacy, practice, research, and education. It was evidence that the PDIA investment in social work and end-of-life care was continuing to have an effect.

This chapter has described in detail two core areas of PDIA-funded activity—research and education—and has tried to show how these contributed to a wider

---

91. K. Walshe-Burke, "Professional Social Work Education in End-of-Life Care Contributions of the Project on Death in America's Social Work Leadership Development Program," *Journal of Social Work in End-of-Life & Palliative Care* 1, no. 2 (2005): 11–36.

92. Grace Christ, interview by David Clark, October 27, 2004.

93. T. Altilio, G. Gardia, and S. Otis-Green, "Social Work Practice in Palliative and End-of-Life Care: A Report from the Summit," *Journal of Social Work in End-of-Life and Palliative Care* 3, no. 4 (2008): 68–86.

goal of strengthening the multidisciplinary field of palliative and end-of-life care as a specialty area of practice. PDIA devoted half of its funds to educational activities and produced a plethora of curricula, programs, and innovations. These contributed to "climate change" in the field, but at a level which has not been assessed or quantified. There were notable successes, however, and the new recognition given to end-of-life care content by those responsible for the training of doctors, nurses, and social workers was a major achievement. At many levels PDIA was able to demonstrate the gaps that existed in the provision of end-of-life care training and drew on a huge pool of experts who could give advice on how these could be filled. The recognition of palliative medicine as a subspecialty in its own right cannot be attributed solely to PDIA influence, but there is no doubt that those who engaged in this challenge and who successfully brought their expertise and energy to bear on it, drew in considerable part from their PDIA experience. We have also seen how, over the lifetime of PDIA, research endeavors in the field became more sophisticated and better organized, and as they did so, they found an audience in newly created specialist journals, as well as in the high impact mainstream scientific literature. If many of the early studies were descriptive and focused on service development and innovation rather than the measurement of outcome, then this can be forgiven as a necessary phase in the evolution of the field, and certainly one being encountered elsewhere in the world, even where specialty status had arrived earlier. PDIA scholars and grantees established themselves over the period as some of the world's leading researchers and innovators in end-of-life care studies, whose influence continued to be felt in the years following the closure of the program. This examination of the development of the specialist field of palliative care puts us in the right position to make some wider assessment of the work of PDIA, which is the subject of the next and penultimate chapter.

8

Assessing the Impact of the Project on Death in America

We have reached the point of making a summative interpretation and assessment of the work of PDIA. This chapter looks at three areas. First, it examines the way in which PDIA was structured and organized and offers some reflections on its administration and management. Second, it explores the special contribution made by the faculty scholars. Third, it considers the impact of the whole PDIA initiative and explores the extent to which the venture was successful in meeting its ambitious goal. This also provides an opportunity to reflect on the role of private philanthropy in endeavors that seek to promote change in society. It concludes that PDIA was a *necessary* but not *sufficient* condition for the transformation of the culture of dying in the United States. The task, as defined, was simply too complex, the parameters too daunting for the goal to be reached in nine years and within the available resources. Over 2.4 million Americans die annually. The patterns of dying, grieving, and mourning that exist across a society as culturally diverse as the United States have so far defied any single analysis. Moreover, the process of dying has become a territory increasingly occupied by conflicting ethical and moral viewpoints to the extent that defining a *culture* of dying and how it might be *transformed* becomes deeply problematic. In this context, it is not surprising that the ambitious goal of PDIA should have proved difficult to achieve. Making sense of the impact of PDIA therefore involves looking at how it was managed over time, how the program strategy changed, and how an exit strategy was forged that would leave behind continuing capacity for development in the field.

There can be no doubt that the PDIA board initially set a very ambitious goal when it embarked upon an endeavor to transform the culture of dying in the United States. Perhaps its weakness in this context was also that pervasive quality of Mr. George Soros himself, as recognized by one biographer: a hubristic orientation and self-confidence that just might be found wanting in the face of complexity and challenge on a grand scale.[1] In the early days particularly, there was perhaps a lack of realism on the part of board members who thought that an ambitious range of grant making across a spectrum of social and cultural issues could make a significant, identifiable, and measureable impact. Culture has a habit of not behaving in a predictable way and can have an obdurate quality that makes it resistant to calculated interventions defined by experts to bring about particular ends.

In the early years, the board supported a wide range of grants that focused on a diverse spectrum of projects. Some of them were conducted by individuals working outside of any obvious institutional arrangement—as filmmakers, poets, writers, and so on. These were the years in which the culture of dying, in its broadest sense, was attended to by PDIA. But going forward, this attention to culture could be seen to diminish as a concomitant rise took place in the engagement of PDIA with the "field" of palliative care and ways to strengthen it. If this was a loss, then it was a necessary one, as limited resources and a shortening timescale quickened the board's resolve to concentrate on a professional and policy agenda in an intentional strategy to promote capacity building in palliative care.

But if the *culture* could not be wholly transformed, then the field of end-of-life care, specifically the emerging speciality of palliative care, was undoubtedly amenable to major change. This indeed began to occur during the lifetime of PDIA and was undoubtedly attributable in significant part to the actions of the program, and especially the work of the faculty scholars. PDIA attempted to do more than it ultimately achieved, but clear success in addressing the professional agenda of palliative care would more than compensate for any other shortcomings born of well-intentioned but, ultimately, unrealistic goals and ambitions. If the culture of dying was not dramatically altered, the specialist area of palliative care certainly was, and PDIA can take much credit for it.

MODUS OPERANDI

The analysis presented here has placed the board at the very center of everything that PDIA did and managed to achieve. By the same token it is the board that can be held to account for what was not done or those things that might have been done differently. Yet the overall judgment on the workings of the board has to be a positive one, and that reflects hugely on the skill, wisdom, and deft handling displayed by its chair, Kathy Foley. It is difficult to avoid cloying praise here, but it is an interpretation that was shared by other key partners who

---

1. M. T. Kaufman, *Soros: The Life and Times of a Messianic Billionaire* (New York: Vintage Books, 2002).

worked with PDIA over the lifetime of its activities, including senior staff at the United Hospital Fund, the Robert Wood Johnson Foundation, and the National Institutes of Health. In Mary Callaway, she had the perfect foil. If Foley could nurture and inspire, Callaway could make sure the job got done. They disagreed at times but shared a common passion for the improvement of end-of-life care in the United States and beyond; and if one brought the accumulated wisdom of the health-care professional and researcher, the other had the lived experience of the family carer, and the unflagging attention to detail and administration that ensured things got done within budget and time frame. Most grantees and scholars found in Kathy Foley and Mary Callaway women of enormous generosity of spirit, with a limitless capacity for work that was inspiring and motivating. The group that made up PDIA staff was never large. Foley and Callaway were there throughout. They were supported over time by a series of able administrative staff: Jerry Garcia, Michael Pardy, and Lori McGlinchey.[2] PDIA seemed capable at times of a work rate way above its human resources capacity. It shifted paperwork on a grand scale, processed voluminous quantities of grant applications, annual updates, and final reports. On the office floor at OSI, it was regarded as a model venture within US programs.

Kathy Foley led a board that, despite some small personnel changes over time, remained active and involved in shaping the strategic direction of PDIA through its nine years. Board members showed huge energy for detailed discussion about strategy and the practical aspects of grant making that would enable policy to be put into practice. Their initial enthusiasm seemed to diminish little and even at the final retreats for faculty scholars and social work leaders that took place in 2003 and 2004, board members could be found actively engaged in the sessions and taking part in energetic discussions at the breakfast, lunch, and dinner table.

It might be observed that several board members received as much as they gave. Susan Block became heavily invested in the Faculty Scholars Program and felt a palpable sense of loss as it came to an end. Bo Burt found the inspiration in his work with PDIA to write a scholarly treatise on American culture, law, and death.[3] Patricia Prem and Ana Dumois appeared to draw great personal satisfaction from their work in promoting the development of social work in end-of-life care. David Rothman captures the sense of this personal engagement in the following:

> I don't think there was ever a selection committee or directors of a project that were as intimately involved with the day-to-day work of the group as

---

2. In addition to Kathy Foley and Mary Callaway, a full list of PDIA staff comprises: Virginia Brannigan; Michael Pardy; Lori McGlinchey; Jerry Garcia; Felicity Aulino; Sarah Cassetta; Kerri Demers; Ronnie Frankel; Nina Gadmer; Natalie Guttmann; Sallie Lynch; Julie McCrady; Abe Rein; Karen Siemenski; Toni Stanton; Diane Stedike; Edward Sunderland.

3. B. Burt, *Death Is That Man Taking Names: Intersections of American Medicine, Law, and Culture* (Berkeley and Los Angeles: University of California Press/Millbank Books on Health and the Public, 2002).

Project on Death in America. Why? I would attribute a good deal of it to the fact that we were doing something genuinely innovative and novel. I mean we were giving out grants, fellowships, in death and dying, and that's not the same enterprise as giving out fellowships to discover the uses of a molecule or to do survey research.... We did retreat—literally retreat a couple of times—and talk about our own feelings, sentiments. There was one particular night at the Stanhope Hotel where Kathy had arranged a dinner for all of us at the top of the Stanhope Hotel looking out on this absolutely glorious scene of Central Park spread out before us and across the park the glittering lights of the West Side. And we—this was not accidental—we subconsciously put ourselves in a glamorous setting because we were going to talk to each other about our own feelings about death and dying. We pledged that we were in absolute total privacy and nothing said that night would ever go out further, and to the best of my knowledge, it never did. But a selection committee, a board, finding the need to sit down and ruminate emotively about the subject matter, that was different. And being on a selection committee about death was different. I can't help but think that this, unlike other selection committees, really had a life-changing effect...a personal as well as professional impact on everybody.[4]

At the board meeting of November 16 and 17, 1999, part of the discussion was transcribed. At one point Bo Burt remarked that "my service on this board, I have come to feel, is the most constructive thing that I have been involved [with] in my career." At another point in the meeting Patricia Prem refers to "this wonderful board." In an interview Bob Butler observed: "I don't think any organization I've been involved with—and I've been on a *lot* of nonprofit boards—has taken as much of my time as the Project on Death in America. And I say that not with resentment, but it's an aberration that we all stuck with it."[5]

PDIA was different to other American programs at OSI. It seems to have been more autonomous, its board more practically engaged and, perhaps to an extent, it was less well understood by senior OSI managers. Head of American programs Gara LaMarche captures some of this:

They have incorporated themselves into the management structure here, but programmatically my relationship with PDIA has been much more hands-off than with anything else. I didn't create it. I've advised them on various things, both organizationally and substantively, and I think they appreciate that. But I have seen myself in a very different relationship to PDIA, partly because of its history and partly because, almost unique among our programs, they set up a governing structure where a substantial amount of responsibility was delegated by George Soros and the OSI board to the PDIA board. So the ordinary process is: grants are recommended to

---

4. David Rothman, interview by David Clark, March 31, 2004.

5. Robert Butler, interview by David Clark, July 23, 2003.

me and then to Aryeh Neier, and I'm involved in the approval of every grant in the place, but with PDIA we haven't done it that way, because the board has had that authority.[6]

David Rothman served both on the PDIA board and also on the central board of OSI. He was able to see how PDIA fared within OSI in relation to other programs. The comparison was favorable. He noted at a PDIA board meeting: "We set the standards for being systematic. And others don't always match us as being as systematic as we are."[7] It is true that the policy of reviewing most applications within the PDIA board created a heavy workload for its members. But their concern, within a small field, was that a wider panel would create greater conflicts of interest and also more variations in opinions and viewpoints. The board, therefore, attempted to define the conflicts of interest, biases, and opinions within it in order to impose a kind of quality rationale upon its decision-making processes.[8] This, the argument went, made for both rigor and efficiency. But elsewhere in OSI, a program director could decide to go with an initiative dependent only on the approval of Aryeh Neier to move it forward. By contrast, in PDIA, "it would be a laborious discussion where we would have to be brought up to speed about the project, and then they'd have to be brought up to speed about the issues, and then you'd have to move forward."[9] This could put the chair of the board and the director of the program—in the one person of Kathy Foley—in a difficult and sometimes frustrating position.

The board was also keen to meet applicants at interview, especially for the professional development programs. It was a model drawn from academia and medicine and was again greedy of time and travel. For many of those attending the interviews, however, the experience was a piece of continuing personal and professional development in its own right, as Harvey Chochinov observes:

> It was one of those interviews where I felt that anything that I could do or say to convince this group of people that they ought to fund me, I had done, and that if they decided that they weren't going to fund me that I could be at peace with that because I had...shown them, I had put my very best foot forward. I had told them exactly what I thought I *could* do, what I *wanted* to do. I had expressed the passion that I felt...and before I left I can recall something like, "There's just one last thing I need to say and that is, if I am funded, I truly believe I can make a difference"...something to that effect.[10]

---

6. Gara LaMarche, interview by David Clark, October 28, 2004.

7. Transcript of part of the PDIA board meeting, November 17, 1999.

8. Kathy Foley, interview by David Clark, October 27, 2003.

9. Kathy Foley, interview by David Clark, October 27, 2003.

10. Harvey Chochinov, interview by David Clark, July 23, 2003.

Tim Keay had failed to be selected for Cohort One of the Faculty Scholars Program, but was interviewed again the following year:

> So as all the scholars will tell you, you go up to this office up in New York City in this high-rise building there, and you're sitting at this round table with the sun shining in your eyes, and Bo Burt on one side with a big smile and Kathy Foley there, and Susan Block, and these attorneys and these well-known names, Joanne Lynn...the top of the crop, as it were, there at the table. And, as I recall, Bo Burt said, "I'll ask you questions first so you feel comfortable." You know, "I feel real comfy now [laughs]—law professor from Yale ask me questions..." But we started talking, talked about the research, some of the work I'd been doing, and I talked about how important it was to deal with an extremely vulnerable population in the United States, which was the elderly in nursing homes, where people dying there will often have terrible deaths unfortunately. I was talking about how in their first cohort the PDIA board had pretty much taken all scholars who were working in hospital end-of-life care, and I said "If you don't take me, take *somebody* who works on end-of-life care in nursing homes—it's so important. I mean one out of five people in the United States dies in a nursing home." And Kathy Foley, who was at the table, said, "No, it can't be that many"...If Kathy Foley, the expert on end-of-life care, if *she* doesn't know how many people die in American nursing homes, how is the average person supposed to know? I mean it's not even on people's radar.[11]

The close engagement of board members, especially with particular projects that were near to their own interests, could also bring problems. Joanne Lynn was receiving considerable PDIA support for her own work program and felt the need to withdraw from the board to avoid a conflict of interest. Bo Burt's promotion of the Bazelon Project led to few tangible outcomes. A project involving David Rothman and Robert Butler in the production of a scholarly volume on the history of death in America did not come to fruition but did lead to a successful National Endowment for the Humanities Summer Seminar.[12] More notable was the success of Susan Block and the Faculty Scholars Program and the tireless efforts of Patricia Prem to see the Social Work Leadership Program get off the ground. Likewise, the Arts and Humanities Program saw David Rothman's contribution to best effect.

---

11. Tim Keay, interview by David Clark, July 24, 2003.

12. This was hosted by David Rothman in 1998 at Columbia University under the auspices of a National Endowment for the Humanities Summer Seminar for faculty across the United States, on the history of death in America, and it led to some tangible outputs: J. W. Green, *Beyond the Good Death: The Anthropology of Modern Dying* (Philadelphia: University of Pennsylvania Press, 2008)—the author acknowledges the 1998 seminar as the inspiration

Board members were not only closely involved with the issues; they also helped to promote what one faculty scholar called a "sentimental" attachment to the issue of end-of-life care that became widely pervaded throughout PDIA, and ultimately led back to the OSI founder:

I think one of the interesting things about end-of-life care generally is it seems to be a career that *most* people embark on after some significant life or medical or professional experience, and it's really not an entry level career: it requires some sort of emotional priming event. So I think to some extent the intensity of the PDIA project reflects the fact that these leaders in the field were brought into the field by some intense priming event—that includes George Soros, who had these interestingly dichotomized deaths in his own family: one parent died the bad, high-tech death, and the other one died the empathic, interpersonal, hospice-style death. And it was the tensions between the two that apparently led him, at least by legend—PDIA legend or folklore—to fund the program.[13]

For Susan Block, this issue of personal orientation was crucial to how faculty scholars were selected, but it also recognized the wider context in which they would be working, acknowledging that the "personal" was also related to the "institutional":

We wanted a personal statement so we could find out who these people were because they were supposed to be transformational people, so we needed to know something about that. We wanted to *hear* in their statements...a capacity for self-reflectiveness...that it wasn't just like, "I'm the greatest and this is why you should give me the money..." It was like, "These are some of the influences that have shaped who I am and why I think I could do this work and where I want to go with it." So that reflective piece was very important. We also wanted to make sure that there was an institution—that they were embedded in an academic institution where they had support so they could go back there and someone would listen to them as they were going to make change in that institution. We wanted them to be *leaders*. I think that was another big point, that these were people who we felt were our representatives out in the academic world, who were going to lead this improvement in end-of-life care. We wanted these people to be in the belly of the beast—the academic medical center—and be able to speak that language but also have this commitment to hospice and palliative care.[14]

for the book; and a paper from Drew Gilpin Faust, pre-figured D. G. Faust, *This Republic of Suffering: Death and the American Civil War* (Random House/Vintage: New York, 2009).

13. Stephen Miles, interview by David Clark, July 24, 2003.

14. Susan Block, interview by David Clark, July 21 and 23, 2003.

It is clear that several members of the board endorsed the confessional style of some of those who sought PDIA funding. It encouraged deep—and public— reflection on the experience of giving and receiving care at the end-of-life, and it maintained a close attachment to the values of palliative care not only in its strategic thinking and action but also in its day-to-day relations and the conduct of its meetings. It was a "therapeutic turn" that served the goals of PDIA very well indeed.

THE SPECIAL ROLE OF THE FACULTY SCHOLARS

Perhaps the most notable achievement of the PDIA years was the creation of the Faculty Scholars Program, which began in 1995 and continued to recruit until 2002. During this time, PDIA invested $13.4 million in the work of 87 faculty scholars who, it was estimated, went on to leverage a tenfold effect in awards made to support research, education, and program development in hospice and palliative care.[15] Board member Bo Burt took the view that "from the very begin- ning we self-consciously and purposefully put our major bet on the Faculty Scholars Program."[16] For Bo Burt, the influence of fellow board member Robert Butler was particularly strong here, since it was Butler who had used a similar approach a decade earlier in helping to forge the specialty of geriatrics. The deci- sion to allocate a major proportion of PDIA resources was made early in the life of PDIA and was never revisited or questioned. As Burt put it, "We carried this conviction throughout the life of PDIA."[17] The goal was a transformational impact through the creation of a new cadre of people (mostly physicians and many in major academic institutions) who would be dedicated to pursuing a career in the care of dying people. Placement in the academy was a key criterion by which PDIA hoped to achieve a "multiplier effect," whereby scholars would teach others, who would then in turn have a wider influence. The decision to do this was undoubtedly shaped by the fact that several of the board were in the academy and that the voice of medicine on the board was also well developed.

Much credit must go here to Susan Block for her success in fostering group cohesion among the scholars and for her commitment to the program as a key element within PDIA. It was she who had first raised the idea of a scholars' pro- gram in a document sent to Aryeh Neier after the first ever meeting on Long Island in September 1993; the response had been to invite her onto the board in order to develop the concept further.[18] She explains:

---

15. *Transforming the Culture of Dying: The Project on Death in America, October 1994 to December 2003* (New York: Open Society Institute, 2004).

16. Bo Burt, email to David Clark, June 19, 2010.

17. Bo Burt, email to David Clark, June 19, 2010.

18. Susan Block, interview with David Clark, July 21, 2003.

I felt really strongly that there needed to be faculty who could become this field. Remember there was no palliative care in the United Stated in 1994. There was none. It didn't exist. There were hospices out in the community doing wonderful work, but it was outside the mainstream of medicine and there was very little communication between the hospice world and academic medicine context. There were exceptions but they were really very, very few of them. So the construct was "let's take the principles and practice of hospice and bring them into the academic mainstream." And that was what the faculty scholars could do. It needs to get brought into the academic centers where students are trained and where residents are trained and where it can have a broader impact. In order to do that there needed to be people in those academic centers who were the *best* embodiments of what this type of care is and who could teach it and bring people along and develop research programs to build a knowledge base. The kind of people who needed to be in it were people who were not just smart, but were wonderful teachers and the kind of role models who would be like pied pipers for students and residents, who had this sort of authenticity about who they were that they could communicate to people that would help build a field. The vision in my mind about the personal qualities of these people was very important, because I have a very strong belief in the power of role models, and I thought these people had to be role models to sort of bring people along and the field along.[19]

In advocating for a Faculty Scholars Program within PDIA, Block had looked at other similar interventions. None were quite like what she envisioned. They often seemed too narrow:

I felt it was really important that there be this breadth. That these people could represent, not just their intellectual side but their spiritual side and their emotional side. I had a strong sense about these as core principles of hospice, that there needs to be this integration. So these *people* need to be *integrated* people. The board collectively had this very high aspiration for the faculty scholars: we thought we wanted these to be transformational people.[20]

Initially funding for the scholars was for three years, later cut back to two. Beyond that, the nature of the "call" changed little over the duration of PDIA. There was a request for personal statements, a need to identify self-reflection in the applicants, a concern to find transformational qualities and understanding of the influences that had shaped the candidates and their goals and aims. It was also important to ensure that the scholars were embedded in an academic institution where they had support for the changes they might wish to foster. In

19. Susan Block, interview with David Clark, July 21, 2003.

20. Susan Block, interview with David Clark, July 21, 2003.

short, the board was looking for leadership capacity in a wide sense. In the first cohort of scholars,[21] it found this in abundance. They were highly successful in capturing resources, so in a sense it was not a matter of changing their approach so much as giving the resources to push forward and make a greater impact. The first cohort was a group comprising pent-up demand, a pipeline that could be activated quickly and with considerable effect.

Accordingly, the individual studies conducted by faculty scholars, which have been described at various points in earlier chapters, were only one component of their experience and of the purpose of the board in supporting them. The program was designed to do more than simply fund grants and projects. It deliberately brought the scholars together into what became an enduring community of interest, described by Burt as "an intense, collaborative learning network with senior people already in the field and with their immediate peers."[22] This was pursued most intensely in the scholars' retreats,[23] where as we have seen, high energy collaborations were fostered and sustained, new skills were taught and learned, and a growing sense was imbued across the cohorts of membership of an elite force of change agents and thought leaders. Susan Block recalls the atmosphere at the first scholars' retreat:

> It was the summer of 1995; there were sixteen faculty scholars and the board members. It was very intimate. I remember putting a lot of effort into planning that retreat, into thinking about the tone and the nonhierarchical relationships that we wanted to develop between the scholars and the board, and the sense of collaboration and safety we wanted to develop within the group of faculty scholars. There was just this sense of closeness and shared purpose in having—of *joyfulness* in having found each other and being together and sharing this common mission. There was I think a feeling of them being special, and we felt very gratified that we had *chosen* well; that these seemed like exactly the people we wanted to be helping and supporting. There was a lot of thinking about the future, getting input about what they needed as faculty scholars, a lot of emphasis on people. We wanted the scholars to have some private time; we wanted them to talk about their personal pathways into palliative care so that it wouldn't just be a head thing. And they were terrific.[24]

As the number of cohorts grew, there were more opportunities—as we have seen at various points—for individual scholars to engage in cross-institutional col-

---

21. It comprised 16 scholars, including one four-person team.

22. Bo Burt, email to David Clark, June 19, 2010.

23. These were held twice each year at the beginning and then annually as budgets became more constrained.

24. Susan Block, interview with David Clark, July 24, 2003.

laborative work and to meet together in other professional settings. For Susan Block, there were some differences between the cohorts:

> The first cohort was people who were already in the field; some of them were already leaders in the field. They had been committed to palliative care before anyone cared about it. A lot of the first cohort were building palliative care programs and developing interns to do clinical practice in palliative care They were more senior, they were older, more mature in a lot of ways—professionally, personally. We got those people in early in a *big* cohort, our first cohort.[25]
>
> Then I think there was sort of a period in the middle where people were getting the idea that it might be possible to make a career in this area, or the awareness that PDIA might stimulate people to move into the field. I think in general these were wonderful people—maybe a little bit less risk-takers than the first cohort; a little more mainstream; a little bit more diverse. Cohorts three and four I would say were good solid people who were brought in I think in large part by the existence of funding in the field. Maybe they'd had a little bit of an interest, but the funding in the field helped them move into the area in a way they might not have otherwise. So I think that brought in new people.
>
> Later on there was more of an emphasis on research and less on clinical innovation. In the third wave, it has been a lot of mentees of our early cohorts: palliative care in emergency medicine; palliative care in neuro-oncology; in the subspecialized areas where people already had a strong allegiance to their primary discipline and probably would continue to, but would also *drag* palliative care into that discipline. So cohorts five, six, seven, and eight are much younger. They are too young to be leaders, in general. But they are people with a lot of potential who are doing wonderful things and often really benefiting from mentoring from some of the more senior cohorts.
>
> But I think *always* we funded the people not the projects. That was very clear, from the get-go.[26]

The scholars, once engaged, were monitored quite closely. Their applications set out key milestones. They submitted annual progress reports that were reviewed carefully. Initially there was an external advisory group to give feedback and recommendations to the scholars. There were some scholars who needed a lot of mentoring and monitoring, and some where representations had to be made to their home institution—for example, where department chairs would not give them the protected time that had been promised. In some cases, there were extensive negotiations with the institutions on behalf of the scholars in which

---

25. Several respondents (board members and faculty scholars themselves) acknowledged that cohort two had been "problematic" in various ways; one even ventured the notion that second cohorts are always challenging on such programs.

26. Susan Block, interview with David Clark, July 24, 2003.

the threat of funding withdrawal had to be invoked. It was $75,000 a year and it was supposed to buy 60 percent of the scholar's time. PDIA was determined that commitments would be honored and that all scholars would be supported as effectively as possible to realize their goals.

Fortunately, such cases were few in number and the overall outcome of the Faculty Scholars Program was positive and clear:

> The leaders in the field are our scholars and that was what we wanted to do. If you talk about content areas, I would say clinical service develop-ment, but then clinical service development was used to develop educa-tional programs, which were then used to develop research programs. It was a snowball thing. I think that there were some scholars who we funded to do research and they have done research and built substantial research *programs*, not just one grant or two grants, where they're mentoring young people in palliative care research—that's terrific! And that's important in helping the field develop a legitimacy in the academic world. I think the other thing that was very successful is the number of collaborations that developed and are developing. There are so many synergies and collabo-rations and publications and shared grants and short educational projects that have come out of this. I don't know of any organization that has had such success in creating the conditions for those collaborations to take place as PDIA has.[27]

A study published in 2009 sets out the achievements of the Faculty Scholars Program in detail and documents the progress made by the scholars from the start of their participation in the program. Key outcome variables included grants awarded in palliative care, peer-reviewed publications, academic promo-tions, editorships held, honors awarded, and certifications obtained since the initial Faculty Scholars Program grant award. The study methods included a self-administered survey in 2003 and an update in 2007 involving the collec-tion of scholars' curriculum vita, as well as a review of literature and websites of national medical palliative care organizations. Of 740 applicants who applied during the granting period 1995–2003, 87 were selected as faculty scholars (in eight cohorts of two to three years each). All scholars responded to the surveys. The results revealed that 40 percent were female, 82.8 percent were physicians, and 12.6 percent were nurses. Scholars reported receiving a total of more than $113 million dollars in grants. As of 2007, the PDIA faculty scholars had pub-lished a total of 2,171 papers in peer-reviewed journals. Sixty percent of the phy-sicians were certified by the American Board of Hospice and Palliative Medicine. In addition, scholars had been represented in the leadership of all major medical organizations related to end-of-life care in the United States, as well as in other national end-of-life care initiatives.

---

27. Susan Block, interview with David Clark, July 24, 2003.

The study authors concluded reasonably that the PDIA Faculty Scholars Program had been successful in accomplishing its objective of developing a core group of clinical and academic leaders to advance the field of palliative care in the United States.[28] Rosemary Gibson of the Robert Wood Johnson Foundation agrees:

> We were so lucky that the Project on Death in America had the Faculty Scholars Program because that provided us with a ready pool of identified people who came forward...we then worked with many of them to do other great work. Susan Block has done a marvelous job with the Harvard Palliative Care Education Center. Diane Meier is leading our Center to Advance Palliative Care. David Weissman did a program to work with faculty and residency training programs. Charles von Gunten was absolutely instrumental in developing the EPEC curriculum and making palliative care a specialty in medicine. We can go on and on.[29]

Faculty development initiatives have been widely used in medicine in the United States and the increasing complexity of medical education and practice has led to interventions to promote leadership roles and responsibilities. A systematic review of such schemes attempts to address the question: what are the effects of faculty development leadership interventions on the knowledge, attitudes, and skills of faculty members and on the institutions in which they work?[30] It identified thirty-five interventions of which only two focused on palliative care; the first of these was the PDIA Faculty Scholars Program itself and the second was a local program run by Andrew Billings, Susan Block, and others.[31]

In general the schemes were found to be effective in relation to their goals. There was high satisfaction from participants, with reported positive changes in attitudes toward their own organizations and their leadership capabilities. A greater sense of community and appreciation of the benefits of networking was also identified, together with a better knowledge of leadership principles and strategies, and a change in leadership behavior. The key program attributes to be valued by participants were experiential learning and reflective practice, individual and group projects, peer support and the development of communities of

---

28. A. M. Sullivan, N. M. Gadmer, and S. D. Block, "The Project on Death in America Faculty Scholars Program: A Report on Scholars' Progress," *Journal of Palliative Medicine* 12, no. 2 (February 2009): 155–159.

29. Rosemary Gibson (Robert Wood Johnson Foundation), interview by David Clark, October 26, 2004.

30. Y. Steinert, L. Naismith, and K. Mann, "Faculty Development Initiatives Designed to Promote Leadership in Medical Education. A BEME Systematic Review," BEME Guide No. 19, *Medical Teacher* 34 (2012): 483–503.

31. A. M. Sullivan et al., "Creating Enduring Change: Demonstrating the Long-Term Impact of a Faculty Development Program in Palliative Care," *Academic Medicine* 80, no. 7 (2006): 657–668.

practice, and mentorship. Areas for future development in such programs should include more theoretical grounding, further articulation of the definitions of leadership, and the use of alternative practices including narrative approaches and peer coaching. All of these points seem to resonate with the mode of operation and reported benefits of the PDIA Faculty Scholars Program.

As we shall see in the final chapter, the legacy of the program continued to resonate long after the PDIA initiative had ended, and scholars could be seen to continue to collaborate, to leverage change, and to achieve success in the development and consolidation of palliative care within the American health-care system.

THE IMPACT

Previous chapters have given insights into the many projects, initiatives, and experiments funded by PDIA, with the goal of improving end-of-life care in American society. These activities crossed disciplinary boundaries, engaged with communities of many kinds, and in some cases sought to articulate with high level public debate across the whole nation. PDIA grant making worked through three distinct funding cycles. These had a cumulative impact and built upon one another to foster a legacy of the whole initiative; but for the PDIA board, there were doubts about the continuation of funding, which meant that plans could only be made for three years at a time and each renewal of OSI funds was preceded by a period of uncertainty and concern. Ultimately, there was an awareness that PDIA would be of fixed duration and would not continue indefinitely; it would have to create an impact that was capable of being sustained and developed after it had ceased direct operations, as Kathy Foley explains:

> PDIA had a vision and a bold approach right from the start. Most of us on
> the advisory board had no firsthand experience as philanthropists, so we
> were willing to attempt things that more experienced foundation profes-
> sionals might have known were too ambitious. The fact that the project was
> not going to continue indefinitely kept us focused on our goal of working to
> make changes at the bedside within the health-care system, so that the work
> would continue beyond us.[32]

In viewing the legacy of PDIA, we need first to take cognizance of the structure of its activities and how these took shape over time. These have been seen, across the nine years, as falling into three key phases of activity.[33]

---

32. K. M. Foley, "An Open Letter to the Grantmaking Community." In *Transforming the Culture of Dying: The Project on Death in America, October 1994 to December 2003* (New York: Open Society Institute, 2004).

33. *Transforming the Culture of Dying, October 1994 to December 2003.*

Developing a Funding Strategy (1994–1998)

From the very beginning, the PDIA board sought to act as a catalyst for change in end-of-life care by fostering cooperation and collaboration among the various professionals already working in nursing, medicine, social work, ethics, policy, financing, and other areas of the field. PDIA sought to hold up a mirror to questions about end-of-life care and mortality in modern American culture. To achieve this, the board was assiduous in identifying experts from different disciplines and bringing them together to map out the territory and determine the most pressing needs. In its first three years, PDIA received more than 2,000 grant requests over four grant cycles and funded 122 projects in the seven priority areas it had identified.[34] The grant amounts ranged from $5,000 to $400,000 and represented many different approaches to the subjects of death, dying, and bereavement—from the medical to the philosophical to the organizational and political. The board and staff used the deluge of grant requests as an opportunity to survey the terrain, to understand the scope of need, the level of interest, and the range of available expertise. In the process of reviewing the grant proposals, the board was also able to form a picture of the emergent and struggling field of palliative care itself. Initially, reflecting this exploratory stage, the board chose to fund a range of initiatives that responded to the complexity of the medical and societal challenge of providing appropriate, compassionate care for dying and bereaved people, but as time went on, the "field" of palliative care itself would become the major focus of strategy and grant making, in an effort to build capacity by strengthening the numbers and the capabilities of individuals working within it. PDIA perceived the best grant applications to come from academics, especially doctors, and it in turn supported them to enhance the emerging field of palliative care. But PDIA was a good deal less successful in attracting the interests of, or partnerships with, major health-care providers and had very little in the way of direct engagement with health-care insurers—examples in which its focus on the professional cohort of individual grantees obscured its ability to think structurally and to impact on major aspects of service provision and financing.

In its second year, 1995, PDIA joined forces with the Robert Wood Johnson Foundation, the Nathan Cummings Foundation, the Rockefeller Family Office, and the Commonwealth Fund to form *Grantmakers Concerned with Care at the End of Life*. This coalition organized conferences and shared information in order to inform funders about the major social, economic, and medical issues in end-of-life care and to encourage them to address those issues in their grant making. It marked a spirit of collaboration and cooperation between foundations

---

34. These priority areas were: the epidemiology, ethnography, and history of dying and bereavement in the United States; the physical, emotional, spiritual, and existential components of dying and bereavement; the contribution of the arts and humanities; new service-delivery models for the dying and their families and friends; educational programs for the public about death and dying; educational programs for the health-care professions; and the shaping of governmental and institutional policy (see chapter 1).

that characterized the whole PDIA enterprise and that outlived PDIA itself. It must be acknowledged, however, that the scale of involvement across these foundations varied significantly. Whereas PDIA invested $45 million over nine years, in a similar period the Robert Wood Johnson Foundation spent around $150 million on end-of-life issues, and this excluded its $28 million investment in the SUPPORT study.[35]

Building Critical Mass (1998–2000)

In 1997, George Soros and OSI's board of directors reviewed the progress of PDIA and endorsed another three years of funding. During this second funding cycle, the board expanded its commitment to professional education. With the guidance of board member Patricia Prem, PDIA created the Social Work Leadership Development Initiative to strengthen professional practice and promote research, training, and policy development for social workers. PDIA also created a special funding initiative to support nursing leadership. These were heavily focused on building professional capacity and on seeking to identify talented individuals beyond the medical profession who had an important role to play in advancing palliative care. As we saw, the results were mixed with nursing. The social work initiative, however, produced a slow burn that was still evident several years after PDIA ceased funding, though no internal analysis was conducted on its "leveraging" effects, akin to that undertaken for the work of the faculty scholars. From a variety of disciplines and perspectives, PDIA was also important in helping the cause of pediatric palliative care to advance and to get a hearing, and, as we observed in chapter 4, in the lifetime of PDIA grant making, the landscape of pediatric palliative care in the United States changed considerably. These years also saw heavy investment in grants and initiatives that stimulated new clinical service developments and educational programs, as well as innovative approaches to matters of clinical practice. There was a rich mosaic of innovation here, some of which was mainstreamed elsewhere. More generally, it can be observed that there was a great deal of collaboration between grantees and scholars funded by PDIA that was not envisioned in their original applications, and which contributed to an overall leveraging effect that made PDIA "punch above its weight."

The mounting professional agenda did not prevent PDIA from launching an arts and humanities initiative in 1998, chaired by board member David Rothman. As we saw in chapter 2, grantees such as Eugene Richards, Meredith Monk, Nancy Mairs, and Deidre Scherer produced video, photography, poetry, essays, dance, and artwork to express individual and community experiences of illness, death, and grief, and to encourage conversation and thoughtful reflection.

---

35. Rosemary Gibson, interview by David Clark, October 26, 2004.

A particular success of the initiative was in selecting projects that required only modest PDIA support to help them toward realization and, in so doing, accomplished much more for PDIA than the scale of its investment. Moreover, some of the works remained alive in the public consciousness long after the initial funding had expired. This and related PDIA work contributed to a growing visibility within American life of issues concerning death, dying, and bereavement. But as always with PDIA, the goal was not simply to depict these issues, but also to address them in an active and reformist manner.

In 1999, PDIA board member Bo Burt led the development of a community grief and bereavement initiative. From interfaith, community-based, and school-based programs to programs for special groups, such as incarcerated youth or union home health-care workers, grantees created programs to support individual and community bereavement; but as we saw in chapter 2, the results were mixed and the legacy unclear. PDIA also chose to address challenging legal and economic barriers, and to improve access to care for particularly vulnerable populations. These underserved groups include children, the elderly, non-English speakers, the incarcerated, the homeless, racial and cultural minorities, and people with physical or developmental disabilities. Here again only partial successes could be noted, and PDIA seemed at times unclear and uneasy in its orientation to matters of social inequality and related policies. At the end of this period, however, in 2000, the Bill Moyers television series aired on public broadcasting and was a major success, and this can be seen as the outcome of some careful lobbying and participation on the part of PDIA personnel. It created huge public interest in end-of-life issues. One year later, after the bombings of September 11, 2001, American society had a still more visceral encounter with death and bereavement, as it struggled to make sense of, and come to terms with, the personal, social, and geopolitical consequences of what had taken place, and as much thinking and debate on matters of death, dying, and bereavement moved into a "post 9/11" framework.

Institutionalizing Change (2001–2003)

In 2000, George Soros and the OSI board had authorized three more years of funding. PDIA now ramped up its attention to building a sustainable field of palliative care with sufficient infrastructure and leadership to make a significant impact on the barriers to better care. In 2002, together with the Emily Davie and Joseph S. Kornfeld Foundation, PDIA formed the *Funders Consortium to Advance Palliative Medicine* to support existing and new palliative care fellowship training programs. The goal was to help increase the numbers of physicians with advanced training in palliative medicine, thereby helping palliative medicine achieve formal recognition as a medical subspecialty through the Accreditation Council for Graduate Medical Education and the American Board of Medical Specialties.

In 2002, Soros announced the reorganization of his international network of foundations. The board knew that PDIA would close at the end of 2003 and devoted a great deal of energy during that final year to developing an exit strategy, reviewing its operation, along with the original funding strategies, goals, and individual initiatives. A series of roundtable discussions and individual meetings was held, actively engaging palliative care leaders—including former board members, faculty scholars, nursing and social work leaders, grantees, cognate organizations and associations, experts in the field, and other funders—to help frame an appropriate conclusion to the PDIA program. The outcome, as we saw in chapter 1, was controversial. Some criticized the disproportionate funds that were allocated to the different disciplines and the fact that the lion's share went to medicine. Others wanted PDIA to find a mechanism to maintain itself at the very least through an annual retreat for scholars and grantees. Some were concerned that the end of PDIA funding coincided with the withdrawal of the Robert Wood Johnson Foundation support for end-of-life care initiatives, compounding a sense that the field's expansive years were coming to an end. But most accepted that difficult decisions had to be made and the test of the whole PDIA initiative would be the extent to which its influence was now embedded in organizational cultures and practices and within the architecture of policy. These issues went beyond the immediate dimensions of an exit strategy and were of more enduring consequence.

One aspect of the approach taken at this time was the call for other philanthropic funders to become involved in end-of-life issues and the recognition that in some areas there were opportunities to make a dramatic difference in the lives of patients, families, and communities, as Gara LaMarche noted in this statement in October 2004:

> Over the past decade, foundations have had an enormous impact on the development of palliative and end-of-life care services in the United States. Thanks to grant makers across the country, people with life-threatening illnesses are now more likely to be cared for by healthcare professionals— nurses, clergy, social workers, and doctors—trained in pain management, knowledgeable about advance care planning, and respectful of how religion or culture can affect a patient's experience of illness and dying. Caregivers and patients are learning that isolation, pain, and inadequate care need not define the dying process.[36]

The final PDIA report[37] asserts that all people with serious or advanced illness should expect and receive reliable, skilful, and supportive palliative care to relieve pain and other physical symptoms and to give patients the highest quality of life possible at all stages of serious illness. It also makes the important assertion that

---

36. PDIA press release (October 1, 2004).

37. *Transforming the Culture of Dying, October 1994 to December 2003.*

palliative care can be delivered alongside potentially curative treatments, by an interdisciplinary health-care team that addresses physical, psychological, and practical problems. This is a very significant point in positioning a discipline that might be seen as exclusively concerned with the care of the *dying* as an active component in the care of the *living*, and not simply as something confined to the last days and weeks of life. Palliative care, thus defined, the report makes clear, supports families *throughout* the patient's illness and is sensitive to the importance of religious, spiritual, and cultural responses to suffering, to death, and to bereavement. Kathy Foley hoped that "funders will use this report to consider how the communities they serve will benefit from improved palliative and end-of-life care services, and how they can integrate palliative care into current and future funding priorities."[38] Certainly the PDIA faculty scholars and social work leaders had been important actors in this process and had done much in their PDIA-funded roles to promote the palliative care model as an integrated form of care.

Reflecting on these wider issues in 2004, Vicky Weisfield of the Robert Wood Johnson Foundation saw three major achievements within the field at that time: in educational initiatives; in the practice and working environment where palliative care is delivered; and in the level of public awareness of end-of-life issues.[39] There is no doubt from the evidence that has been reviewed in earlier chapters that PDIA made a significant contribution to each of these areas. In so doing, its efforts complemented and strengthened those of other funders and, in particular, they seem to have worked in harmony with the Robert Wood Johnson Foundation initiatives. David Gould of the United Hospital Fund adds to this:

> I think what PDIA has done is it has helped create this network, this national network of leaders around the country that build a sense of community, and a reality of community that will make an enormous difference going forward.[40]

He continues:

> Kathy was instrumental in reminding us to stay focused on palliative care. I've always called it palliative care, and in talking with my boss Jim Tallon, he said, "well, you just try to bring hospices into hospital" and I said "no," because I don't think that's the answer. I think hospices are a programmatic component of a larger palliative care universe and we've got to figure out what those other services are and how they integrate with inpatient care and outpatient services and home-care services and hospice as a piece of

---

38. PDIA press release October 1, 2004.

39. Vicki Weisfield (Robert Wood Johnson Foundation), interview by David Clark, October 25, 2004.

40. David Gould, interview by David Clark, October 27, 2004.

that. At one point we started to move away from palliative care because the American culture around aversion to death or anything death and dying in those days was very profound, and while the Project on Death in America was tackling it head on, it had quite a substantial body to tackle head on, and I remember at one point thinking, well, maybe we should sort of call this our special-care hospital initiative and then we—[the United Hospital Fund] said "Don't do that. Call it palliative care, stay with palliative care, keep it in the title." And it was a helpful reminder to stay focused and let people know what it is that you're about.[41]

Such comments raise the question of whether the palliative care field reached a tipping point *during* the PDIA years?[42]

In 2000, Daniel Callahan had seen a "mixed record of reform" in the promotion of better quality end-of-life care efforts over recent decades and maintained that initiatives to improve the care of patients at the end of life had been only fitfully successful. He set much store by the "imperative" of medicine to defeat death and found that, in the face of this, those seeking to make death acceptable as a part of life and to ameliorate the suffering of the dying would struggle to promote their cause.[43] The following year three US experts—Joan Teno, Marilyn Field, and Ira Byock—also commented on how difficult it can be to achieve change and improvement in end-of-life care.[44] For example they cited how, in 1986, the World Health Organization declared the undertreatment of pain to be a public health crisis, yet there remained evidence that pain continues to be badly assessed and managed and the SUPPORT study showed that nearly a half of the intervention patients were in severe pain in the last three days of life.[45] These three experts also observe that the first American hospice was founded in 1974, yet thirty years later the majority of hospice services were seeing ever-shorter lengths of stay among their patients, with less opportunity to reduce suffering for dying patients and those close to them. Likewise, the 1998 Dartmouth Atlas of Health Care revealed significant variation in where people spend their days before death. In some regions of the United States, as many as 30 percent of those who died had been

---

41. David Gould, interview by David Clark, October 27, 2004.

42. M. Gladwell, *The Tipping Point: How Little Things Can Make a Big Difference* (Boston and New York: Little Brown, 2000).

43. D. Callahan, "Death and the Research Imperative," *New England Journal of Medicine* 342 (2000): 654–656.

44. J. M. Teno, M. J. Field, and I. Byock, "The Road Taken and to be Traveled in Improving End-of-Life Care," *Journal of Pain and Symptom Management* 22, no. 3 (2001): 713–716.

45. A controlled trial to improve care for seriously ill hospitalized patients. The study to understand prognoses and preferences for outcomes and risks of treatments (SUPPORT). The SUPPORT Principal Investigators [published erratum] appears in *Journal of the American Medical Association* 274 (1995): 1591–1598.

admitted to an ICU in the last six months of life,[46] whereas the figure was under 10 percent in other regions. They point out that the slow pace of progress in improving end-of-life care contrasts with the rapid change that often follows the introduction of new procedures and medications elsewhere in medicine and suggest that a number of factors may retard the rate of improvement in end-of-life care. These include the place of death within the prevailing health-care culture, which is also fragmented and often leaves patients and their family caregivers confused, overwhelmed, and feeling that they have fallen through the cracks. Likewise, they state, financing policies undervalue palliative care and provide scant support for case management, while at the same time important gaps remain in the evidence base needed to provide effective symptom management, sensitive psychosocial and spiritual care, and practical and emotional support for family caregivers. Teno, Field and Byock suggest the need for taking stock, for learning lessons from other examples of culture change in health and medicine. They see this as based on three key steps and apply these to end-of-life issues. First, those committed to improving care must create the necessary public awareness and consensus on the need to improve poor end-of-life care and to reform the practices and policies that lead to such care. Second, health-care professionals and health-care institutions must have ready access to the necessary knowledge, skills, and tools for improving care. Third, organizational and other systems must be created to sustain or extend change once desired behaviors and results have been achieved initially. These authors took the view that a long road still remained to be traveled and that the time frame and commitment of those involved should be in years, not months. Writing just as PDIA was preparing to close, they looked ahead to a decade where an array of private and government organizations would continue to work together in strategic efforts to ensure high quality end-of-life care, but saw no quick fixes or magic bullets.

The PDIA contribution to the development of a palliative care research agenda was also an important component of these debates, though as we saw in chapter 7, there were some who felt that progress had not been rapid enough. Indeed by 2008, faculty scholar Sean Morrison was still highlighting the inadequate levels of support for palliative care research. In a study that set out to identify funding sources of palliative medicine research published between 2003 and 2005, and to examine National Institutes of Health (NIH) funding of palliative medicine research from 2001 to 2005, the authors identified 388 palliative medicine research articles and 2,197 investigators. Of these papers, 72 percent received extramural funding: 31 percent from the NIH, 51 percent from foundations, and 16 percent from other sources. Only 109 investigators received NIH funding, and the National Cancer Institute (NCI), National Institute of Nursing Research (NINR), and National Institute on Aging (NIA) funded 85 percent of all NIH

---

46. J. E. Wennberg., *The Dartmouth Atlas of Health Care 1998* (Dartmouth, NH: American Hospital Association 1998).

awards.[47] Research in palliative care had expanded significantly since the start of the PDIA program, but there remained doubts about the commitment of the palliative care community to research issues and its potential to develop a rigorous research culture and evidence-based approach, elements considered essential to placing palliative care on a level playing field with other medical specialties.

Nevertheless, some PDIA scholars and grantees were increasingly recognized in the early years of the twentieth century as among the world's leading figures in palliative care research.

Faculty scholar Stephen Miles, commenting in 2003 as PDIA was coming to a close, was struck by how his colleagues had forged themselves into a coherent *community* of professionals working together. He took the view that while the PDIA funding stream was ending, this would not mean the demise of the community. In this he seems to have been proven right. By the end of the decade, six years later, there was plenty of evidence of ongoing contact and collaboration between the scholars and grantees. But he did note that there were still relatively few academic clinicians interested in having a high level of engagement with end-of-life issues and with palliative care. Indeed he thought there was a danger among some of the later cohorts of PDIA scholars of overestimating the size and scale of the field to which they were committing themselves long term. For Miles, PDIA was a "micro-community" of no more that three hundred to four hundred people that formed part of a cadre of institutions and initiatives that over a twenty-five-year period combined to shape the end-of-life and palliative care field. These included the hospice groups that lobbied for Medicare recognition, the bioethics societies that constructed the theoretical underpinnings to the treatment plans that were brought into palliative care, the professional programs promoted by the Robert Wood Johnson Foundation, and also the wider public forces of consumerism, the debates about the "denial" of death in America, and the widespread media interest in matters to do with death, dying, and bereavement which served as a form of public education.[48] In short, the PDIA effort was crucial but should be seen within a longer and more broad-based history of end-of-life reform in late twentieth-century America. As another commentator put it when referring to PDIA, Last Acts, and related initiatives, "These educational programs [were] produced as an effective response to a rapidly emerging moral imperative for improving end-of-life care. They expanded the palliative care workforce and provided the field with the momentum and financial resources required to enter its next developmental state.[49]

It can be concluded that in the PDIA years the conditions necessary to reach a tipping point had been recognized, if not realized. At the same time, the role of PDIA in the wider history of end-of-life care in the United States can

47. L. Gelfman and S. R. Morrison, "Research funding for palliative medicine," *Journal of Palliative Medicine* 11, no. 1 (2008): 36–43.

48. Stephen Miles, interview by David Clark, July 24, 2003.

49. C. D. Kollas, "Palliative Care Advocacy in the United Sates: Are There Lessons for Geriatric Psychiatry?" *American Journal of Geriatric Psychiatry* 20, no. 4 (2012): 284–290.

be overemphasized and is not necessarily recognized by all commentators. For example, in the 2007–2008 edition of the journal *Omega*, Stephen Connor of the National Hospice and Palliative Care Organization reviewed the historical development of hospice and palliative care services in the United States and made no mention at all of the PDIA program.[50] Likewise PDIA could be grandiose at times in the claims it made for itself—for example, the assertion that "death is no longer the taboo subject that it was when George Soros established PDIA three years ago," which appeared in its first triennial report.[51] PDIA was *of* its time as much as it *shaped* its time, and this can be seen in relation to public debates about care of the dying that occurred in these years, as well as in the involvement of other philanthropic organizations with cognate missions.

As we have seen, a related issue is the tendency for PDIA to be misrepresented by some commentators as an organization in favor of, and actively promoting, euthanasia. Much Internet commentary on the life and times of George Soros, a good deal of it openly hostile to the man and his activities, depicts him, and in turn the Project on Death in America, as pro-euthanasia and assisted suicide. There is in fact no evidence to suggest that any PDIA program sought to support euthanasia or physician-assisted suicide, though several PDIA board members, grantees, and scholars did engage in the associated debates and also published work on these subjects. PDIA coincided with some major debates and events in America relating to legal and ethical issues at the end of life. These were the years in which assisted dying was legalized in Oregon, in which Jack Kevorkian's activities came to prominence, and in which cases such as that of Terri Schiavo led to widespread debate and publicity. Despite the critiques surrounding euthanasia and assisted dying, it is important to see the more significant contribution of PDIA in the ethics field, which was about defining the ethical landscape of palliative care itself and how this could be shaped to relieve suffering at the end of life. Here many PDIA-funded works generated rich insight and commentary that strengthened the ethics of palliative care and did much to promote its goals.

Other critical voices were directed to the political correctness of PDIA, with its "Dear Mr. Death" letters and support to create a hospice for Native Americans.[52] Here the protagonists usually orient their arguments to George Soros, in all his aspects, as well as to PDIA. So, for example, his involvement with debates about how Americans should die is seen as just another illustration of the financier philanthropist's high-handed tendency to make prescriptive statements about the lives of others and how they should be lived. The Internet debates of this type were still raging in 2009. Fueled by opposition to the Obama health reforms,

---

50. S. Connor, "Hospice and Palliative Care in the United States," *Omega* 56, no. 1 (2007–2008): 89–99.

51. *Project on Death in America, July 1994–September 1997, Report of Activities* (New York: Open Society Institute, 1998), 8.

52. Forbundet Mot Rusgift, "George Soros' Agenda for Drug Legalization, Death, and Welfare": http://www.fmr.no/george-soros-agenda-for-drug-legalization-death-and-welfare. 78404-10285.html (accessed December 22, 2009).

some commentators, on belatedly discovering the existence of the PDIA, saw in it an attempt to save money for "big government" by prematurely ending the lives of older people who would otherwise be a high cost to the health-care system.[53] Such misrepresentations and blatant parodying of PDIA itself seem set to continue, though they appear to have caused little concern to the PDIA board, its scholars, and its grantees.

The breadth of interest on the part of George Soros and the range of issues with which he has engaged undoubtedly resonate with a style of philanthropy that is much more than simple grant making to worthy causes. It acknowledges the interrelations between the private and the public, the personal and the professional. It is emblematic of the new forms of philanthropy that are so well illustrated by PDIA and reveal some of the particular qualities of philanthropic intervention in late twentieth-century America. This occurs where political systems show evidence of a shift from hierarchically organized and unitary systems of government to arrangements that are more horizontal in character and relatively fragmented,[54] and where considerable scope emerges for the role of nongovernmental and philanthropic endeavor, often focused on single issues. When this is combined with high concentrations of individual wealth in the hands of elite donors, as became increasingly the case in the United States from the 1980s, then the scope for private philanthropy to influence the activities of the public domain becomes more evident. One hallmark of such philanthropy is a concern with issues of personal misfortune, suffering, and disadvantage, seen as matters that require new models of intervention. Philanthropy may have the potential to act as a transformative agent in this context[55] and might engage in complex areas of social and public interest that cut across the jurisdictions of specific departments of government or particular service organizations. Much of the activity of the Open Society Institute can be seen in this context and the work of PDIA is a particularly good example of it.

This approach can be distinguished from, and is wider than, traditional modes of charity that are oriented primarily at the poor and at immediate needs. The new philanthropy encompasses charity but represents a broader range of private giving for public purposes.[56] George Soros's Open Society Institute falls squarely into this domain and has been engaged in programs for community

---

53. Threedonia.com, "The Project on Death in America," http://www.threedonia.com/archives/9911 (accessed December 22, 2009).

54. A. M. Eikenberry and P. M. Nickel, "Towards a Critical Social Theory of Philanthropy in an Era of Governance" (unpublished manuscript, 2006), available at the Institute of Policy and Governance at Virginia Tech, http://www.ipg.vt.edu/Papers/EikenberryNickelASPECT.pdf (accessed September 24, 2009).

55. A. M. Eikenberry and P. M. Nickel, "Towards a Critical Social Theory of Philanthropy in an Era of Governance."

56. F. Ostrower, *Why the Wealthy Give: The Culture of Elite Philanthropy* (Princeton: Princeton University Press, 1995).

development, as well as for policy and legal change. It has been concerned with advocacy and challenges to vested interests, and it has at times had a strongly political character, especially focused on human rights issues. It has not been associated with major capital ventures or with the acquisition of art or land for social purposes. Nor has it involved direct fund-raising, since the resources have come from George Soros's own personal wealth. In this sense, OSI can be seen as part of an emergent cadre of New York–based philanthropy that developed in the city from the 1980s. It is also consistent with a wider view of elite philanthropy as something that constitutes a beneficial social institution, which forms an expression of identity and a way of being within an elite culture.[57] Interestingly, the board of PDIA was not charged with raising funds but with spending them. This has a bearing on its composition over the lifetime of the program. The members were experts in their chosen field, not well-meaning outsiders. In addition, the PDIA board was small, which despite some individual differences, created a cohesive approach. There do not appear to have been any subgroups within it. Moreover, it was chaired by a woman, and women were always well represented on it. These factors combined to make the board effective in pursuing its strategy. As the board members became more accomplished over time in their role as philanthropic agents, and as their agenda shook down to concentrate on professional issues of palliative and end-of-life care, so they became more effective in their approach and impact. When the time came, they also proved capable of forming a robust exit strategy which would go on resonating within the field in the years that followed.

The debate about the person of George Soros will doubtless continue as long as his influence persists. Wider academic reflections on the role of his particular style of philanthropy will also evolve as commentators seek to make sense of the role of such endeavors in shaping contemporary society and culture. For present purposes, the task is more limited: to offer some final evaluation of the work of the Project on Death in America, as seen some half dozen years from the point when its funding programs ended.[58] We can conclude that PDIA was a well-developed example of the new philanthropy that emerged in the late twentieth-century. It was able to make use of private wealth to address a range of public issues hitherto largely ignored by government, the professions, and the media. Some might be uncomfortable that philanthropic interventions were necessary to draw attention to the need for improved care of the dying. It might be argued that philanthropy should not be required to stimulate the medical establishment to do its work appropriately. Yet there is no doubt that such philanthropy did leverage change. Many PDIA grantees and scholars found that their "Soros funding" opened doors for them within their organizations and professional groups. At the same time, such philanthropy sat easily with the elite model of change espoused by the PDIA

---

57. F. Ostrower, *Why the Wealthy Give.*

58. This chapter was finished in December 2009.

board. This made for effective work in confronting the medical establishment, in promoting research, and in fostering publications in the scientific and professional literature. Yet it seemed less successful in dealing with grassroots activism at the community level and when dealing with disadvantaged and underserved populations. Nor did it wholly connect with the world of policy, policy making, and politics, and there was no major policy initiative in PDIA, though the desire to move in that direction was often expressed. Ultimately, the PDIA program was most effective when it remained on the home ground of its key board members— the professional field of palliative and end-of-life care. Although it struggled here to fully embrace an interdisciplinary model of care, its achievements were nevertheless considerable. Most tangibly, these could be seen in the innovative service programs that it funded and coaxed into being, in the widely disseminated research work, the major publications, and in the research grants. Most visible of all was the contribution it made to the recognition of the speciality of palliative medicine. But sitting above all of these, less concrete and more conceptual in character perhaps, was a far more significant achievement. PDIA, building on the experiences that Kathy Foley had gained in her work with the World Health Organization, was instrumental in defining end-of-life care in terms of a new language—that of public health. This evolved gradually over the lifetime of PDIA and by the conclusion of the program was an explicit dimension of its thinking and practice. It created a lasting legacy that would assist subsequent efforts to improve end-of-life care in the United States—and further afield.

We have seen that Kathy Foley did so much to help initiate PDIA, to manage it through nine years of activity, and then to nurture its legacy and promote ongoing development. In a 2003 journal editorial, she set out the state of end-of-life care in the United States, acknowledging the barriers to progress, highlighting the major landmarks of achievement, many of which have been reviewed in detail here, and the specific contributions of philanthropic funders. She concluded as follows:

> The future looks promising. There is increasing professional and public interest, and a growing leadership of healthcare professionals and a strong incentive for change. Yet policy and systems change, particularly for reimbursement, occurs slowly; however, the remarkable achievements to date provide tangible benchmarks to measure the integration of palliative care into our public health system.[59]

59. K. Foley, "Advancing Palliative Care in the United States," *Palliative Medicine* 17 (2003): 89–90.

9

A Culture Transformed?
Post-PDIA Progress in Palliative
and End-of-Life Care

In this final chapter, we have an opportunity to reflect on the words of Kathy Foley and to explore how "promising" the future proved to be, at least in the decade after PDIA formally ended. It is clear that the program produced a momentum that was maintained in many ways. Sources of funding seemed to grow, and the key leaders and their mentees continued to pursue their endeavors. Palliative care services expanded and penetrated deeper and wider into the hospital system. Research consolidated and produced new and potentially game-changing findings. There was a growing sophistication about policy matters and how to influence them. The understanding of public attitudes became more nuanced, and the implications of that understanding fed into the language and strategy for palliative care development. Three areas are explored here.[1] First, there is an assessment of the continuing role of philanthropy in shaping the field that was defined by PDIA and other interventions. Second, we look at key actions, studies, publications, and debates that infused the field in the post-PDIA decade—and find many rich examples of activity, innovation, and growth. Third, and in conclusion, there is an opportunity to review the continuing challenges that face the field in the American context—and the various propositions about how they might be addressed.

---

1. I regard this as a wide-ranging, but not necessarily fully comprehensive review of the field in the period. I cover the years after PDIA ended in 2004 up until the chapter was finalized in the summer of 2012.

CONTINUING ROLE OF FOUNDATIONS

We have seen that PDIA was one of a number of philanthropic grant makers that had engaged in promoting palliative care in the United States, going back over several decades. Widely acknowledged as the most significant player, the Robert Wood Johnson Foundation (RWJF) funded the SUPPORT study beginning in 1988. Concerned by its findings, RWJF invested $148 million in end-of-life related initiatives between 1996–2003.[2] Like PDIA, the focus of this initiative was a self-consciously elite approach to *strategic philanthropy* in which carefully selected areas of work became the focus for building a field of specialist activity, expertise, and critical mass. For RWJF, three areas were prioritized: improving the education of practitioners; building model palliative care programs, especially in hospitals; and raising public awareness. RWJF staff and those at PDIA worked closely together to leverage their investments in these areas, to complement their activities, and to engage with a pool of grantees, some of whom were benefitting from support from a number of foundations. For example, of the eighty-seven PDIA faculty scholars, twenty individuals were further supported by RWJF in assuming major roles in its programs.[3]

These interconnections make the success of specific philanthropic interventions difficult to evaluate. PDIA shared similar goals to RWJF but had to pursue them with fewer resources. The staff members of both organizations appeared to have good working relations and were able to combine their efforts to enhance effectiveness. The wider synergy between them did not go unnoticed. A *New York Times* reporter commented in 1997 on the PDIA and RWJF involvement: "Foundation giving has often helped create academic and public interest in a topic...But the sharp increase in research on death demonstrates the growing power of philanthropy almost to create an academic field."[4] Given this close interworking, it was unfortunate that both foundations simultaneously reduced their financial commitment to the field. As the RWJF president and CEO subsequently acknowledged, "That we dialed down our funding of end-of-life care at the same time that OSI did, was a mistake...we must always be cognizant of our role relative to other funders."[5]

Despite this late stage error, the combined efforts of the two foundations were enormously influential. In an evaluation of the work of the RWJF programs

2. E. Bronner, "End-of-Life Programs." In S. L. Isaacs and J. R. Knickman (eds.), *To Improve Health and Healthcare*, vol. 6 (San Francisco: Jossey Bass, 2003).

3. P. Patrizi, E. Thompson, and A. Spector, *Improving Care at the End of Life: How the Robert Wood Johnson Foundation and Its Grantees Built the Field* (Princeton, NJ: Robert Wood Johnson Foundation, 2011), 29.

4. J. Miller, "When Foundations Chime in, the Issue of Dying Comes to Life," *New York Times* (November 22, 1997).

5. R. Lavizzo-Maurey, Preface. In P. Patrizi, E. Thompson, and A. Spector, *Improving Care at the End of Life: How the Robert Wood Johnson Foundation and Its Grantees Built the Field* (Princeton, NJ: Robert Wood Johnson Foundation, 2011).

relating to end-of-life care, Patrizi, Thompson, and Spector[6] show how the staff of the two foundations began to articulate a perspective on the ways in which change occurs in medicine. This involved an emphasis on three things: legitimacy, peer relationships, and money. An emergent field in medicine needs high level institutional and personal support, research evidence, standards, quality assurance, and certification. Physicians listen best to other physicians and will respond to effect change. At the same time, new clinical practices require reimbursement streams or must be demonstrably cost effective if institutions are to adopt them.

These are complex and nuanced mechanisms. Accordingly, it was clear in the years after PDIA ended and when RWJF was also reducing its investment in palliative care and end-of-life issues that the role of philanthropy and private grant making in support of palliative care development was not yet concluded. The fragile field would continue to rely on third party and philanthropic funding for some time to come. It was important, therefore, that during its period of operation and afterwards, PDIA was able to contribute to the *culture* of grant making for palliative and end-of-life care in the United States. This culture continued to evolve into the second decade of the twenty-first century and went considerably beyond the immediate preoccupation with disbursing funds to specific grantees. Both on the home front and internationally, the PDIA legacy was in evidence wherever issues around support for end-of-life care initiatives came onto the agenda. In a sense, the entire period of PDIA operations and the subsequent decade represent only one extended phase in a cycle of American philanthropy in support of hospice, palliative, and end-of-life care that stretches back to the 1970s. Diane Meier, in 2010, provided a comprehensive description of philanthropic funding for palliative care in the United States, noting that "the number and diversity of foundation and philanthropic investments in the field of palliative care is remarkable."[7] She provides an extensive inventory of activities—from research to leadership development, professional education, capacity building, guidelines, standards, and public outreach—detailing in each instance the relevant funder. This impressive list goes well beyond the twin pillars of OSI and RWJF, the foundations that in many ways opened up a space for other funders to occupy. Moreover, as we shall see in due course, even with the closure of PDIA, OSI was not yet done with a major commitment to palliative care in the United States.

The establishment of the National Palliative Care Research Center (NPCRC) is a good example of the enduring role of philanthropy in supporting American palliative care initiatives. Under the leadership of PDIA faculty scholar Sean Morrison, the NPCRC was established in July 2005 with a $3.25 million grant

---

6. Patrizi, Thompson, and Spector, *Improving Care at the End of Life.*

7. D. Meier, "The Development, Status, and Future of Palliative Care." In D. E. Meier, S. L. Isaacs, and R. G. Hughes (eds.), *Palliative Care: Transforming the Care of Serious Illness* (San Francisco: Jossey Bass for the Robert Wood Johnson Foundation, 2010), 146.

over five years from the Emily Davie and Joseph S. Kornfeld Foundation.[8] This
was a challenge grant that covered half of the five-year budget, and the new center
was required to raise matching dollars. After its establishment, the NPCRC also
received additional funding from the Brookdale Foundation, the Olive Branch
Foundation, the American Cancer Society, the American Academy of Hospice
and Palliative Medicine, and the National Institute on Aging. It used these funds
to (1) help support research projects conducted by committed and successful palliative care investigators throughout the United States; (2) to develop talented
young investigators and research leaders through competitive national career
development awards; and (3) to provide an organizing and strategic home for
researchers working in relative isolation in medical centers and universities
throughout the country.[9]

NPRC works closely with the Center to Advance Palliative Care (CAPC),
which was established by another PDIA faculty scholar, Diane Meier, in 1999
(see chapter 4) as a National Program Office of the Robert Wood Johnson
Foundation. CAPC has received support from a large consortium of funders[10]
and provides health-care professionals with the tools, training, and technical
assistance necessary to start and sustain successful palliative care programs in
hospitals and other health-care settings. It takes on a national role to promote
increased availability of quality palliative care services for people facing serious illness. As the nation's leading resource for palliative care program development, CAPC offers comprehensive training for palliative care programs at
every stage, from strategic planning and funding to operations and sustain-
ability. It also provides seminars, audio conferences, tools, reference materials, a website, and has established the Palliative Care Leadership Centers as a
major training and mentoring initiative across the United States. CAPC also
sponsors a website for patients and families about how to access palliative care
and attends to improved public understanding of palliative care practices and
services.[11]

---

8. The Kornfeld Foundation was established by Emily Davie Kornfeld in 1979. Ms. Kornfeld's
personal philanthropy supported medical research in the control and treatment of pain,
as well as efforts directed at enhancing individual choice in medical treatment and dying.
Subsequently the Foundation evolved its interests to include bioethics, palliative care, medical research, and education.

9. National Palliative Research Center, "Supporting NPCRC," http://www.npcrc.org/about/
about_show.htm?doc_id=376154 (accessed June 10, 2012).

10. This consortium included Atlantic Philanthropies, the Open Society Institute, Brookdale
Foundation, John A. Hartford Foundation, Y.C. Ho/Helen and Michael Chiang Foundation,
Archstone Foundation, Donaghue Foundation, Partnership for Palliative Care, Olive Branch
Fund, New York State Health Foundation, New York Community Trust, Mill Park Foundation,
Fan Fox and Leslie R. Samuels Foundation, the Altman Foundation, the American Cancer
Society, Cameron and Hayden Lord Foundation, and the Veterans Administration (as part of
its palliative care/end-of-life initiative).

11. Get Palliative Care.org, http://www.getpalliativecare.org/ (accessed July 9, 2012).

Continuing philanthropic support on a large scale has been a key element in the success of both CAPC and the NPCRC. The OSI pledged a $10 million challenge grant to the NPCRC and CAPC. For every three dollars raised from additional sources, OSI made a one dollar contribution. Additionally, Atlantic Philanthropies committed $7 million to the two centers in response to the OSI challenge. These initiatives were facilitated by the work of the Partnership for Palliative Care. Founded in 2008 by a group of national leaders in medicine and philanthropy (with Kathy Foley as one of its board members), the partnership is another nonprofit with palliative care goals. It promotes and focuses on palliative care service expansion, research, advocacy, and public education. The overarching mission of the partnership's work is to raise public awareness of palliative care so that more people living with chronic disease and serious illness can benefit from its effects. The view of the partnership is that without public demand for palliative care, access to relevant specialists and services is likely to remain marginalized, and further expansion will be impeded at a time when need is escalating and there are growing numbers of people with chronic illness. Since its inception, the partnership has helped to raise over $20 million to support the work of CAPC and NPCRC.

It should be acknowledged that a further example of post-PDIA engagement in the area of philanthropic support can been seen in the ongoing participation of Kathy Foley and OSI in the Collaborative to Advance Funding for Palliative Care (CAFPAC). This group takes the view that philanthropy has played a critical role in advancing hospice and palliative care in the United States and that, collectively, philanthropists have been important in funding the establishment of programs, supporting the development of models that can be replicated, and in offering recommendations for other funders. CAFPAC maintains that more philanthropists are needed to advance funding for palliative care and to seize the excellent opportunities for impact. CAFPAC is a growing group of funders, from across the United States, committed to sharing palliative care grant-making concepts and success stories and to stimulating higher levels of funding in palliative care. Its steering committee includes Kathy Foley of OSI as well as Rosemary Gibson of the RWJF.[12]

In December 2009, drawing on work conducted over the previous two years, CAFPAC published a "snapshot report" on palliative care grant making in the United States,[13] as well as a "toolkit" of advice for grant makers new to the

---

12. The CAFPAC steering committee consisted of the following in 2012: Rosemary Gibson, the Robert Wood Johnson Foundation (former), co-chair; Bobye List, the Emily Davie and Joseph S. Kornfeld Foundation, co-chair; Carol A. Farquhar, Grantmakers in Aging; Kathleen Foley, Open Society Institute; Karen Rosa, Altman Foundation; Christina Spellman, the Mayday Fund; Julio Urbina and Lauren Weisenfeld, the Fan Fox and Leslie R. Samuels Foundation; Pamela Lehman, administrator.

13. "Palliative Care Grantmaking Snapshot Report," commissioned by the Collaborative to Advance Funding for Palliative Care (December 2009), http://www.capc.org/old-tools-for-palliative-care-programs/fundraising/grantmaking-snapshot.pdf (accessed October 15, 2012).

field.[14] The report was commissioned in order to learn about private foundation support for palliative care as well as perceptions of related grant making. By these means, CAFPAC sought to identify ways to engage new funders and support those already involved in palliative care grant making. The resulting study revealed three major trends:

- The number of grants and the number of foundations making them is growing, but palliative care still receives a very small percentage of philanthropic support for health care.
- The number of grants made in palliative care has risen and the range of types of palliative care that are supported has grown, with hospice the primary type of palliative care that receives support.
- While the number of foundations making grants in palliative care has grown, a small number of foundations provide most of the funding.

Those who participated were of the opinion that the three current realities act as barriers to expansion of the field: (1) the focus of contemporary medicine on cure, (2) the lack of understanding of palliative care by both health-care professionals and the public, and (3) insufficient funding from public and private sources. At the same time they considered that demand for palliative care will grow and that grant making in the field should also increase. The findings suggest ways in which private foundations can support the development of the field of palliative care grant making and, in so doing, help overcome the barriers to accessing palliative care services. The report took the view that philanthropists now have an opportunity to build on existing efforts around the United States, including the more than $200 million in grants that the RWJF and PDIA had made to support the development and expansion of palliative care. By continuing to advance palliative care grant making, private foundations could thereby increase the well-being of people with serious illnesses and contribute meaningfully to improving the delivery and impact of health care in the United States.[15] It is important to note in the discussion here that the implications of this go far beyond the borders of the United States.

In the context of a global aging population and the growing demand for end-of-life care services, one influential report has referred to a worldwide *race against time* to improve standards of care at the end of life.[16] In the years following the closure of PDIA, and led by the same team, the OSI International

14. The Collaborative to Advance Funding for Palliative Care, "Palliative Care Grantmaking Toolkit," (December 2009), http://www.capc.org/old-tools-for-palliative-care-programs/ (accessed October 15, 2012).

15. "Palliative Care Grantmaking Snapshot Report," http://www.capc.org/old-tools-for-palliative-care-programs/fundraising/grantmaking-snapshot.pdf (accessed October 15, 2012).

16. Economist Intelligence Unit, "The Quality of Death: Ranking End of Life Care Across the World" (2010), http://www.eiu.com/site_info.asp? info_name=qualityofdeath_lienfoundation&page=noads.

Palliative Care Initiative (IPCI) was a key element in this race and a significant provider of funds, resources, and stimulus.[17] The formation of IPCI in 2000 grew out of experience in supporting palliative care developments in Eastern Europe and Central Asia. Its vision was to go beyond these regions, supported by OSI funds and with a global orientation. IPCI was thus ideally positioned to take its place at the table of a newly formed cadre of international players in palliative care development emerging at that time.

As PDIA closed, IPCI was coming into being. In the overlap there was much continuity between the two—most visibly in the leading personnel (Kathy Foley and Mary Callaway) and, crucially, in the thinking and strategy. A decade after it started, IPCI continued to be the only philanthropic endeavor in palliative care with a global reach. IPCI had clearly accelerated the development of the palliative care field, especially in sub–Saharan Africa, as well as through ongoing work in Central and Eastern Europe. In the opening years of the twenty-first century, IPCI sought to empower individuals and organizations championing the development of palliative care in many countries and jurisdictions, often of limited resources. It also advanced awareness and understanding of palliative care issues and supported the establishment of palliative care friendly laws, policies, and standards. As one respondent to an evaluation report noted, "IPCI created an inspirational piece of history," especially in traditional Open Society territory—among transitional states, in the aftermath of communism, and in the face of dictatorial regimes.[18]

From the outset, IPCI achieved a great deal with relatively modest funding, again drawing on the best traditions of PDIA. Until 2004, its annual budget hovered around the $500,000 mark. The budget more than doubled in 2005, and again in 2007, and in 2010 IPCI had $2.5 million per annum at its disposal. This marked increase in available funds (though not commensurate with those available to PDIA) shows a growing recognition of palliative care within the OSI Public Health Program (OSI-PHP) and an acknowledgement of the success and impact of the work of IPCI. Like PDIA, IPCI got by on the work of a small and dedicated staff group, which increased only slightly after 2005. In early 2010, IPCI had four staff members, three full time and one part time. At the same time, the IPCI leadership commands enormous admiration and respect among peers. The standing of its senior staff, combined with their unquestioned and palpable passion for palliative care, sets IPCI apart from other like-minded donors in the field.

In 2000, IPCI began by giving large numbers of small grants to a wide range of individuals and projects. This allowed its staff to identify key players in the field in countries and regions of the world where palliative care activity was not well

---

17. The following paragraphs are summarized from a commissioned evaluation report about the work of IPCI by Kim Brice, Tom Lynch, and David Clark, which was submitted to OSI in autumn of 2010.

18. K. Brice, T. Lynch, and D. Clark, "An Evaluation of the Open Society Institute's International Palliative Care Initiative" (unpublished report, 2010).

documented—again a striking parallel with the early work of PDIA. This same approach to funding a range of initiatives with relatively small grants was to continue for a few years after 2005, at which time IPCI went global. After 2005, IPCI appears to have moved away from interventions that are primarily concerned with service development in localized areas and toward those that have had a greater impact on policy, advocacy, and system change across whole jurisdictions. Such initiatives appear much more targeted to build capacity, to enhance knowledge and expertise in a specific region, and to create the champions who will bring about systems change.

Again, like PDIA with the Faculty Scholars Program, IPCI has adopted a self-consciously elite approach to grant making. It seeks to develop high profile, high status individuals who can make an impact on palliative care development through their professions, within the policy architecture, and by building a coherent argument for palliative care that incorporates human rights imperatives and economic benefits. IPCI has significantly empowered individuals that have gone on to champion change in the palliative care field at national, regional, or global levels. Within the OSI-PHP, IPCI is considered a forerunner in the area of leadership development. IPCI has supported two sustainable models in the area of education. The first is ensuring that a center or beacon of excellence exists within a geographical region; these centers conduct a range of activities including training and advocacy. To date, IPCI has supported them in Hungary, Mongolia, Poland, Romania, Croatia, Slovenia, Singapore, South Africa, and Uganda. The second model is the development of palliative care curricula in undergraduate and postgraduate medical schools, and IPCI has supported such projects in Bulgaria, Poland, Romania, Tajikistan, and South Africa.

IPCI has also facilitated an array of educational courses and seminars, including the End-of-Life Nursing Education Consortium (ELNEC) training of trainers, with instruction provided by the San Diego Hospice and the Institute for Palliative Medicine, as well as the regular Salzburg and OSI palliative care seminar series. Many of these offerings continue to involve former PDIA faculty scholars and grantees. IPCI has also invested in two flagship projects, the Pain and Policy Studies Group's International Pain and Policy Fellowships (IPPF), and the International Palliative Care Leadership Development Initiative, which it also conceptualized from the beginning.

In the area of capacity building, IPCI has supported many organizations that have pioneered the development of the palliative care field either nationally, regionally, or globally. These include hospice and palliative care associations, cancer centers and institutes and, from time to time, government institutions. IPCI investments in organizations have led to four distinct achievements: (1) establishing new and important organizations in the field; (2) contributing to the growth of national, regional and global palliative care associations; (3) implementing activities that are central to its partners' core business, especially advocacy; and (4) enhancing fundraising capacities. Indeed, IPCI is often lauded for supporting nascent organizations from which many donors shy away. These have included the Foundation for Hospices in sub-Saharan Africa, the Palliative Medicine Unit at Mulago Hospital in Uganda and several palliative care units in cancer hospitals around the world.

IPCI has sought to advance palliative care friendly laws, policies, and standards in many countries around the world, as well as at the global level. IPCI is commended for its investments in the policy area since many argue that sustainable change can only start when strong and supportive laws and policies are in place. Nearly half of its spending has targeted policy changes to increase drug availability; the rest has been spread among several themes, most notably health economics and human rights related issues. In these ways, IPCI has undoubtedly contributed to its partners' ability to mobilize resources. There is ample evidence of how IPCI funding has created a snowball effect and helped several partners attract funding (sometime quite substantial) from other donors. This has been possible because of the legitimacy that comes not just from OSI's reputation but from the visibility and status of the IPCI leadership—recognized experts in the global palliative care field among donors and activists alike. In short, IPCI is a worthy legacy of the work of PDIA and testimony to the enduring power of philanthropy in the field of palliative care.

ONGOING WORK OF PDIA FACULTY SCHOLARS, LEADERS, AND GRANTEES

There was plenty of evidence after PDIA closed that its key scholars and grantees remained active in furthering the field of palliative care. The PDIA board had chosen well in many respects. In numerous achievements and initiatives, the fingerprints of PDIA—and particularly the earlier cohorts of faculty scholars, grantees, and social work leaders—could be clearly detected. In reviewing developments in palliative care in the United States since the closure of PDIA in 2003, it is not difficult, therefore, to find examples of the PDIA legacy and of ways in which the PDIA approach to things continued to shape the field and its aspirations.

Center to Advance Palliative Care and National Palliative Care Research Center

As we have seen, a clear example of such involvement is the work developed by CAPC and the NPCRC, where the powerful combination of Diane Meier and Sean Morrison[19] continues to be much in evidence. The work of CAPC has been about driving palliative care into the American hospital system. It has argued for this on the twin pillars of quality and cost reduction. CAPC was established in 1999 to provide operational and technical assistance to hospitals developing

---

19. Cohort one PDIA faculty scholars in a team of four.

palliative care programs and has produced an array of products for hospital leaders seeking to establish sustainable palliative care services. As early as 2004, CAPC was attracting significant praise. Here is some from Risa Lavizzo-Mourey, president and CEO of the Robert Wood Johnson Foundation:

> · The American Hospital Association reports a 90 percent increase in palliative care programs in the last five years; today one in five hospitals has a program. *US News and World Report* now considers palliative care as a criterion in its annual ranking of the country's top hospitals. These are significant outcomes for director Diane E. Meier, MD, and the center's partners.[20]

From 2000 to 2011, hospital palliative care programs in US hospitals more than doubled in number to 1600, and in 2011 more than 60 percent of hospitals reported the presence of a palliative care program, a figure rising to over 80 percent for the country's medium-to-large–sized hospitals (over 300 beds).[21]

CAPC has also established particular focused initiatives built around specfic aspects of hospital medicine. Launched in 2010, the IPAL (initiative to improve palliative care) Project[22] is a CAPC intervention designed to provide a central venue for sharing expertise, evidence, tools, and resources essential to the integration and improvement of palliative care in *specific* health-care settings. Each IPAL project has been developed using a similar process and involves the following: an oversight board of nationally recognized interdisciplinary leaders; a catalog of most-needed tools and resources to help spur systems-change work that will integrate principles of palliative care into daily practice; the identification of existing tools and resources from established and emerging teams across the country; the development of new peer-reviewed tools representing best practice; and updates for the website as new tools become available.

The initiative's first offering was IPAL-ICU (Improving Palliative Care in the ICU), launched in June 2010, and led by former PDIA faculty scholar Judith Nelson,[23] with support from the National Institutes of Health. This project starts with the premise that, from time of admission into the ICU, all critically ill patients and their families should benefit from palliative care, which should be provided concurrently with intensive care therapies. IPAL-ICU is designed to provide a central venue for sharing expertise, evidence, and tools, along with links to colleagues, organizations, and informational materials. The goal

---

20. "President's Message on Health Care 2004," from the Robert Wood Johnson Foundation, http://www.rwjf.org/files/publications/annual/2004/RWJFAR04_PresLetter.pdf (accessed June 21, 2012; site discontinued).

21. S. Morrison and D. E. Meier, "The National Palliative Care Research Center and the Center to Advance Palliative Care: A partnership to Improve Care for Persons with Serious Illness and Their Families," *Journal of Pediatric Hematology and Oncology* 33 (October 2011): S126–S131, doi: 10.1097/MPH.0b013e318230dfa0.

22. The iPal Project, http://www.capc.org/ipal/ (accessed June 20, 2012).

23. Judith Nelson joined the Faculty Scholars Program in 1999.

is to assist ICU and hospital leaders, as well as clinicians across disciplines, to integrate palliative care and intensive care successfully.

The second initiative is IPAL-EM (Improving Palliative Care in Emergency Medicine), led by Tammie Quest,[24] with support from the Olive Branch Foundation. This starts from the premise that some patients with serious or life-threatening illness may find themselves in an emergency department in the course of their illness, and they should expect to receive high-quality palliative care in that setting. Emergency medicine has increasingly taken a central role in the early implementation of palliative care. Widespread integration of palliative care into the day-to-day practice of emergency medicine, however, is often jeopardized by the demands of many competing priorities. IPAL-EM has been designed to address this issue and to offer a central portal for sharing essential expertise, evidence, tools, and practical resources to assist clinicians and administrators with the successful integration of palliative care and emergency medicine.

It should be noted that the focus of CAPC has not been relentlessly on the hospital setting. In 2007, it published *Navigating Palliative Care*, in collaboration with the National Hospice and Palliative Care Organization, to document the status of hospice-based palliative care initiatives and to identify the opportunities and barriers hospices face in establishing non-hospice palliative care programs across the country. The guide details the lessons hospice organizations have learned when framing or implementing palliative care models and describes firsthand the possibilities and challenges others have observed and experienced.[25]

If CAPC is a home to direct care providers, then NPRC provides the same function for researchers. NPRC seeks to establish priorities for palliative care research; to develop a new generation of researchers in palliative care; and to coordinate and support studies focused on improving care for patients and families living with serious illness. It also endeavors to take research findings and rapidly translate them into effective clinical practice. Prior to the establishment of the NPCRC, there was no organizing force promoting and facilitating the conduct of palliative care research. Because departments or divisions of palliative medicine do not yet exist in most medical schools, palliative care research is mainly conducted by a small number of investigators working in relative isolation from each other at a handful of medical schools in the United States. The NPCRC provides an administrative home to promote intellectual exchange, the sharing of resources, and access to data from ongoing studies to plan and support new research. It does this within a collaborative approach to establishing its funding priorities.

The center has a scientific advisory board comprised of internationally prominent scientists—three of whom were active in PDIA. The board gives

---

24. Tammie Quest joined the Faculty Scholars Program in 2002.

25. National Hospice and Palliative Care Organization, Navigating Palliative Care: CD and Manual, http://iweb.nhpco.org/iweb/Purchase/ProductDetail.aspx?Product_code=821136 (accessed June 21, 2012).

final approval for all research grants, collaborative projects, and junior faculty career development awards based upon recommendations made by the NPCRC's Scientific Review Committee, which likewise includes former PDIA activists. The NPCRC focuses on three specific areas of research: (1) pain and symptom management, (2) improved communication between providers and patients through rigorously designed clinical studies, and (3) health services research, specifically the evaluation of models of care for palliative care delivery.

It emphasizes the need to explore the relationship of pain and other distressing symptoms to quality and quantity of life, independence, function, and disability, as well as to develop interventions directed at their treatment in patients with advanced and chronic illness. It also promotes methods for improving communication between adults or children living with serious illness, their families, and their health-care providers. In addition, it takes the view that current systems of care and reimbursement fail to address many of the needs of patients with serious and chronic illness, and the evaluation of models and systems of care for patients living with serious illness should have some priority. To this end, NPCRC supports pilot and exploratory project grants, junior faculty career development awards, infrastructure support for collaborative studies, and assistance with research design and statistical support. In a collaborative parallel initiative, the American Cancer Society (ACS) also supports pilot projects in palliative and cancer care that are modeled on the NPCRC program. In its first five years, seventeen NPCRC/ACS investigators were funded, leading to seventeen subsequent NIH grants.[26] The center also holds an annual Kathleen Foley Palliative Care Retreat and Research Symposium to provide an opportunity for interdisciplinary palliative care researchers to come together to network, learn from each other, discuss the science of palliative care, and develop new research ideas and collaborations.[27]

These two centers are described in a paper by Morrison and Meier.[28] Both contribute to the development of research as a knowledge base for good clinical care and associated programs. Both seek to disseminate such knowledge widely to patients, families, and professionals, and to ensure integration in mainstream care. Both make use of social marketing approaches, have developed sensitivity to their target audiences, and employ websites and social media to good effect. Both work to influence and collaborate with policy makers, regulatory bodies, and federal funding agencies to ensure the continued growth of palliative care. Focused on service development and knowledge creation and united by a desire to use best evidence as a driver for change, the two centers are concrete and con-

26. National Palliative Care Research Center, "5th Annual Kathleen M. Foley Palliative Care Research Retreat and Symposium," http://www.npcrc.org/usr_doc/retreat_intro_and_overview_2011.pdf (accessed July 16, 2012).

27. Ibid.

28. S. Morrison and D. E. Meier, "National Palliative Care Research Center and Center to Advance Palliative Care."

tinuing evidence of palliative care recognition, and they serve as platforms for further innovation and development.

Specialty Recognition and Consensus Guidelines

Also of major significance in the years immediately following the closure of PDIA has been the work to achieve formal recognition for the specialty of hospice and palliative medicine. This recognition was gained in 2006 through the Accreditation Council for Graduate Medical Education (ACGME), which accredits physician training programs, and the American Board of Medical Specialties (ABMS), which sets the standards for specialists in its member boards. Lupu et al note the importance of this achievement:

> Both certification and accreditation elevated standards within a nascent specialty, and adherence to high principles ultimately convinced those in organized medicine that a formal specialty status for hospice and palliative medicine was warranted.[29]

This involved a transition in the physician certification process from the independent American Board of Hospice and Palliative Medicine (ABHPM) to the ABMS, and thereafter in the accreditation of training programs from another independent organization to the ACGME.[30] In this process, hospice and palliative medicine became a subspecialty of no less than eleven primary specialties, a first in the history of the ABMS. Formal certification of physicians and accreditation of training programs began in 2008.[31] It had been a complex route, but journey's end had been reached and PDIA Cohort One faculty scholar Charles von Gunten chose a baseball analogy to make the point, likening the process to a home run. In an editorial published in October 2006, he observed the following:

> At some baseball games, they set off a round of fireworks when something like this happens. It is always spectacular—multiple fireworks going off simultaneously, so you don't know where to look. It is enough to sit back and enjoy it. That's what I am doing now. As an adult you know the fireworks will end, and it will be time to go back to doing the work that is still

---

29. D. Lupu et al., "Hospice and Palliative Medicine in the USA: The Road to Recognition," *European Journal of Palliative Care* 16, no. 3 (2009): 136–141.

30. R. Schonwetter, "Hospice and Palliative Medicine Goes Mainstream," *Journal of Palliative Medicine* 9, no. 6 (2006): 1240–1242.

31. Meanwhile, in Canada, a country that has played a major role in the development of modern palliative care, specialty status for palliative medicine has not been attained, to serious detrimental effect in the eyes of at least one senior commentator. See N. Macdonald, "The Development of Palliative Care in Canada." In E. Bruera et al. (eds.), *Textbook of Palliative Medicine* (London: Hodder Arnold, 2006), 22–28.

to be done. But, it would be a shame not to sit back, childlike, and enjoy the sense of spectacle, bedazzled.[32,33]

Once again it seemed to be evidence of the effective collaboration of PDIA and RWJF. The Robert Wood Johnson Foundation had supported ACGME to develop standards for postresidency fellowship programs in hospice and palliative care and then to accredit programs as they came on line. PDIA supported ABHPM's leadership role in gaining formal recognition. The result was specialty recognition in near record time.[34]

Linked to these achievements was the decision to have the specialty association of physicians, the American Academy of Hospice and Palliative Medicine (AAHPM), join the American Medical Association officially as part of its specialty section. This growth and maturation of the AAHPM to a professional association that went far beyond the interest of hospice medical directors is certainly important, and there is no doubt that PDIA scholars played a key role in the process. One of the big issues within PDIA was whether to splinter and form a new group of "academic" doctors or to try to work within the AAHPM and have it move to, or at least include, an academic thrust. Diane Meier and Charles von Gunten argued for the latter and that view ultimately prevailed.

Another key area of development that merits acknowledgment is an initiative to produce national clinical practice guidelines for quality palliative care through the National Consensus Project (NCP).[35] This collaboration between major palliative care organizations is an attempt to further define and underscore the value of palliative care and to improve upon its delivery in the United States. A major objective of the NCP is to heighten awareness of palliative care as an option in treating those with a life-limiting or chronic debilitating illness, condition, or injury, and to raise public understanding of the growing need for such care. The development of palliative care consensus guidelines was discussed during a national leadership conference coordinated by the Center to Advance Palliative Care convened in December 2001 at the New York Academy

---

32. C. F. von Gunten, "Bedazzled by a Home Run," *Journal of Palliative Medicine* 9, no. 5 (2006): 1036–1036.

33. Joanne Lynn, in commenting on the manuscript of this book, took a more cautious viewpoint. "The support of PDIA and others for making palliative care a specialty of medicine is a key part of the work. I still wait to see whether that effort turns out to be, on the whole, a good thing. It has allowed substantial expansion of the number of paid practitioners, which is a good thing, but the professional gains are still tenuous and perhaps are coming at the cost of undercutting geriatrics and even primary care. I hope that eventually our palliative care specialty will develop a stronger commitment to training practitioners in the skills needed for local delivery system reform and that we will become part of strategic planning on behalf of our patients and their caregivers." Joanne Lynn, personal communication, July 3, 2010.

34. Patrizi, Thompson, and Spector, *Improving Care at the End of Life*, 14.

35. National Consensus Project for Quality Palliative Care, "Welcome," http://www.national-consensusproject.org (accessed June 21, 2012).

of Medicine. Participants at the conference were identified through a national peer nomination process. This meeting served as the genesis of the NCP and its core aims:

- To define an effective national consensus process for establishment of clinical practice guidelines for quality palliative care in the United States
- To develop such guidelines through an evidence-based review process involving major US palliative care organizations and a large number of professionals in diverse disciplines
- To disseminate the guidelines to all stakeholders involved in the delivery of health care to persons with life-threatening illnesses
- To promote formal recognition, stable reimbursement structures, and accreditation initiatives in palliative care

This endeavor was supported by a coalition of national palliative care organizations to oversee and ensure its success. An original twenty-member steering committee provided leadership in the writing and completion of the consensus document, along with communication and dissemination of progress reports. Additionally, the committee was charged with the responsibility to secure necessary financing to support the project. Nearly one hundred nationally recognized palliative care experts reviewed and contributed to the development of the guidelines, ranging from physicians to nurses, to social workers, chaplains, therapists, and other critical palliative care support professionals. To augment the dissemination of the guidelines, more than one hundred organizations, representing significant national constituencies, were invited to review and endorse the guidelines.

The NCP is based in Pittsburgh, Pennsylvania, at the Hospice and Palliative Nurses Association, one of four partner organizations comprising the Hospice and Palliative Care Coalition. The other partners are the American Academy of Hospice and Palliative Medicine (AAHPM), the Center to Advance Palliative Care (CAPC), and the National Hospice and Palliative Care Organization (NHPCO). The NCP has been structured to maximize the participation and input of a broad range of palliative care professionals, health-care organizations, policy and quality review entities, consumers, and payers. A series of working groups has been formed to ensure a comprehensive, transparent, and representative consensus process underpinning the development of *Clinical Practice Guidelines for Quality Palliative Care.*[36]

The NCP has implemented a strategic communications and dissemination plan designed to inform, educate, and influence critical constituencies—from health-care professionals to the general public—on the importance of palliative care as a viable option for patients of any age who are diagnosed with life-threatening

---

36. National Consensus Project for Quality Palliative Care (2009), *Clinical Practice Guidelines for Quality Palliative Care,* 2nd ed., http://www.nationalconsensusproject.org/Guidelines_ Download2.aspx (accessed October 15, 2012).

illness or a chronic debilitating condition or injury. Endorsement and voluntary adoption of the NCP's clinical practice guidelines will inaugurate a national initiative that aspires ultimately to quality and performance assessments, and a universal approach to ensuring quality palliative care across the nation.

Landmark Texts

During the period of the program, numerous PDIA scholars and grantees demonstrated an appetite for the production of major collections and textbooks that helped to shape and establish the field of palliative and end-of-life care, many examples of which have been described in earlier chapters. In reviewing the output since the closure of PDIA, there is continuing evidence of the production of such works. It is encouraging to see that these range not only across the preoccupations of academic medicine, but also engage more fully with interdisciplinary perspectives, something that was always challenging for PDIA.

In 2009, the second edition of the *Handbook of Psychiatry in Palliative Medicine* was published, edited by PDIA faculty scholars Harvey Chochinov and William Breitbart.[37] Eight years after the first edition, this book shows how psychiatric (or psychosocial) palliative care has evolved and the effect this has had on palliative medicine. Its twenty-eight chapters and sixty-seven contributors make it clear that palliation that neglects psychosocial dimensions of patient and family experience fails to meet contemporary standards of comprehensive palliative care. While a focus on somatic issues has sometimes overshadowed attention to psychological, existential, and spiritual end-of-life challenges, the book shows the growing interest in a multidisciplinary approach to care for the dying beginning to take hold. One reviewer described the editors as "well-known sensitive giants in a field that requires a balance of scientific evidence-based thinking and empathic humaneness."[38]

In 2010, Diane Meier, with colleagues Stephen Isaacs and Robert Hughes, produced an edited volume within the Robert Wood Johnson Foundation series on health policy. Entitled *Palliative Care: Transforming the Care of Serious Illness*,[39] the book begins with a major essay by Meier on the development, status, and future of palliative care in the United States. This is followed by twenty-five reprinted chapters and landmark publications from major figures in the field, going back to the work of Elisabeth Kübler-Ross in the 1960s. Described by one

---

37. H. M. Chochinov and W. Breitbart, *Handbook of Psychiatry in Palliative Medicine*, 2nd ed. (New York: Oxford University Press, 2009).

38. M. Blumenfield, review of *Handbook of Psychiatry in Palliative Medicine*, 2nd ed. In *American Journal of Psychiatry* 167 (2010): 355–356, http://ajp.psychiatryonline.org/article. aspx?articleID=102152 (accessed 13 July 2012), doi: 10.1176/appi.ajp.2009.09071056.

39. D. E. Meier, S. L. Isaacs, and R. G. Hughes, *Palliative Care: Transforming the Care of Serious Illness* (San Francisco: Jossey Bass, 2010).

reviewer as "a whirlwind tour of the history of the hospice and palliative care movement and how it is reshaping the care given to those with serious illnesses,"[40] the book has quickly become essential reading for those entering the field, as well as a remarkable record of achievement over a forty-year period.

In 2011, the *Textbook of Interdisciplinary Pediatric Palliative Care*, edited by Joanne Wolfe (a faculty scholar), Pamela Hinds (a PDIA grantee), and Barbara Sourkes broke new ground.[41] Across 44 chapters and written by more than 120 contributors, the book addresses language, communication, symptoms, quality of life, and the full spectrum of life-threatening illness in children, showing the benefits of a collaborative interdisciplinary strategy. The book's innovative format includes an electronically searchable electronic text. One reviewer took the view that "the interdisciplinary focus of the new book sets it apart."[42] Another wrote: "This outstanding volume is a must for pediatric palliative care specialists," going on to describe its relevance for pediatricians generally, as well as for adult palliative care specialists.[43] This was a major milestone for a specialized field of endeavor whose champions had at times felt slightly marginal to the main thrust of PDIA.

In 2011, two members of the PDIA Social Work Leadership Development Program, Terry Altilio and Shirley Otis-Green, edited the first edition of the *Oxford Textbook of Palliative Social Work*. This monumental work contains eighty-four chapters, many of them authored by PDIA grantees.[44] In an early chapter, Susan Blacker and Grace Christ define social work's role and leadership contributions in palliative care. They detail the contributions made by the PDIA social work leaders and draw attention to subsequent developments that came out of their program. Primary among these is the Social Work Hospice and Palliative Care Network, which was established in December 2007. Intended as a parallel venture to the Hospice and Palliative Care Nurses Association and the American Academy of Hospice and Palliative Medicine, the network includes practitioners, educators, researchers, and policy advocates, and it has an international membership. This "virtual community of practice" has gone on to organize major conferences and to contribute expertise in analyzing, influencing, and implementing policy change to improve care of those with life-limiting illness and those who are dying or bereaved.

---

40. Geripal, "A Geriatrics and Palliative Care Blog" (April 26, 2010), http://www.geripal.org/2010/04/palliative-care-transforming-care-of.html (accessed July 10, 2012).

41. J. Wolfe, P. Hinds, and B. Sourkes, *Textbook of Interdisciplinary Pediatric Palliative Care* (Philadelphia, PA: Elsevier Saunders, 2011).

42. R. Woodruff, *IAHPC News* (May 5, 2011), http://www.hospicecare.com/news/11/05/reviews.html (accessed July 16, 2012).

43. S. Weinstein, review of *Textbook of Interdisciplinary Pediatric Palliative Care*. In *Journal of Pain and Symptom Management* 42, no. 6 (2011): 972.

44. T. Altilio and S. Otis-Green (eds.), *Oxford Textbook of Palliative Social Work* (New York: Oxford University Press).

Key Studies Post-PDIA

Several studies stand out in the post-PDIA decade for their importance in shedding light on the delivery of palliative care, for how that care is perceived on the part of patients and families, and for evidence of its effectiveness.

In 2004, Joan Teno and others established good evidence of the quality of hospice care in the United States. This was the first attempt in the country to examine the adequacy or quality of end-of-life care in institutional settings compared with deaths at home. It used Teno's favored "mortality follow-back" method to survey family members or other knowledgeable informants representing 1,578 decedents, with a two-stage probability sample used to estimate end-of-life care outcomes for 1.97 million deaths from chronic illness in the United States in the year 2000. Informants were asked over the telephone about the patient's experience at the last place of care at which the patient spent more than 48 hours. Family members of patients receiving hospice services were more satisfied with overall quality of care—70.7 percent rated care as "excellent," compared with less than 50 percent of those dying in an institutional setting or with home health services. The study concluded that many people dying in institutions have unmet needs for symptom amelioration, physician communication, emotional support, and being treated with respect, and that family members of decedents who received care at home with hospice services were more likely to report a favorable dying experience.[45]

This was complemented in 2007 by a publication involving PDIA faculty scholar James Tulsky, which for the first time provided solid evidence of the cost-reduction benefits of hospice care. The authors point out that since their inclusion in US Medicare, hospices have been expected to reduce health care costs, but the literature on their ability to do so has been mixed. The contradictory findings of earlier studies may have been due to selection bias and the period of cost comparison used. Accounting for these possibilities, the 2007 study focuses on the length of hospice use that maximizes reductions in medical expenditures near death. The authors used a retrospective case-control study of Medicare decedents (1993–2003) to compare 1,819 hospice decedents with 3,638 controls, matched through their predicted likelihood of dying while using a hospice. The variables used to create matches were demographics, primary medical condition, cost of Medicare-financed care prior to the last year of life, nursing home residence, and Medicaid eligibility. The study showed that hospice use reduced Medicare program expenditures during the last year of life by an average of $2,309 per hospice user: $7,318 in expenditures for hospice users compared to $9,627 for controls. On average, hospice use reduced these Medicare costs during all but two of the hospice users' last seventy-two days of life; about $10 on the seventy-second day prior to death; and with savings increasing to more than $750 on the day of death. Maximum cumulative expenditure reductions differed by primary condition. The maximum reduction in Medicare expenditures for each

---

45. J. M. Teno et al., "Family Perspectives on End-of-Life Care at the Last Place of Care," *Journal of American Medical Association* 291, no. 1 (2004): 88–93.

user was about $7,000, which occurred when a decedent had a primary condition of cancer and used a hospice for their last 58 to 103 days of life. For other primary conditions, the maximum savings of around $3,500 occurred when hospice was used for the last 50 to 108 days of life. Given the relatively short length of hospice use observed in the Medicare program, the authors argued that increasing the length of hospice use for seven in ten Medicare hospice users would increase savings to the program.[46]

A study published in August 2010[47] produced findings that rocked both palliative care specialists and generalists alike. Advanced cancer patients who received early palliative care in conjunction with standard care for their disease not only reported better quality of life, but lived a few months longer than patients who received only standard care. The research included 151 patients diagnosed with metastatic non-small cell lung cancer who were randomly assigned to one of two treatment plans. At twelve weeks, 86 percent of those who were still alive filled out assessments of their quality of life and mood. Those who received palliative care—which included addressing physical and psychosocial symptoms, establishing goals of care, assisting with decisions about treatment and coordinating care—on top of standard treatment, scored significantly higher on a quality-of-life scale and reported fewer depressive symptoms than those having regular care alone. Moreover, in the palliative group median survival was 11.6 months, versus 8.9 months, and fewer of them received aggressive care at the end of life. The new findings were widely seen as endorsing the view that palliative care is not synonymous with renouncing all attempts to cure the disease and demonstrating that cancer care and palliative care can be concurrent.

The following year another study, led by several PDIA veterans, found that using well-established palliative care teams to coordinate the care of seriously ill Medicaid patients can save money, at least in the hospital, where their use reduced inpatient costs by about $6,900 per admission for the average patient.[48] The study looked at data from 2004 to 2007 covering 485 Medicaid patients who received palliative care. Patients included people with metastatic cancers, HIV/AIDS with one of several secondary diagnoses, and congestive-heart failure patients with frequent hospitalizations, among others. Of those patients receiving palliative care, 296 patients were discharged alive (some went to hospice and others went back to home care) and 189 died in the hospital. Researchers matched those patients with 1,576 similar patients who received usual care. Then they compared the hospital costs incurred by the two groups. The difference was $4,098 per admission for patients discharged alive and $7,563 for those who died

46. D. H. Taylor et al., "What Length of Hospice Use Maximizes Reduction in Medical Expenditures Near Death in the US Medicare Program?" *Social Science and Medicine* 65, no. 7 (2007): 1466–1478.

47. J. A. Temel et al., "Early Palliative Care for Patients with Metastatic Non–Small-Cell Lung Cancer," *New England Journal of Medicine* 363 (2010): 733–742.

48. R. S. Morrison et al., "Palliative Care Consultation Teams Cut Hospital Costs for Medicaid Beneficiaries," *Health Affairs* 30, no. 3 (2011): 454–463.

in the hospital. The study found that in New York State alone that could mean a savings of between \$84 million and \$252 million annually, depending on the percentage of Medicaid patients receiving palliative care, if every hospital with 150 or more beds had a palliative care team. *Where do the savings come from?* asked the *Wall Street Journal's* Health Blog?[49] Sean Morrison's reply was that palliative care teams "listen to what patients want to achieve from the health-care system, listen to their goals and what they want to accomplish, then match their treatment to those goals. Some patients might want to pursue all treatment options, while others want to be comfortable and to minimize symptoms. In the setting of this very complex, very sick population, you're eliminating misutilization."

By 2011, the *Washington Post* could report that while Americans still had a poor understanding of palliative care, its availability in hospital settings was becoming better established.[50] At that time, only 24 percent of the US population claimed to be familiar with the term palliative care, but 58 percent of hospitals with more than 50 beds now had palliative care services.[51] The findings of the opinion poll cited here were instructive. By a wide margin, Americans believe it is more important to enhance the quality of life for seriously ill patients, even if it means a shorter life (71 percent), than to extend life through every medical intervention possible (23 percent)—a result consistent across all political affiliations. More than half of Americans (55 percent) believe that the health-care system has the responsibility, technology, and expertise to offer treatments and to spend whatever it takes to extend lives. This is compared to 37 percent who believe the health-care system spends far too much trying to extend the lives of seriously ill patients. Americans are unfamiliar with the term palliative care (24 percent say they are "familiar"), especially compared to end-of-life care (65 percent) and hospice care (86 percent). Nearly two out of every three Americans (63 percent) have had personal or family experience with palliative care, end-of-life care, or hospice care. A strong majority believe there should be more of an open debate about public policies regarding palliative care options (78 percent agree). Respondents also agree that educating patients and their families about these issues is important (97 percent) and they think a public dialogue will provide more information about care options (86 percent). Yet roughly half (47 percent) of respondents across all political affiliations say they worry that emphasizing palliative and end-of-life care options could interfere with doing whatever it takes to help patients extend their lives as long as possible.[52]

49. *Wall Street Journal*, Health Blog, "Study: Palliative Care for Medicaid Patients Reduces Their Hospital Costs," Katherine Hobson, http://blogs.wsj.com/health/2011/03/08/study-pall iative-care-for-medicaid-patients-reduces-their-hospital-costs/ (accessed June 21, 2012).

50. "Hospitals Increasingly Offer Palliative Care," *Washington Post* (March 28 2011).

51. Center to Advance Palliative Care, "Analysis of U.S. Hospital Palliative Care Programs: 2010 Snapshot," http://www.capc.org/news-and-events/releases/analysis-of-us-hospital-palli ative-care-programs-2010-snapshot.pdf (accessed June 21, 2012; data reported was for 2008).

52. Red Orbit, "New Poll: Americans Choose Quality Over Quantity at the End of Life, Crave Deeper Public Discussion of Care Options," *National Journal* (March 2011), http://www.

Another study conducted in the same year for CAPC and with support from the American Cancer Society was designed to produce a roadmap for communicating with consumers and policy makers on the benefits and future direction of palliative care.[53] It too found a lack of awareness among potential consumers and patients with serious illness that palliative care services exist.

Likewise, the term palliative care had little or no meaning to consumers, with many inside the health-care industry framing it as end-of-life care. However, once informed, consumers are extremely positive about palliative care and want access to this care if they need it: 95 percent of respondents agreed that it is important that patients with serious illness and their families be educated about palliative care; 92 percent of respondents say they were likely to consider palliative care for a loved one if they had a serious illness; 92 percent of respondents say it is important that palliative care services be made available at all hospitals for patients with serious illness and their families. The study developed and tested a new language definition of palliative care and suggested it should be used when defining or describing palliative care for consumers:

Palliative care is specialized medical care for people with serious illnesses. This type of care is focused on providing patients with relief from the symptoms, pain, and stress of a serious illness—whatever the diagnosis. The goal is to improve quality of life for both the patient and the family. Palliative care is provided by a team of doctors, nurses, and other specialists who work with a patient's other doctors to provide an extra layer of support. Palliative care is appropriate at any age and at any stage in a serious illness, and can be provided together with curative treatment.[54]

redorbit.com/news/health/2008599/new_poll_americans_choose_quality_over_quantity_at_the_End/?storylink=digger-topic (accessed October 12, 2012).

53. Center to Advance Palliative Care, "2011 Public Opinion Research on Palliative Care," http://www.capc.org/tools-for-palliative-care-programs/marketing/public-opinion-research/ 2011-public-opinion-research-on-palliative-care.pdf (accessed June 21, 2012).

54. Center to Advance Palliative Care, "2011 Public Opinion Research on Palliative Care," 13, http://www.capc.org/tools-for-palliative-care-programs/marketing/public-opinion-research/2011-public-opinion-research-on-palliative-care.pdf (accessed June 21, 2012). On this evidence, Diane Meier and other leaders in the palliative care field set out to seek funding for an ambitious five-year, multimillion-dollar social marketing campaign to increase public awareness regarding palliative care. "We've recognized that we're not going to see policy change without public support," Dr. Meier said. Among the policy changes she and her colleagues seek is a big boost in the palliative care workforce, which at present is so small as to constitute a major barrier to access.... Another priority is to develop a midcareer board certification track in palliative care across all medical disciplines.... Starting in 2013, the specialty will require fellowship training for board certification in palliative care. See The Oncology Report, "Palliative Care Specialists Ponder Public Awareness Campaign," http://www.oncologypractice.com/oncologyreport/single-view/palliative-care-specialists-ponder-public-awareness-campaign/4ef71705c9e7b4f8c1a4803880a51cd1.html (accessed July 16, 2012).

Evidence from studies such as these was welcomed by palliative care activists and marked a sense of growing confidence in the community of palliative care leaders. Here were data to support the case that palliative care has beneficial effects and can reduce costs. Moreover these findings achieved the twin success of being published in respectable medical journals and, at the same time, of gaining wider publicity in the mass media. Palliative care seemed to be coming of age. The aspirations so often articulated at PDIA retreats over the years were beginning to be realized. Investment in research and capacity building was paying off and the supporters of palliative care were now taking the argument onto the central ground of American health-care policy, with all its challenges and contradictions. The president of the Association of American Medical Colleges remarked as follows in June 2011:

> Patients with multiple chronic conditions often require the highly specialized and individualized care academic medical centers provide, including an interdisciplinary team of health care and social service providers, pain management, and increased communication with at-home caregivers. All these elements are aspects of palliative care, a subspecialty aimed at improving the quality of life for patients with one or more chronic conditions. Contrary to the perceptions of many, palliative care is often administered alongside curative treatments and has been shown to extend the lives of some patients. Interestingly, multiple studies have shown that this is exactly the kind of care patients want, even if they are not familiar with the term *palliative care.*
>
> The increased national focus on palliative care could not come at a better time. According to the Centers for Disease Control and Prevention, chronic conditions, such as heart disease, cancer, and diabetes, are the leading causes of death and disability in the United States, accounting for 70 percent of all deaths in the country. The U.S. population also is aging, with nearly one in five Americans expected to be age 65 or older by 2030. With both chronic disease and higher rates of health care utilization associated with aging, and more Americans having access to regular health care through the Affordable Care Act, the need for palliative care is only likely to increase...Palliative care and related fields, like geriatrics, are a microcosm of the larger health care system. Everything is amplified when the patient in front of us is managing multiple chronic conditions, from the need for us to work seamlessly with other health professions to placing the patient and their family's needs truly at the center of our efforts. For all these reasons, palliative care is a high-impact specialty that will see increased demand moving forward and will require some of medicine's brightest minds to choose it as their career path.[55]

---

55. D. G. Kirsch, "A Word from the President: Embracing the Value of Palliative Medicine,"Association of American Medical Colleges (June 2011), https://www.aamc.org/newsroom/reporter/june2011/250904/word.html (accessed July 9, 2009).

Further Reverberations

A key element in much of PDIA's ambition was the creation of leaders who could forge and then transform a field of endeavor. It is clear from the examples given here that many faculty scholars, leadership award holders, and grantees continued to influence the shape of palliative care in the United States over many years after the PDIA concluded its programs. One indicative measure of this can be seen in a set of awards made annually by the American Academy of Hospice and Palliative Medicine: the Project on Death in America Palliative Medicine Community Leadership Awards. These recognize physician leaders who have advanced the field of palliative care by the education of the next generation of palliative care leaders. The award promotes the visibility and prestige of physicians in both academic and clinical settings who are committed to mentoring future leaders and serving as role models for other health professionals engaged in improving the care of the dying. The awards began in 2006 and have been given to eight individuals, seven of whom were beneficiaries of PDIA funding and five of whom were faculty scholars.

The Academy's Award for Excellence in Scientific Research in Palliative Care reveals a similar picture. It recognizes meaningful, exemplary research contributions to the field of hospice and palliative care, and the recipient is expected to present his or her research within the broad context of the field of hospice and palliative care. These awards began in 2004, and by 2012, three had gone to former PDIA faculty scholars and three more to PDIA grantees.[56]

In the social work arena, 2007 saw the inaugural PDIA Social Work Leadership Award. This goes to social workers who demonstrate outstanding leadership and who have advanced the field in end-of-life, hospice, and palliative care. The goal of the award is to acknowledge and increase the visibility of social workers' contributions to the field and to encourage future generations to continue providing quality care to the seriously ill, dying, and bereaved. By 2010, two of the four awards had been given to former PDIA social work leaders.[57]

It is possible to see the model of PDIA reverberating in initiatives that seek to build leadership and improvement in medicine and health care as well. For example, in 2012, a $2.6-million, three-year grant from the John Templeton Foundation got underway in which former PDIA faculty scholar Daniel Sulmasy and Farr Curlin co-direct the Program on Medicine and Religion at the University of Chicago to create a *Clinical Scholars Program*, designed to provide the essential infrastructure for the spiritual renewal of the medical

56. In 2012: J. Randall Curtis, MD, MPH; in 2011: Harvey Chochinov, MD, PhD, FRCPC; in 2010: Sebastiano Mercadante, MD; in 2009: Vincent Mor, PhD; in 2008: Irene Higginson, BMedSci, BMBS, FFPHM, PhD; in 2007: Betty Ferrell, PhD, RN, FAAN; in 2006: James Tulsky, MD; in 2005: Joan Teno, MD, MS; in 2004: Eduardo Bruera, MD, http://www.aahpm.org/about/default/awards.html (accessed October 15, 2012).

57. Social Work Hospice & Palliative Care Network, http://www.swhpn.org/award/ (accessed July 10, 2012).

profession.[58] Also in 2012, the Templeton Foundation made a $1.5million grant to the Health Care Chaplaincy (a national leader in advancing the role of chaplaincy care within palliative care and a former beneficiary of PDIA funds) to support six research projects on the role of chaplaincy care. Likewise, in the same year, the Cicely Saunders International Faculty Scholars initiative was established to encourage individuals who will be future clinical leaders and investigators in end-of-life and palliative care.[59]

Future Challenges

Hospice, and then palliative care, was a "small rebellion" that got underway in the United States in the early 1970s.[60] Forty years on, the achievements have been considerable. This book has focused on the particular contributions made by the PDIA during the nine years of its operations (1994–2003). In this final chapter, I have also reviewed some of the ongoing developments in palliative care that have taken place in the United States, in many of which PDIA scholars and grantees have continued to have a major role long after the closure of PDIA itself. It is fitting to conclude with some consideration of where palliative care now sits in the American context and the challenges that it will face in the future.

A global report on the quality of death published in 2010 placed the United States in ninth position in terms of the quality of its end-of-life care provision.[61] The report states as follows:

This reflects the high overall cost of healthcare in the US, where expenditure has risen sharply in recent years, now accounting for one dollar in every six spent. The US ranks better in terms of infrastructure—at positions 7 and 8 for Quality and Availability of End-of-Life Care respectively (and top of the list when it comes to healthcare spending as a percentage of gross domestic product). However, this is offset when considering the financial burden to patients, driven up by the low availability of public funding and social security spending on healthcare.[62]

58. University of Chicago, Arete, "Clinical Scholars Program Delves into Physician Spirituality" (December 19, 2011), http://arete.uchicago.edu/features/curlin.shtml (accessed June 29, 2012).

59. Each will study at the Cicely Saunders Institute at King's College London for three to four years before moving out to take senior positions around the world; http://www.csi.kcl.ac.uk/faculty-scholars.html (accessed June 21, 2012).

60. S. Connor, "Hospice and Palliative Care in the United States," *Omega* 56, no. 1 (2007–2008): 89–99.

61. Economist Intelligence Unit, "Quality of Death," The countries ahead of it were: United Kingdom, Australia, New Zealand, Ireland, Belgium, Austria, Netherlands, Germany, and Canada.

62. Economist Intelligence Unit, "Quality of Death," 13.

Financial considerations remain central to thinking about the provision of hospice and palliative care in the United States. Medicare reimburses hospice providers at a flat daily rate, based on four levels of home and inpatient care, assuming patients have a terminal illness and an estimated six months or fewer to live. The Medicare Payment Advisory Commission (MedPAC) recommended amendments to the system, starting in 2013, to give relatively lower payments the longer the treatment lasts. In a 2009 report to Congress, the agency suggested that the present system provides incentives for hospice providers to admit long-stay patients and claimed this may have led to inappropriate utilization of the benefit among some hospices.[63]

Seen this way, the question arises as to whether Medicare's per diem payment structure may create financial incentives to select patients who require less resource-intensive care and have longer hospice stays. For-profit and nonprofit hospices may respond differently to such financial incentives. A study published in 2011 in the *Journal of the American Medical Association*, the world's most widely circulated medical journal, set out to compare patient diagnosis and location of care between for-profit and nonprofit hospices and to examine whether the number of visits per day and the length of stay vary by diagnosis and profit status. Using 2007 data from the National Home and Hospice Care Survey and a representative sample of 4,705 patients discharged from hospice, the main outcome measures were diagnosis and location of care (home, nursing home, hospital, residential hospice, or other) by hospice profit status, hospice length of stay, and the number of visits per day by various hospice personnel. The results proved to be of major import and showed that when compared, for-profit hospices had a lower proportion of patients with cancer and a higher proportion of patients with dementia and other non-cancer diagnoses. After adjustment for demographic, clinical, and agency characteristics, there was no significant difference in location of care by profit status. However, for-profit hospices compared with nonprofit hospices had a significantly longer length of stay and were more likely to have patients with stays longer than 365 days, and less likely to have patients with stays of less than seven days. Compared with cancer patients, those with dementia or other diagnoses had fewer visits per day from nurses and social workers. The study concludes that compared with nonprofit hospice agencies, for-profit hospice agencies had a higher percentage of patients with diagnoses associated with lower-skilled needs and longer lengths of stay.[64] Commenting on these results, Charles von Gunten captured the thoughts of many working in the field:

This article in JAMA confirms all the whispers, and the previously published preliminary evidence. The for-profit agencies whose shares are traded

---

63. MedPac, "Report to the Congress: Medicare Payment Policy," (March 10, 2009).

64. M. W. Wachterman et al., "Association of Hospice Agency Profit Status with Patient Diagnosis, Location of Care, and Length of Stay," *Journal of the American Medical Association*. 305, no. 5 (2011): 472–479.

publicly on the stock exchanges and report large profits do, in fact, "cherry pick" less expensive patients who live longer.[65]

To this is added another dimension, highlighted by the *Quality of Death* report:

In the US, appropriate end-of-life care is often trumped by the "cure at all cost" attitude of doctors, along with the strong religious views many families hold on the sanctity of life...Meanwhile, recent healthcare reform debates in the US—provoking talk of "death panels," and with references in some quarters to a "euthanasia bill"—have forced the issue of end-of-life care into the background. "Everyone has been terrified about talking about palliative care until health reform passed," says Diane Meier, director of the US-based Center to Advance Palliative Care. The inflammatory nature of the US debates has highlighted the biggest cultural barrier to delivering palliative and hospice care—the fact people associate it with dying rather than providing quality of life when suffering terminal illness. Dr Meier views this as a social marketing challenge. "The problem with hospice is that it's firmly linked in everyone's minds with giving up." The irony, she says, is that to promote higher quality and better access to palliative care, the services need to go by another name. "We force people to wear the scarlet letter in order to get the care," she says.[66]... "Until we can get across to the public and health professionals that palliative care is about living, as well as possible, for as long as possible, with a serious illness," she says, "patients will continue to suffer unnecessarily."[67]

As Morrison and Meier note, "sizeable challenges remain if care for seriously ill people and their families is to improve in the United States."[68] They list these challenges as (1) a lack of public understanding of what palliative care is about, (2) an inadequate knowledge base to underpin clinical practice across the core elements of pain and symptom management, communication skills, spiritual support, and co-ordination of care, and (3) a lack of integrated and adequately supported palliative care programs in hospitals, nursing homes, and homecare agencies—the latter being heavily tied up with systems for reimbursement.

It is in this nexus of issues that the debate now sits. We see within it some enduring elements of PDIA's mission, but arguably a retreat from engaging with the "culture of dying" that was so central to PDIA. In this context, the "good death" is seen as something that can only be constructed retrospectively, since prospectively what Americans are seeking is cure and, failing that, high quality

---

65. C. Von Gunten, "Did you ever?" *Journal of Palliative Medicine* 14, no. 5 (2011): 534–535.

66. Economist Intelligence Unit, "Quality of Death," 16.

67. Ibid., 19.

68. S. Morrison and D. E. Meier, "National Palliative Care Research Center and Center to Advance Palliative Care."

symptom control. This so-called reframing from *end-of-life* to *palliative* care, involves the creation of a demand to provide care "upstream"—reflecting the concern of patients and families that physicians abandon them if hospice care is recommended. Thus it is observed:

> The notion of a "good death," which hospice effectively enables for many people, has greatest salience *after* [my emphasis] a loved one has died. Most people and families facing a serious illness do not want a good death; they want a cure. The frame of palliative care allow[s] patients, families, and physicians to accept care and amelioration of pain while they pursue active treatment.[69]

Is this now the proposed direction for palliative care in the United States? If so, then the key orientation is to work from the *facts* of what patients and families want, rather than the *values* of what is believed to be good for them. We might call this a shift from a reformist to a consumerist position. This should then be supported in turn by the *evidence* of effective care, rather than the *rhetoric* of a social movement. In this culture, the inspirational figures become not the clinical idealists and founders of hospice and palliative care, but rather the business entrepreneurs, the marketing leaders, and the inspirational stars of sport and popular culture. At the 5th Annual Kathleen M. Foley Research Retreat and Symposium of the National Palliative Care Research Center in the autumn of 2011, a key quote in the introductory presentation came from the Canadian ice hockey player, Wayne Gretzky: "I skate to where the puck is going to be, not where it has been." Reflecting this idea, the introduction set out the goals for 2020: First, all patients and families will know how to request palliative care in the setting of serious and life-limiting illness. Second, all health-care professionals will have the knowledge and skills to provide palliative care. Third, all health-care institutions will be able to support and deliver high quality palliative care.[70] The message of the retreat was that palliative care is presently linked to end-of-life care in the minds of professionals and (to some extent) policy makers. The argument is that this is a bad thing and creates a barrier to gaining access to high quality medical care for persons with serious illness—even those who are dying. It also states that many people in need of palliative care are not dying and, even among those who are, very few (including their clinicians) are able to accept that fact until death is imminent. The message is clear: "We need to de-couple palliative care from end-of life care, terminal care, and care of the dying."[71]

---

69. Patrizi, Thompson, and Spector, *Improving Care at End of Life*, 27.

70. National Palliative Care Research Center, "5th Annual Kathleen M. Foley Palliative Care Research Retreat and Symposium," http://www.npcrc.org/usr_doc/retreat_intro_and_overview_2011.pdf (accessed July 16, 2012).

71. Ibid.

What will be the effects of this de-coupling? Some commentators see considerable benefit and argue that this is entirely consistent with prevailing social
norms.

> In fact one could argue that because as a modern society we have succeeded
> so well at prolonging lives, we have a moral obligation to increase the qual-
> ity of those prolonged lives. An emphasis on the acceptance by a patient
> that he or she is dying, prior to the initiation of palliative care, creates a
> dichotomous model where patients must choose between two extremes.
> In order to serve *all* patients with life-threatening illness rather than only
> those who acknowledge that they are dying, we must develop novel ways of
> delivering palliative care. This begins with redefining palliative care, as the
> World Health Organization did recently, with an emphasis on early iden-
> tification and prevention of suffering. It must continue with education of
> patients and families, as well as health-care professionals from disciplines
> outside palliative care, that palliative care is an integral part of good care
> for those with life-threatening illness, not an alternative, optional, ideologi-
> cally based form of care, where patients must accept that they are dying.
> And there must be greater efforts at integrating palliative care with other
> medical disciplines. The denial of death thesis may have served a purpose at
> the beginning of the hospice and palliative care movements, where one aim
> was to advocate for dying people and give them a voice. However, the con-
> tinued emphasis on the presumed denial of death in modern society is not
> only dated but may also exclude from palliative care a large population of
> patients who need and deserve such services. Many terminally ill patients
> are not ready to be labelled as dying, but all wish to stop suffering.[72]

Not surprisingly, some continue to equate palliative care with the care of the
dying and fear it will further reinforce the tendency to the medicalized death
that has been such a feature of American life in modern times. At the University
of St Louis, Jeffrey Bishop, physician and ethicist, has drawn attention to the
dangers that might result from greater involvement with palliative care as death
approaches. In this scenario, the reforming and humanizing aspects of palliative
care are themselves exposed as a force of power and surveillance:

> Palliative care must achieve the level of a science, with instruments of
> assessment, in order to be true care. Palliative care extends the reach of the
> expert into the crevices of the patient's psyche, into the fissures of his social
> relations, into the caverns of his religious life. It extends beyond the grave
> into the familial space left empty by the patient's death. Medicine becomes
> at best totalizing, at worst totalitarian.[73]

---

72. C. Zimmermann and G. Rodin, "The Denial of Death Thesis: Sociological Critique and
Implications for Palliative Care," *Palliative Medicine* 18 (2004): 121–128.

73. J. P. Bishop, *The Anticipatory Corpse: Medicine, Power, and the Care of the Dying* (Notre
Dame: University of Notre Dame Press, 2011).

The evidence presented here suggests that even if this latter view is a theoretical possibility, it remains a long way short of realization in the US context. The palliative care field is still small and has yet to become a major source of attraction to doctors in training. It is generally seen as fairly marginal to much of modern medicine. For these reasons, it seeks to become more integrated with the mainstream and views this as a future measure of success. Some of the greatest accomplishments of those involved in PDIA seem to have been focused on this goal. Great human benefit should flow from better public understanding of palliative care and easier access to it. But one should always beware of the unintended consequences of action. To paraphrase Levi Strauss, palliative care may not only be good to do, but it may also be *good to think*—for it can nourish the human experience in the process.[74] A key question then becomes, how can the ideals of palliative care be preserved as its practices are extended?

The publication of this book coincides with the twentieth anniversary of the meeting in the home of Mr. George Soros, at which the ideas were forged that led to the creation of the Project on Death in America. In turn we are ten years on from when I first took the train up into the Rocky Mountains, heading for the faculty scholars' retreat. I have tried here to capture the nine active years of the PDIA program, as well as the legacies and out-workings that occurred in the decade following. All categorizations of time are to some extent arbitrary. But there is some clear evidence here that the progress of palliative care has been enhanced in the last decade as the result of interventions made by PDIA and other organizations in the ten years before that. Those involved will look back and view these years through many different lenses. I trust that in this book I have captured some insights into their achievements, struggles and breakthroughs along the way—and, of course, the challenges that remain.

---

74. C. Levis Strauss, *The Savage Mind* (Chicago: University of Chicago Press, 1968).

PDIA Faculty Scholars Program

Cohort One
1995–1996

J. Andrew Billings, MD
Palliative Care Service at Massachusetts General Hospital

William Breitbart, MD
Training and Education in the Psychiatric Dimensions of Palliative Care

Nicholas Christakis, MD, PhD, MPH
Physicians' Prognoses about Death and Their Relation to Patient Referral to Hospice

Stuart Farber, MD
Curriculum on Dying for a Family Medicine Residency Network

Gerri Frager, RN, MD
Pediatric Supportive Care Program for Children with a Life-Threatening Disease

Carlos F. Gomez, MD
Narrative Database in a Palliative Care Program

Sarah J. Goodlin, MD
Care of Dying Patients in the Connecticut River Valley

Cohort Two
1996–1997

Harvey Max Chochinov, MD, FRCPC
Psychiatric Dimensions of Palliative Medicine

Timothy J. Keay, MD, MA-Th
End-of-Life Medical Care in Nursing Homes

David R. Kuhl, MD
Spiritual and Psychological Issues at the End of Life

Marcia Levetown, MD
Cross-Disciplinary Model for Teaching Palliative Care

Michael Lipson, PhD
Attentional Dynamics Training: Personal Death Awareness for Health Professionals

Susan J. McGarrity, MD
The Role of the Academic Institution in Palliative Care

Cohort Three
1997–1998

Janet L. Abrahm, MD, FACP
Disease Management Program for the Care of the Dying

Robert Mark Arnold, MD
Teaching Physician Change-Agents to Communicate with Terminally Ill Patients about Psychosocial and Ethical Aspects of Care

J. Randall Curtis, MD, MPH
Quality of Communication about End-of-Life Care

Joseph J. Fins, MD
Reconstructing the Care of the Dying through the Integration of Clinical Ethics and Palliative Care

Laura C. Hanson, MD, MPH
Martha Henderson, MSN, DMin
Improving Nursing Home Care for the Dying

Nancy Hutton, MD
Completing the Circle: End-of-Life Care for Children with AIDS

Cohort Four
1998–2000

Anthony Back, MD
Robert Pearlman, MD, MPH
Evaluating and Ameliorating End-of-Life Suffering

Jeffrey H. Burack, MD, MPP, BPhil
Exploring the Transition to Terminal Illness

James F. Cleary, MB, BS, FRACP
Introducing Graduate, Postgraduate, and Continuing Medical Education in Palliative Medicine with Practice Changes in Inpatient, Clinic, and Remote Settings

Lewis M. Cohen, MD
The Renal Palliative Care Initiative

Frank D. Ferris, MD
Consensus-Building as a Process to Effect Change in Care of the Dying

Cohort Five
1999–2001

LaVera M. Crawley, MD
Barbara Koenig, RN, PhD
Improving End-of-Life Care for the Underserved through Targeted Continuing Education for African American Physicians

Lachlan Forrow, MD
Expanding a Palliative Care Initiative at Beth Israel Deaconess Medical Center and CareGroup

Judith Eve Nelson, MD, JD
Integrating Palliative Care in the Intensive Care Unit

Steven D. Passik, PhD
The Oncology Symptom Control and Research Program: Creating a Palliative Care Clinical, Educational, and Research Initiative in a Community-Based, Rural, Oncology Setting

Diane E. Meier, MD, PhD; Judith C. Ahronheim, MD; Jane Morris, RN; Steven H. Miles, MD
Curriculum on End-of-life Care in a Managed Care Program

Thomas J. Smith, MD
Efficacy and Cost Effectiveness of End-of-life Care

James A. Tulsky, MD
Model for Improving Physician Communication with Dying Patients

Charles F. von Gunten, MD, PhD
Visiting Palliative Care Education Program for Health Care Professionals

David E. Weissman, MD
Death Education Curriculum in Primary Care Residency Programs

Walter M. Robinson, MD, MPH
Terminal Care for Children Dying of Noncancer-related Causes

John Lee Shuster Jr, MD
Curriculum for Neuropsychiatric Complications of Terminal Illness

Daniel P. Sulmasy, OFM, MD, PhD
Quality Time: Measuring and Improving the Quality of Care Rendered to Inpatients at the End of Life

Sharon M. Weinstein, MD
Palliative Intervention in Tertiary Cancer Care

Betsy MacGregor, MD
Project on Dying and the Inner Life

Marianne LaPorte Matzo, PhD, RN, CS
Care for the Dying Patient: An Educational Program for the Associate Degree Nursing Student

Peter A. Selwyn, MD, MPH
Care of Patients with Late-Stage AIDS in a Skilled Nursing Facility

Wayne A. Ury, MD
A Palliative Medicine Curriculum for an Internal Medicine Residency Program

Neil S. Wenger, MD, MPH
Measuring and Improving the Quality of Care for Seriously Ill Inpatients toward the End of Life

Linda Ganzini, MD
Legalization of Physician-Assisted Suicide in Oregon

Jean A. Linzau, MD; Michelle Grant Ervin, MD
End-of-Life Care Provider Education in an Ethnically and Spiritually Diverse Community

Steven Z. Pantilat, MD
A Palliative Care Curriculum for Medicine Residents and Hospitalist Trainees

Samuel K. Payne, MD
The Development and Evaluation of Telemedicine Applications in Palliative Care

Deborah Witt Sherman, PhD, RN, ANP, CS
Implementation, Evaluation, and Refinement of an Advanced Practice Palliative Care Nursing Program

Thomas J. Prendergast, MD
Improving End-of-Life Care within the Intensive Care Unit

Myles N. Sheehan, SJ, MD
Improving Care of the Dying in the American Catholic Community

Joanne Wolfe, MD, MPH
Improving Care at the End-of-Life for Children with Cancer

(continued)

Appendix 1 Continued

Cohort Six 2000–2002	Cohort Seven 2001–2003	Cohort Eight 2002–2004
Victor T. Chang, MD *Study of Outcome Measurement in Terminal Cancer Patients*	**Richard Brumley, MD Kris Hillary, RNP, MSN** *Transferring End-of-Life Knowledge in Clinical Culture*	**F. Amos Bailey, MD** *Integration of Palliative Care Training into the Curricula of Medical Oncology and Geriatric Medicine Fellowship Training*
Anthony N. Galanos, MD *A Study to Determine Specific Barriers to a Good Death at a Tertiary Care, Academic Medical Center, and to Initiate Change*	**Christopher Daugherty, MD** *Decision Making, Information Seeking, and Awareness of Prognosis among Dying Cancer Patients and Involved Physicians*	**Bruce Himelstein, MD** *Rapid-Cycle Quality Improvement in Pediatric Palliative Care Education*
R. Sean Morrison, MD *Palliative Medicine in the Acute Care Hospital: A Model for Education, Professional Development, and Clinical Care*	**Joanne M. Hilden, MD** *Children's Oncology Group: Pediatric Advanced Illness Care Coordination*	**Eric Krakauer, MD, PhD** *Clinical Policy Development for Optimum End-of-Life Care*
Anne C. Mosenthal, MD, FACS Patricia A. Murphy, PhD, RN, CS, FAAN *Palliative Care in an Inner City Trauma Service*	**Daniel C. Johnson, MD** *Decreasing Symptom Distress at the End of Life through Evidence-Based Education*	**Terri Maxwell, RN, MSN** *Health System-Wide Quality Improvement Initiative for Palliative Care*
	Judith A. Kitzes, MD, MPH *Native American End-of-Life Care*	**Susan C. Miller, PhD, MBA** *Timely Access to Hospice Care: Understanding Barriers and Influencing Change*

J. Cameron Muir, MD
Development of Interdisciplinary Outpatient Palliative Care Services: Enhancing the Continuum of End-of-Life Care

Kendra Peterson, MD
Quality of Life/Quality of Death: Living and Dying with a Malignant Brain Tumor

Kathleen Puntillo, RN, DNSc, FAAN
Improving Symptom Assessment and Management during Palliative Care of Dying Patients in Intensive Care Units

Kenneth E. Rosenfeld, MD
Pathways: An Institutional Quality Improvement Program in End-of-Life Care

Laurie Jean Lyckholm, MD Patrick Coyne, RN, MSN
Improving End-of-Life Care for the Medically Underserved by Defining Barriers to Access and Developing an Educational Curriculum

Mary E. Paulk, MD
Palliative Care for Indigent and Minority Patients and Investigation into the Constitutionality of Current Government Funding Practices for End-of-Life Care

Michael A. Weitzner, MD
Increasing Clinicians' Awareness and Screening for Clinical Depression in Home Hospice Cancer Patients

Holly G. Prigerson, PhD
Psychiatric Disorders in Dying Patients and the Family Caregivers Who Survive Them

Tammie E. Quest, MD
A Palliative Care Curriculum for Emergency Medicine Residents

Michael W. Rabow, MD
Between the Blackboard and the Bedside: An Examination of the Hidden Curriculum in End-of-Life Care

Joseph S. Weiner, MD, PhD
Emotional Distress of Physicians Discussing Advance Care Planning: Impact of a New Training Program for Fellows, Interns, and Medical Students

PDIA Social Work Leadership Development Award Program

Cohort One, 2000	Cohort Two, 2000	Cohort Three, 2001	Cohort Four, 2002	Cohort Five, 2003
Joan Berzoff *Developing a Certificate Program and Textbook in End-of-Life Care*	**Terry Altilio** *A Multidimensional Intervention for Social Workers in Palliative and End-of-Life Care*	**David A. Cherin** *The University of Washington's School of Social Work End-of-Life Care Knowledge Institute*	**Mercedes Bern-Klug** *Psychosocial Concerns at the End of Life for Nursing Home Residents: The Role of Social Work*	**David Browning** *Developing a Pediatric End-of-Life Care Curriculum for Social Workers*
Susan Blacker *Social Work and End-of-Life Care: An Educational Initiative*	**Elizabeth Mayfield Arnold** *Unmet Patient Needs at the End of Life: The Hospice Social Work Response*	**Ellen L. Csikai** **Mary Raymer** *The Social Work End-of-Life Care Educational Program (SWEEP)*	**Sheila R. Enders** *Creating a Handbook for Advance Care Planning and Decision Making at the End of Life in Populations with Low Literacy, Mild Learning Disabilities, or Mild Cognitive Deficits*	**Karen Bullock** *Resource Enrichment Center*
Iris Cohen *Multidisciplinary Care Tools: Teamwork and Family Conferences in Palliative Care*		**Judith Dobrof** *Caregivers and Professionals Partnership: Assessing a Structured Support Program*		**Elizabeth Chaitin** *Interdisciplinary Specialty Team Training in Palliative Care*
Barbara Dane *University/Agency Collaboration to Advance Training in End-of-Life Care*	**John F. Linder** *Fostering Interdisciplinary Cooperation in the Delivery of Enhanced End-of-Life Care Through a Collaborative Social Work/Clergy Graduate Curriculum*	**Betty J. Kramer** *Strengthening Social Work Education to Improve End-of-Life Care*	**Richard B. Francoeur** *Palliative Care in an Inner-City Minority Population: The Impact of Chronic Disease, Material Deprivation, and Financial Burden*	**Nancy Cincotta** *A National Initiative to Unite Social Workers and Families in the Interest of Dying Children*
			Barbara L. Jones *Psychosocial Protocol and Training Program for End-of-Life Care for Children with Cancer: A Social Work Curriculum*	**Elizabeth J. Clark** *Building Social Work Practice and Policy Competencies in End-of-Life Care*

Jim Keresztury
Social Work End-of-Life Training—A Network Approach

Mary Sormanti
State-of-the-Art Psychosocial Care for the Dying and Those Who Love Them

Gary L. Stein
The Excellence in End-of-Life Care Fellowship for Social Workers

Margo Okazawa-Rey Norma del Rio
Multicultural Social Work Practice with Clients at the End of Life

W. June Simmons
End-of-Life Social Work Field Education Project

Susan Taylor-Brown
Enhancing the Care of Families Living with HIV/AIDS: A Clinical, Educational, and Research Initiative in a Community-Based HIV Care Facility with a Family Camping Component

Katherine Walsh-Burke
Internet-Based Continuing Education Curriculum

Shirley Otis-Green
Proyecto de Transiciones: Enhancing End-of-Life and Bereavement Support Services for Latinos within a Cancer Center Setting

Amanda Sutton
Yvette Colon
The End-of-Life Internet Forum

Jane Lindberg
Social Worker Bereavement Training Program

Susan Murty
Developing Social Work Leadership in End-of-Life Services in Rural Communities

Bruce A. Paradis
End-of-Life Care: Birth through Old Age

Sherri Weisenfluh
The Kentucky Project, Enhancing End-of-Life Care: A Social Work Manual for Students and Practitioners

Nancy Contro
Latino Families in Pediatric Palliative Care

Rita Ledesma
Loss and Bereavement in an American Indian and Alaska Native Community

Bonnie Letinich
Pediatric Palliative Care Education for Social Workers

Aloen Townsend
Family Assessment Collaboration to Enhance End-of-Life Support

Terry A. Wolfer Vicki Runnion
Casebook on Death and Dying for Social Work Education